D1776637

PROGRESSIVE CASTING AND SPLINTING for LOWER EXTREMITY DEFORMITIES in Children with Neuromotor Dysfunction

by
Beverly D. Cusick, M.S., P.T.

Illustrations done under contract by
Charles Ortenblad III

Therapy Skill Builders
A division of
Communication Skill Builders ®
3830 E. Bellevue/P.O. Box 42050
Tucson, Arizona 85733/(602) 323-7500

About the Author

Beverly (Billi) Cusick, M.S. RPT, received her Bachelor of Science in Physical Therapy from Boston Bouve College at Northeastern University in 1972. She received NDT training in 1974 and took refresher and baby courses in 1978 and 1980-81. Since 1978 she has written or co-authored numerous publications including *Serial Casts: Their Use in the Management of Spasticity-Induced Foot Deformity* and *Splints and Casts: Managing Foot Deformity in Children with Neuromotor Disorders*—the latter by invitation of the editors of *Physical Therapy* for the December 1988 special issue on the foot and ankle. She frequently conducts workshops on the management of foot deformity in neurologically impaired children and adults and has guest lectured at annual conferences of the APTA, the NDTA, and the AACPDM in the United States and Canada.

Ms. Cusick worked for nine years on the physical therapy staff of Children's Rehabilitation Center (now the Kluge Center) in Charlottesville, Virginia. She then served for three years on the Physical Therapy Education faculty of the College of Health Related Professions at the Medical University of South Carolina (MUSC) in Charleston. She also directed physical therapy services for the Division of Developmental Disabilities (MUSC) in Charleston. She received her Master of Science in Clinical and College Teaching at the University of Lexington, Kentucky, in 1988. She is currently affiliated with Children's Hospital at Stanford University, consulting and practicing privately in California.

© 1990 by

Therapy Skill Builders
A division of
Communication Skill Builders
3830 E. Bellevue/P.O. Box 42050
Tucson, Arizona 85733/(602) 323-7500

ISBN 0-88450-454-9   Catalog No. 4182

10 9 8 7 6 5 4 3

Printed in the United States of America

Contents

CHAPTER 1
Early Development of the Legs and Feet— Biomechanical Terminology

• Sagittal plane • Frontal plane • Transverse plane •
Axis of motion • Triplane motion

• Transcondylar axis (TCA) • Tibial plafond •
Talocrural joint • Transmalleolar axis (TMA—Axis of
mortice) • Lateral pillar • Medial pillar • Hindfoot •
Forefoot • Subtalar joint (STJ) • Talar trochlea •
Midtarsal joint (MTJ) • Ray • Metatarsal break

Symmetry • Valgum • Varum • Version • Torsion

• Anteversion • Antetorsion (femoral) • Coxa valga

• Genu valgum ("knock-knee") • Genu varum ("bowed
legs") • Genicular position • Apparent tibial varum •
Tibiofibular torsion • Talar torsion

• Open-chain motion • Closed-chain motion • Disassociation • Adduction • Abduction • Inversion • Eversion • Supination • Pronation

• Angle of gait (angle of progression) • Subtalar joint
neutral position (STN) • Neutral foot position •
Relaxed calcaneal stance • Calcaneal midposition •
Functional calcaneal midposition • Hindfoot varus •
Hindfoot valgus • Forefoot varus • Forefoot valgus

• Crouch posture • Genu recurvatum • calcaneus
deformity • Equinus deformity • Equinovalgus •
Equinovarus • Pes planus (or planovalgus) • Flexible
pes planus

CHAPTER 2
Identifying Developmental Issues 19

CHAPTER 4
Common Features of Alignment in Children
with Neuromotor Disorders 175

CHAPTER 7
Splinting the Foot and Ankle—The Basics of
Fabrication and Implementation 313

CHAPTER 8
Research Considerations **365**

If you would be interested in ongoing information from the author directly, please send your name and address to:

Beverly Cusick
Therapy Skill Builders
3830 E. Bellevue
Tucson, AZ 85716

Preface

"Science may someday discover what faith has always known."

—Ashley Brilliant

This text is a station, a place to pause and to account for the developments that have occurred in an ongoing process of learning about the workings of the pediatric foot and leg. The process continues, even as these pages go to press. There is no definitive point of view regarding the concepts and methods offered here. Rather, writing this book was an effort to synthesize and apply recent scientific advances as they contribute to effective management of problems of foot deformity in children with neuromotor impairment.

Written for therapists, orthotists, podiatrists, physiatrists, orthopedists, and orthopedic technicians, this text is also a call for more effective collaboration among team members who manage children with chronic "challenges"; it issues an invitation to collectively comprehend and thus to create new solutions to old problems. There are no rules. No single approach is correct for everyone. There are encouraging signs of progress, however, and these pages are a tribute to just that—progress.

Therapists who read this manual and/or attend my related workshops should use this information to try to understand better the roles of the orthotist and the podiatrist. I welcome the cooperation of orthotists who share my interest in improving foot deformity management methods. We all seek a fuller understanding of the biomechanical issues of pediatric lower extremity alignment and function. Knowledgeable orthotists and podiatrists possess skills and materials that are essential resources for the child who needs effective and durable foot support systems.

In March 1977, Joan Mohr, a consulting pediatric therapist, trained me and other members of the staff of Children's Rehabilitation Center (CRC) in Charlottesville, Virginia. The class included several therapists, an orthopedic technician, and Michael Sussman, M.D., an orthopedist. We learned a cast application procedure developed in England for use in conjunction with the neurodevelopmental treatment approach to the management of cerebral palsy. The rationale at that time was to achieve inhibition of functional hypertonus, while providing a therapist with what amounted to an extra pair of hands through increased distal stabilization. The casts were used to help elicit more successful antigravity responses in the trunk and proximal joints. The casts were contraindicated if the triceps surae group exhibited fixed contracture. We were also instructed that bivalving of casts was contraindicated because "parents cannot reapply them appropriately."

From this, our "casting program" was launched. The first preliminary report by Sussman and Cusick was published in the *Johns Hopkins Alumni Journal* in 1979. Within two years we performed over 140 casting procedures (including reapplications) on more than 90 children. We initiated most of these procedures during an admission to CRC for comprehensive therapeutic and educational programming and parent training. The only post-cast follow-up intervention available to us was the polypropylene ankle-foot orthosis. This high-volume demand on the orthotists created some serious problems in the areas of workload and production. The result was that those children for whom braces were ordered remained in solid casts until the braces were delivered; many had to undergo cast changes at intervals of three to four weeks in the interim.

In 1979, Linda Yates, supervisor of Therapy Services at Good Samaritan Hospital in Puyallup, Washington, expanded our horizons by introducing us to bivalving and to her method of inserting a contoured plaster and wood footboard into the sole of the cast. I was excited by this new option, which allowed us to discontinue using solid casts. With this technique, the staff members and I felt that we had been granted a needed measure of control over cast-use intervention. We soon determined that, for many of the children who used them, the bivalved casts were adequate to address the primary problem of positioning the functionally contracted foot and ankle. In this way, while maintaining an uninformed but instinctive concern for achieving normal alignment within the foot structure, we drastically reduced the number of solid cast interventions and replaced them with bivalved casts, often while awaiting the delivery of follow-up orthoses.

Nevertheless, we experienced considerable difficulty once the orthoses were delivered, primarily in three respects:

1. Skin breakdown often occurred over the talus and the navicular tuberosity.
2. The sole of the orthosis was typically flat, providing inadequate support for the longitudinal arches.
3. The forefoot commonly slipped off the floor of the orthosis.

I was not yet aware of the criteria that I might have applied to determine the appropriateness of specific support features in an orthosis, particularly as they related to the pediatric foot at varying ages. I was therefore not equipped with the specific principles needed to request that braces be produced from a mold that had been taken for the primary purpose of achieving optimum biomechanical alignment.

In late 1980, Mary Clark, M.D., an orthopedic surgeon who had worked with therapists at Children's Hospital in New Orleans, suggested a technique to Mike Smith, CRC's orthopedic technician. Mike began using Aquaplast-T® splinting material to make foot splints for children with spina bifida. By August 1981, the advantages of Aquaplast-T® over plaster in managing foot and ankle deformity related to cerebral palsy had become apparent. We began to use splints to address directly the post-cast and post-operative management concerns regarding functional alignment of the foot and ankle. Because CRC's caseload of children with cerebral palsy totalled over 600 at the time, we gained experience in the area of lower-extremity splint fabrication at a staggering rate.

From the spring of 1979 through 1983, the CRC staff provided 835 plaster casts, 356 solid ankle-foot splints (SAFSs), 34 crouch-control ankle-foot splints (CAFSs), and 58 stabilizing foot splints (SFSs). The shift from the use of plaster casts to the use of splints was under way.

In May 1983, I attended a three-day symposium during which R. Paul Jordan, Jeffrey Cusack, and Barbara Resseque (all podiatrists with the Langer Biomechanics Group in Deer Park, New York) discussed the normal and abnormal biomechanics of the leg and foot in the developing infant and child. This was an invaluable learning experience for me, particularly because I learned some of the ways structural alignment of children varies from that of adults. I was able thereafter to approach the deforming foot with an elementary body of facts and to appreciate better the fundamental significance of the subtalar and midtarsal joints in foot alignment and lower extremity function.

My interest in developmental biomechanics was sparked during the symposium; it was fanned when I read an article written by Barney LeVeau and Donna Bernhardt in *Physical Therapy* (December 1984). After studying all the articles in that issue of *Physical Therapy*, I gained a greater understanding of the impact of structural alignment on neuromotor function, along with the skills to communicate that information to others.

In 1984, CRC's production figures for foot-support alternatives to polypropylene orthotics were as follows: 127 casts, 596 solid ankle-foot splints (SAFSs), 20 crouch-control ankle-foot splints (CAFSs), and 77 stabilizing foot splints (SFSs). Cast applications were dropping rapidly, and in that year, Smith and I encountered the hinged ankle-foot orthosis with an overlap stop. Hanger Orthotics Lab in Chicktawaga, New York, was involved in fabricating hinged orthoses for children enrolled at the United Cerebral Palsy Association (UCPA) of Western New York in Syracuse. We have no idea who originated this device and have failed ever since to find the inventor. However, we had been given a model for developing a similar device out of Aquaplast-T®. The concept of using dynamic support systems for the foot and ankle entered the splinting arena with an enthusiastic reception.

At the end of 1984, I left CRC for Charleston, South Carolina, to take a faculty position in the pediatrics department and the physical therapy education program at the Medical University (MUSC) and to launch a physical therapy service for a new developmental disabilities clinic on campus. I was interested in applying my expanding knowledge of serial casting as a means of restoring lost mobility to the ankle joint. I encountered substantial success: of 38 children who used 176 casts in a three-year period, only two children went on to undergo tendo-Achilles lengthening. In 1987, I began using long-leg serial casts to reduce hamstrings contracture, with similar results though on a smaller scale: three children who underwent long-leg serial casting (totalling 13 casts) showed reductions in knee flexion contracture ranging from 30-45 degrees. In those three years (1985 through 1987) I attended Gary Gray's seminar on the biomechanics of the foot and gained more layers of understanding of this intricate topic. I also made over 250 splints, continued to develop and modify designs, and incorporated the hinged ankle into my repertoire of splinting options.

I have continued to learn from seminar participants and the literature, continually adapting and modifying my concepts, information pool, and methods. This has led, finally, to the status of management methods and rationale as they are presented in this text. In December 1988, Patrick Agnew, a pediatric podiatrist from Norfolk, Virginia, shared with me his copy of the *Symposium on Podopediatrics—Clinics in Podiatry,* and a still deeper swath was cut in the path of my education.

Like most clinical practitioners, I am continually in training. As an educator, I am always learning. I do not regard this book as the definitive word on the use and fabrication of casts and foot splints in the treatment of children with central nervous system deficit. It is instead an invitation to readers to share my knowledge base, resources, and techniques, and to expand on them. This book is a way to begin.

So, let us begin.

Since the completion of *Progressive Casting and Splinting*, several issues of terminology, calcaneal structure, and assessment have been resolved. Bev Cusick felt it imperative to pass along these notes—written in her own words.

Subtalar vs. talonavicular neutrality
Subtalar neutral position (STN) is commonly determined by palpating the talar head and the talonavicular joint, with the implication that the subtalar joint congruity is thereby derived accurately. John H. Weed, DPM, warns against palpating the talar head because of the variable normal and immature configurations of the talus, and because of varying normal alignments of the talus in the low-arched and high-arched foot.

Instead, Weed recommends using a variety of other techniques for determining STN. Information on these techniques has been included in the notes for Chapter 3. References to the "talonavicular congruity" should be converted to STN.

Calcaneal torsion in the newborn foot
This obscure finding (one citation in the literature) is of great significance in understanding the prevalence of hindfoot varus in subtalar joint neutral position in children and adults.

Specific terms for weightbearing and non-weightbearing deformity
The orthopedic literature commonly uses the terms *varus* and *valgus* to describe weightbearing hindfoot deformities, and so they were incorporated into this text. However, instructors for the American Physical Rehabilitation Network (APRN) have pointed out that varus and valgus are **open-chain** deformities of the congruent foot structures. In the closed-chain foot structures, calcaneal deviations can be more accurately described as *inverted* or *everted* from the sagittal plane. The reader should convert the terms used in the text within the same contexts wherever possible.

Acknowledgments

My deepest thanks go out to the children I have known, whose challenges and patience, struggles and victories have contributed to the insights and suggestions I have come to share with others in seminars and various publications. Thank you for all that you have taught me, and for all that I will continue to learn by working for and together with you.

Thanks also, equally heartfelt, go to the parents and caregivers of those children, who have understood that my efforts to help are sincere. They have endured my frustrations and shortcomings with faith that I give them the best of my knowledge in the midst of an ongoing learning process.

Among my mentors and professional competency models, of whom there are several, I take this occasion to mention those who gave me the tools for practical and creative clinical thinking in the area of managing foot deformity in children with cerebral palsy. They include Berta Bobath, Joan Mohr, Rene Leimgruber, Barbro Salek, Lois Bly, Paul Jordan, Nancy Hylton, Sandy Brooks, Gary Gray, and Susan Coram. You all share in each of my professional judgments and in all ensuing successes.

To Dan Grogan of Charlottesville, Virginia, thanks for your keen perception and special skill in photographing infants and children with and without special needs. Your exemplary work remains a lasting contribution to my educational efforts, both in this text (most of the line drawings in Chapter 2 are taken from your photographs) and in the slides I use during seminars. I still and probably always will miss working with you.

And to the therapy staff of Project Child in Hamilton, New Jersey, thanks for your assistance and indulgence in allowing me to take photographs for use in this text during a workshop practicum.

Donald Burgis of Mount Pleasant, South Carolina, contributed many hours and considerable talent to generating line art for this text and for other instructional purposes. For your time and generosity, Donald, I remain grateful.

I hold a special place in my heart for Bill Pfeifle and Davis Gardner, my advisors in the Allied Health Educational and Research program at the University of Kentucky in Lexington. Your flexible, sensible, and joyfully collaborative guidance helped me attain a graduate degree, and you contributed substantially to the momentum that brought this project to press. I hope that within its pages you can find evidence of your influence on my education. You're wonderful people. I feel privileged to know you.

I offer gladly unfading gratitude for the abundance of information, observations, insights, direction, and experience that my colleagues in physical therapy, podiatry, orthotics, orthopedics, physiatry, and occupational therapy have shared with me over the years. These colleagues have contributed substantially to the development of this text. I look forward to learning more along with and through you all.

Finally, the most profound thanks go to Lee, my husband and real love, my guide into the wondrous labyrinths of the written word, the shorter sentence, and the word processor. You are my source of strength and humor, tolerance and balance. Without you, this text would still be my daydream. It is now a contribution. Our contribution.

Introduction

Chapter 1 is a review of terms that apply primarily to developmental biomechanics, a subject that needs unambiguous and consistent definitions. Some authors or clinicians use vague terms or disregard the mechanical issues in favor of such unsubstantiated and unquantifiable entities as "tone." These people often muddy the waters of communication with other professionals, including their own team members.

In the interest of preventing ambiguity, for example, this book has routinely avoided using the term "inhibitory" to describe the casts used in managing spasticity. Instead, they are named "cast boots," "below-knee casts," or "serial casts" because there is little or no data that proves that they "inhibit" tonus. Observations of improved mobility and reduced resistance to passive motion have been reported and quantified by both clinicians and researchers. It is generally accepted that the actual mechanism involved is related to physiologic growth of muscle and lengthening of connective tissue cells rather than to neurologic influences.

Language that connotes "hokus-pokus" and eludes substantiation clouds the area of biomechanical intervention by discouraging rational collaboration. Not only must professionals use terms carefully, accurately, and consistently, but we should also confine ourselves to selecting labels that accurately represent the process. In my reading of the literature, I have found dual definitions of such terms as "subtalar joint neutral position." I have chosen a single definition for each term used in this text for the sake of consistency and clarity.

Chapter 2 is devoted to a study of the changes in lower extremity structural alignment that normally occur within the first seven years of life. The discussion of developmental biomechanical issues of bone modeling and joint alignment is then followed by an analysis of outstanding features of gait as it develops in infants and preschoolers. This chapter is a foundation upon which to build specific principles useful in the assessment of factors influencing closed-chain biomechanics in the lower extremities. The content should help in selecting optimum interventions and in anticipating limitations on their effectiveness.

Chapter 3 reviews several assessment procedures designed to reveal pertinent features of structure, joint alignment, and mobility in the trunk and lower extremities. The chapter discusses the basic anatomy of the foot and the workings of the lower extremity's closed kinetic chain. The writings of Merton Root, John McCrea, Ronald Valmassy, and Michael McDonough contain a more detailed review of the principles and recommended procedures for assessment of leg and foot alignment in the child.

Chapter 4 contains an exploration of the problems of joint alignment and function as they commonly occur in children with central nervous system deficit. This chapter distinguishes specific normal from abnormal biomechanical features and their apparent functional consequences.

Chapter 5 considers intervention measures for the deformities and functional limitations described in Chapter 4. This chapter goes into the historical perspectives of orthotic management and alternative approaches to managing deformity in the foot and ankle. The chapter discusses criteria for splint selection and provides specific indications, contraindications, and limitations of these procedures. Five basic splint designs and some modifications are described.

Chapter 6 reviews the history of the use of casts in managing problems related to hypertonus in the lower extremity. It focuses on the results of clinical research and on using plaster in serial applications to reduce static soft tissue contracture. This chapter discusses indications, precautions, and principles of application, care, and treatment in casts, as well as suggestions for follow-up to casting treatment.

Chapter 7 addresses the general principles of using elastic thermoplastic splinting material as a medium. It also reviews the process of molding the foot and ankle into optimum alignment. This chapter discusses the features to look for in a well-made device, as well as some common questions raised in seminars by experienced clinicians.

Chapter 8 is devoted to research. It offers many questions that yearn for answers. The chapter calls for quantifiable data about the influence of splint systems on structural alignment and on functional efficiency, both in short-term and long-term applications.

CHAPTER 1

Early Development of the Legs and Feet— Biomechanical Terminology

In order to discuss effectively the structural and biomechanical features of the developing child's legs and feet, there must be a common ground of terminology. Unfortunately, the available literature is unclear about the proper use of many terms; it is not unusual to find different authors using dissimilar terms to describe the same motion or position.

For example, the motion of ankle dorsiflexion is variously described as either flexion or as extension of the ankle—although clearly it cannot be both (Kapandji 1970; Mann 1985). Considering the flexor and extensor synergies in the lower extremities (the "total" patterns of hip/knee/ankle flexion and extension), *dorsiflexion* best describes flexion of the ankle and *plantarflexion* best refers to an extensor function. However, not all authors see it this way, so confusion over terminology persists.

Rodgers and Cavanagh (1984) suggested that the lack of precision in the use of biomechanics terminology reflects two shortcomings: a lack of formal training in biomechanics as a component of professional preparation, and the relative infancy of the field. They responded by publishing "a collection of frequently used biomechanical terms that have consistent meanings across the various disciplines." Their list, however, features mechanical terms rather than those that describe structures and joint alignment features. The main sources for the latter terms are the writings of Root et al. (1971 and 1977), McCrea (1985), Gray (1986), Tachdjian (1985), and Crouch (1985). Where I have discovered conflicting definitions or a lack of consistency in the use of terms in the literature, I have selected the usage that offers the most clarity. Certainly, an interdisciplinary collaboration on a new list of terms and definitions is in order. I hereby volunteer to serve on such a committee.

Although every attempt has been made to use terms accurately and consistently throughout this book, the reader is advised to review these terms with any and all attending and associated physicians, orthotists, podiatrists, physiatrists, therapists, and orthopedic technicians prior to treatment. This will help confirm that the members of the management team agree on the meaning of the terms they all use. Besides causing confusion, an apparent misuse of terms might unfairly suggest ignorance of the subject under discussion. Some time spent ascertaining the accepted use of terminology could avoid such a misunderstanding while facilitating both interteam communication and collective problem-solving skills.

The next chapter will use these terms in an analysis of the biomechanical influences on the developing skeleton in children, with emphasis on the lower extremities.

Body Planes and Motions

Any discussion of posture and biomechanical issues must refer to the three body planes. These provide the examiner with a frame of reference for observing and measuring features of structural alignment and specific movements, and the application of forces during movement.

The body planes are flat and pass through the body while it is in its anatomical position. They describe the direction of motion of a body segment and of the body as a whole. They also describe the location of an axis of motion (Crouch 1985).

Sagittal plane

Any plane that divides the body longitudinally into left and right sides. The motions of flexion and extension of the limbs and trunk occur on the sagittal plane. The feet are parallel when anatomically aligned on the sagittal plane. The median sagittal plane divides the body into equal left and right halves, and is also known as the midsagittal plane. The concept of "midline" incorporates the median sagittal plane.

Frontal plane (also known as "coronal")

Any plane that divides the body or body segment longitudinally into anterior and posterior portions. The motions of abduction and adduction at the hip and shoulder occur on the frontal plane. The foot motions of "pure" inversion and eversion also occur on the frontal plane (Crouch 1985).

Transverse plane (also known as "horizontal")

Any plane that is at right angles to both the sagittal and frontal planes and that divides the body into superior and inferior portions. The motions of rotation within the neck, the trunk, and the legs occur on the transverse plane, as do abduction and adduction of the foot (Crouch 1985).

Axis of motion

An imaginary line that passes through the center of a moving joint or body segment, aligned perpendicular to the plane on which the motion occurs (Crouch 1985; Gray 1986).

Triplane motion

A motion that consists of components that occur on all three body planes simultaneously. The axis of motion also falls through all three planes, perpendicular to the triplane motion executed (Gray 1986).

The following lists of terms are limited to those that pertain directly to the concepts discussed in this book. (For more extensive definitions, see the references at the end of this chapter.) Where appropriate, each list describes terms in a proximal-to-distal sequence.

Anatomical Features

Transcondylar axis (TCA)	A line parallel and adjacent to the posterior surface of the femoral condyles (McCrea 1985).
Tibial plafond	The distal surface of the tibia. The plafond articulates with the talar trochlea within the talocrural joint.

- **Upper segment**—The talus, distal tibia, and distal fibula.
- **Lower segment**—All the bones of the foot that are distal to the talus.

Talocrural joint	The ankle joint; that is, the articulation between the talus and the tibia and fibula. The motions of supination and pronation, which consist primarily of dorsiflexion and plantarflexion, occur at this joint, with secondary eversion and inversion as well as abduction and adduction. This happens because of the triplane location of its axis (Oatis 1988; Root et al. 1971).
Transmalleolar axis (TMA; also "the axis of mortice")	The axis of the talocrural joint. It can be located by extending the knee joint, aligning the tibial crest on the sagittal plane, palpating the bases of the medial and lateral malleoli, and comparing a line connecting them with the frontal plane.
Lateral pillar	The point of stability for the weight-bearing foot. The lateral pillar consists of the calcaneus, the cuboid, and the fourth and fifth rays.
Medial pillar	The point of mobility for the weight-bearing foot. The medial pillar includes the talus, the navicular, and the medial three rays.
Hindfoot (rear foot)	The calcaneus and the talus only (Gray 1986; Root et al. 1977; Jordan et al. 1983; Root et al. 1971).
Forefoot	The navicular, the cuboid, and all bones distal to them; essentially the entire foot, excluding the talus and the calcaneus (Root et al. 1977; Jordan et al. 1983). Some authors identify the cuboid and navicular and the cuneiforms as the midfoot. However, the forefoot motions occur primarily at the midtarsal joint, which lies proximal to the cuboid and navicular.
Subtalar joint (STJ)	The articulation between the talus and the calcaneus. The STJ allows supination and pronation, with the typical primary motions of calcaneal inversion and eversion, secondary abduction and adduction, and minimal dorsiflexion and plantarflexion (Root et al. 1977; Jordan et al. 1983; Root et al. 1971). When operating together, the STJ and the talocrural joint allow motion to occur on all three planes.
Talar trochlea	The most proximal surface of the body of the talus. The trochlea articulates with the tibial plafond within the talocrural joint (Riegger 1988; Oatis 1988).
Midtarsal joint (MTJ)	A combination of two joints: the calcaneal-cuboid and the talo-navicular joints. Both articulations share oblique and longitudinal

functional axes of motion. The MTJ allows supination and pronation at both axes. The primary motion of the oblique axis is forefoot dorsiflexion and plantarflexion, with secondary abduction and adduction and minimal inversion and eversion. The longitudinal axis primarily allows forefoot inversion and eversion, with minimal abduction and adduction and minimal dorsiflexion and plantarflexion (Root et al. 1977; Root et al. 1971). Together, the two axes of the MTJ allow forefoot motions to occur in all three planes.

Ray

A component of the foot structure that operates as a unit. A ray includes a metatarsal bone. Each of the medial four rays consists of a metatarsal and its adjacent tarsal bone. The fifth ray consists only of the fifth metatarsal.

Metatarsal break

The oblique axis that comprises the metatarsophalangeal (MTP) joints, from the head of the second through the head of the fifth metatarsal (Crouch 1985).

Postural, Joint, and Structural Alignment

Symmetry

A feature of trunk alignment that maintains an equal distance between the shoulders and hips when there is a comparison of right and left sides. Strength, control, and mobility generally appear to be equally distributed around a midline orientation during a comparison of left and right sides (Bly et al. 1980; Bly 1983).

Valgum

A position in which the distal segment is everted (directed laterally) distal to the joint.

Varum

A position in which the distal segment is inverted (directed medially) distal to the joint.

Version

A positional change in the direction of a part such as the head and neck of the femur relative to the frontal plane (McCrea 1985). The concept of version also pertains to inversion and eversion of the foot, and to the acetabulum and its orientation relative to the frontal plane.

Torsion

A twist within the shaft of a long bone, along its longitudinal axis (McCrea 1985; Jordan et al. 1983).

Hip and Femur

Anteversion

A positional change in which either the acetabulum or the head and neck of the femur are directed anteriorly, relative to the frontal plane. The head and neck of the femur are maintained in this alignment by soft tissue, including ligament, muscle, and joint capsule (McCrea 1985). Femoral neck anteversion is normally sustained in infancy by lateral rotation contracture of soft tissues surrounding the hip joint

(Jordan et al. 1983; Pitkow 1975). Persistence of this lateral rotation contracture beyond the age of two years sustains the anteverted alignment of the femoral head and neck. When the lateral rotation contracture resolves in early childhood, anteversion resolves. The femoral neck aligns closer to the frontal plane to allow the head of the femur to assume its optimum *closed-packed* (congruent) position for weight-bearing.

Anteversion is not associated with alignment of any other part of the femur. It is a feature of the hip joint alone (McCrea 1985; Jordan et al. 1983).

Antetorsion (femoral)

A medial twist of the shaft of the bone, distal on proximal. When the transcondylar axis (TCA) is aligned on the frontal plane, the femoral head and neck are directed anteriorly (McCrea 1985). This finding at the femoral neck is usually misnamed "anteversion" when in fact it is a feature of alignment that occurs only when the condyles are parallel to the frontal plane. It indicates the existence of torsion in the femoral shaft.

Persistent antetorsion becomes evident with reduction of the contracture that maintains anteversion in early life. As the proximal femoral head and neck align on or near the frontal plane and gain maximal congruity with the acetabulum (the closed-packed position) for weight-bearing, the distal TCA pitches medial to the frontal plane. The result is a medially displaced patella. More distally, the feet align either in a noncompensatory in-toed stance or in a compensatory out-toed stance.

Coxa valga

An increase in the angle of inclination between the femoral neck and shaft, greater than 130 degrees. This angle is measured relative to the sagittal plane with the femoral neck aligned on the frontal plane (McCrea 1985; Jordan et al. 1983).

The term valga (valgus, valgum) implies that the segment that is distal to the joint deviates laterally (Tachdjian 1985). Here the proximal segment of the femur, rather than the hip joint, is included in the description of "coxa valga."

Coxa valga combines with lateral rotation and hip flexion contractures to displace the distal femur laterally in the young infant.

Knee and Tibia

Genu valgum ("knock-knee")

A condition in which the segment distal to the knee joint deviates laterally when measured relative to the sagittal plane. Genu valgum occurs in the frontal plane.

Genu varum ("bowed legs")

When measured relative to the sagittal plane, this deviation occurs in the frontal plane in such a way that the lower leg deviates medially under the knee joint (Tachdjian 1985; Gray 1986).

Genicular position

A position in which adaptations in length in the soft tissues surrounding and within the knee joint result in an abnormal distribution of rotary mobility of the lower leg relative to the femur. When the rotation of the lower leg is medial, this deformity is often mistaken for medial tibial torsion. Internal (medial) genicular position increases when the knee is flexed (loose-packed) and reduces when the knee is fully extended (McCrea 1985).

Apparent tibial varum

An apparent lateral bowing of the distal lower leg (including the tibia and fibula) that usually occurs in the lower third of the segment (Root et al. 1977). In fact, the tibia and fibula are straight. The evident "bowing" is caused by medial *rotation* of the lower leg that displaces posterior muscle bellies laterally, in combination with the underdevelopment of the head of the gastrocnemius muscle (McDonough 1984; Wilkins 1986).

Tibiofibular torsion

A twist in the shaft of the tibia along the longitudinal axis (McCrea 1985). In lateral tibial torsion, the fibula is twisted as well, in the same direction as the tibia. The fibula is included in the clinical measurement to detect torsional deformity in the lower leg.

Internal (medial) torsion, which can be detected accurately only with appropriate roentgenographic methods, is a rare deformity (Bleck 1982).

Talar torsion

Normal immature configuration of the talus in infancy, whereby the talar neck is elongated, laterally twisted, and adducted relative to the sagittal-plane bisection of the talar trochlea. The talar head, which articulates with the navicular, is inverted on the frontal plane by the lateral twist in the talar neck (Tachdjian 1985; Bleck 1982).

Joint Motions

Open-chain motion

A combination of several joints united successfully where the end segment is free, such as when the foot is in the swing phase of its gait, unloaded (Gray 1986; Root et al. 1977). In the open chain, motion of the distal segment occurs with little or no effect on the position of adjacent proximal segments.

Closed-chain motion

A combination of several joints united successfully where the end segment is not free. An example is when the foot is bearing body weight and the head is maintained in a midline orientation relative to the base of support (Gray 1986; Root et al. 1977). In the ideal closed chain, both ends of the chain are relatively fixed in space, and the motion of any body segment, bone, or joint that forms a link in the chain affects the position of the other segments within the chain. The segments are predictably interrelated, like stacking blocks linked by joints.

Disassociation

A feature of the maturation of movement skill, during which the neck and extremities reveal controlled motion separate from the trunk and/or from the opposite extremity; isolated, deliberate movements (Bly et al. 1980; Bly 1983).

Calcaneal torsion

A normal immature configuration of the calcaneus in which the posterior segment is inverted relative to the anterior segment, averaging 10 degrees at birth (Sgarlato 1971; Jordon et al. 1983).

Adduction (within the foot)	A component of triplanar motion in which the longitudinal axis of the segment is directed medially. Pure adduction would occur on the transverse plane. Triplanar axes prohibit pure adduction from occurring (Root et al. 1977).
Abduction (within the foot)	A component of triplanar motion in which the longitudinal axis of the segment is directed laterally. Pure abduction would occur on the transverse plane. Triplanar axes prohibit pure abduction from occurring (Root et al. 1977).
Inversion	A component of triplanar movement that occurs in the frontal plane and allows the plantar surface of the foot to be directed toward the midsagittal plane. With inversion, the distal calcaneus moves medially under the talus (Root et al. 1977; Brooks 1985; Root et al. 1971).
Eversion	Lateral deviation of the distal segment of a part. In the foot, eversion is a component of triplanar movement that occurs primarily in the frontal plane. In the everted position, the plantar surface of the foot is directed outward from the midsagittal plane. The distal calcaneus moves laterally under the talus with eversion.
Supination	Triplanar movement that occurs in the talocrural or foot joints. Supination features various proportional combinations of adduction, inversion, and plantarflexion (Gray 1986; Oatis 1988).
Pronation	A triplanar movement that occurs in the talocrural and foot joints. Pronation features various proportional combinations of eversion, abduction, and dorsiflexion.

Biomechanical Assessment

Angle of gait (angle of progression)	The angle formed by a longitudinal bisection of the foot and the sagittal plane (or line of progression) while walking; often a result of alignment of the knee or the structure of the tibia and fibula.
Subtalar joint neutral position (STN)	A position of maximal congruency at the subtalar joint. This alignment feature is clinically evaluated by palpating the talonavicular joint while supinating and pronating the lower segment. When the talar head is maximally seated into the navicular, the STJ is presumed to be congruent as well. STN position is measured as the resulting angle formed by the posterior vertical bisections of the calcaneus and the distal third of the lower leg (Jordan et al. 1983; Gray 1986; Giallonardo 1988; Oatis 1988).
Neutral foot position	A position in which the STJ and talonavicular joint are congruent and rays 4 and 5 are gently dorsiflexed, or "loaded." As a result, the forefoot is "locked" on the hindfoot in a position of maximum congruity of the joints.

Relaxed calcaneal stance

The angle formed by the vertical bisection of the posterior calcaneus and the sagittal plane in relaxed standing position, at the patient's typical angle and base of gait (Root et al. 1971; Gray 1986).

Calcaneal midposition

Closed chain: In relaxed stance, and during the midstance phase of the gait cycle, the balanced foot reveals a vertical calcaneal bisection that aligns within 2 degrees of the sagittal plane and parallel with the distal lower leg bisection. (This definition corresponds to the terminology used by Root et al. in 1971 to describe STN.) *Open chain:* for the purpose of assessment of STJ mobility, the vertical bisection of the calcaneus is placed in parallel with the bisection of the distal lower leg, and both are aligned on the sagittal plane.

Functional calcaneal midposition

Sometimes the ideal parallel arrangement between the calcaneal and lower leg bisections described above does not exist, and lower leg varum is evident in standing when the calcaneal bisection is aligned within 2 degrees of the sagittal plane. If this happens, the resulting angle of eversion between the calcaneus and the lower leg, described as functional calcaneal midposition, is recorded and implemented in molding for splints or orthoses.

Hindfoot (or calcaneal) varus

A fixed position of calcaneal heel inversion under the talus, when measured relative to the vertical bisection of the distal third of the lower leg when the STJ is aligned in neutral position (Gray 1986; Root et al. 1977; Oatis 1988).

Hindfoot (or calcaneal) valgus

A fixed position of calcaneal eversion when the STJ is aligned in neutral position. Hindfoot valgus is measured as the angle formed by the bisections of the calcaneus and the distal lower leg with STN. This is a rare deformity (Gray 1986; Jordan et al. 1983).

Forefoot varus

A fixed position in which the forefoot is inverted relative to the neutrally aligned foot. Open-chain assessment of the foot with forefoot varus reveals inversion of the plantar surface of the metatarsal heads. The result is a lack of a perpendicular relationship between the plantar plane of the metatarsals and the vertical calcaneal bisection (Gray 1986; Root et al. 1977; Tiberio 1988; Giallonardo 1988).

Gray (1986) suggests that the term "varus," which is used most commonly to describe this feature of alignment, pertains to osseous deformity, while "supinatus" describes a reducible, acquired soft-tissue deformity. Both deviations occur in the frontal plane.

Forefoot valgus

A fixed position in which the forefoot is or can be passively everted relative to the neutrally aligned hindfoot. Open-chain assessment reveals the lack of a perpendicular relationship between the forefoot and the calcaneal bisection. The first metatarsal head aligns distal to the fifth metatarsal head. This deviation is caused either by a fixed, plantarflexed first ray or by excessive dorsiflexion mobility of the fourth and fifth rays (Gray 1986; Root et al. 1977; Root et al. 1971; Tiberio 1988).

Abnormal Leg and Foot Alignment and Function

Crouch posture

A leg position in which the hip, knee, and ankle retain a position of flexion throughout the swing and stance phases of gait. The hip and knee are flexed, often in excess of 30 degrees, and the ankles are hyperdorsiflexed. Crouch posture is usually associated with bilateral lengthening of the heel cords, which results in a calcaneus deformity due to weakness of the triceps surae muscle groups, particularly in the presence of contracture of the hip flexors and hamstrings (Sutherland 1978).

Genu recurvatum

Abnormal hyperextension of the knee, either congenital or acquired. True genu recurvatum is measured at approximately 20 degrees or more, relative to the frontal plane (Tax 1985). Acquired recurvatum is generally associated with hypotonia and ligamentous laxity. Limitation of ankle dorsiflexion mobility (equinus) often results in knee hyperextension, which may not develop into true recurvatum (Root et al. 1977; McCrea 1985).

Calcaneus deformity

Exaggerated ankle dorsiflexion, often accompanied by contracture of long muscles that cross the anterior ankle joint.

Equinus deformity

A fixed or functional limitation of the range of ankle dorsiflexion that occurs with the foot structures aligned in neutral (closed-packed) position. Mild equinus lacks the normal minimum of 5-10 degrees of dorsiflexion beyond zero; in severe equinus, the weight-bearing calcaneus is plantarflexed and elevated from the ground by tightness in the plantar flexors (Root et al. 1977; McCrea 1985). Equinus requires that the knee and/or foot joints adjust by compensating for the forces imposed by the ankle joint's limitation of motion (Root et al. 1977; McCrea 1985; Jordan et al. 1983; Gray 1986).

Equinovalgus

A combination of equinus and pronation (Root et al. 1977; Jordan et al. 1983; Gray 1986).

Equinovarus

A combination of equinus and supination (Root et al. 1977; Jordan et al. 1983).

Pes planus (or planovalgus)

Abnormal pronation of the foot and ankle joints (Franco 1987). Among those children with developmental disability, this deformity is usually seen in the presence of hypotonia, either alone or together with laxity of the supporting ligaments on the medial aspect of the foot (McCrea 1985; Jordan et al. 1983; Tax 1985). Pure pes planus is not initially associated with equinus deformity. Equinus deformity commonly develops secondarily as a long-term result of creep.

Flexible pes planus

Pronation that is evident only in the closed chain; when not in weight-bearing, the foot structures align more normally.

Mechanical Terms

Unless otherwise indicated, the mechanical terms in this section and all of the terms in the following section concerning structural adaptation are drawn from Harold Frost's *Intermediary Organization of the Skeleton, Vol. 2* (1986).

Mechanical usage   The sum of the pull of gravity on the body's mass plus the varied muscle pulls that move, accelerate, and decelerate that mass against multiple resistances of its inertia, its weight, the disadvantageous lever arms, and the resistance of other muscles (Frost 1986, Vol. 1).

Compliance   The opposite of stiffness. The ability to yield or deform under an applied load. For example, cartilage is compliant; mineralized bone is not. Young cartilaginous bone is more compliant than old ossified bone.

Force   Something that can displace matter. Two categories are recognized in biomechanics: *loads* (applied from without) and *stresses* (internal resistance to a load within a structure). See also the definition of *load* that follows.

Load   An outside force that deforms a structure when it is applied. Loading induces strain and causes stresses within the structure.

Strain   Any deformation or change in the shape or dimensions of a structure that is caused by any kind of load applied to it (this does not include strength or stress). The three principal strains do the following: *Compression strain* presses two points within a structure together. *Tension strain* pulls two points within a structure apart. *Shear strain* shifts successive layers laterally over each other in opposing directions.

Stress   The internal force in matter that resists strain or deformation by an applied load of any kind. Stresses include compression, tension, and shear in response to the same types of strain. However, the magnitude of the response to strain might differ from that of the strain itself, depending upon the stiffness and strength of the strained material.

Flexure strain   Bending. This type of strain combines all three principal strains in patterns specific to the point at which the structure is loaded.

Cantilever flexure   Bending produced by longitudinal compression applied to a curved structure, such as weight-bearing on a bowed femur. Cantilever flexure elicits tension, compression, and shear stresses in the bone.

Torque   A twisting load. Like flexure, torque includes all three principal strains, primarily shear strain.

Fatigue   The failure of a material as a result of chronic loading (Rodgers and Cavanagh 1984).

Structural Adaptation

Periosteum

A fibrous, two-layered membrane that encases living bone except where the bone is covered by articular cartilage. The outer layer is strong and fibrous and contains blood vessels. The inner layer is looser and more elastic than the outer layer. The fibers of tendons or ligaments where they attach to bones via periosteum are continuous with the fibers of the periosteum (Crouch 1985). Periosteum generates bone tissue that thickens the shaft in diameter in response to chronically increased loads.

Lamellar bone

This bone type comprises over 99 percent of bone in adults and has a characteristic fiber-like pattern (Crouch 1985; Frost 1986, Vol. 1).

Compact (cortical) bone

Dense, ivory-like outer layer of bone tissue. It is thickest around the hollow diaphysis (shaft) of long bones (Crouch 1985).

Cancellous bone (spongiosa)

Spongy, light, elastic inner bone tissue. Cancellous tissue fills the epiphyses and collects at the enlarged ends of long bones. The trabeculae, which are products of ossification, are arranged in such a way that they withstand strains sustained by compression, tension, and direct impact, with a minimum of weight (Crouch 1985).

Hyaline cartilage

One of three types of cartilage in the body. Hyaline cartilage is the one that forms articular cartilage, epiphyseal plates, and perichondral rings. It lies at the bony attachments of tendons, ligaments, and fascia. Twenty percent of its volume comprises organic matrix, and extracellular water makes up most of the remainder.

Modeling

The process by which agents that are external to a growing tissue influence its speed and direction of growth and its fiber grain in ways that create its microscopic and gross architectures. This process is primarily confined to *growing* skeleton only and is subdivided into micromodeling and macromodeling mechanisms. Modeling occurs through the combined processes of bone formation and resorption.

Micromodeling

The process by which agents external to an actively forming tissue determine its fiber grain and the orientation of its cells and capillaries as they are deposited.

Macromodeling

The process by which agents external to an actively growing bone or connective tissue shape the direction and rate of growth to produce specific, observable architectural features. Lamellar bone macromodeling occurs most rapidly in infancy, slows in adolescence, and stops in adults. Apparently a growth-dependent form of cellular proliferation supports this process.

Remodeling

This process maintains in part the functional competence of already existing tissues and structures. It often occurs in fracture healing.

Minimum effective strain (MES)	The threshold (a range of strain magnitudes) above which the feedback signals for macromodeling evoke a response and affect the modeling system. Strains below MES are considered ineffective in activating the modeling process.
Dynamic strain	Deformation of a structure in response to forces that are applied in changing rates, magnitudes, and direction, such as during movement.
Strain-averaging mechanism	The mechanism by which modeling systems of both bone and fibrous tissue somehow average out the peak strains and strain rates that they endure over a period of time, perhaps between one and twelve months of their application. Then they produce the changes in the tissue's bulk strength that are needed to fit that history of mechanical usage.
Resorption	The removal of an already elaborated tissue such as bone, mineralized cartilage, or ligament by special, usually multinucleated, cells called clasts (for example, osteoclasts and fibroclasts). The process of resorption results not in a net loss of tissue but only in the removal of elaborated tissue.
Drift	An apparent unidirectional motion through tissue space of a bone surface, an intact cortex, or an intact diaphysis. Drift usually occurs with bone macromodeling and involves the processes of bone formation and resorption.
Flexure drift axiom	Repeated nontrivial dynamic cantilever flexure strain evokes those kinds of drifts that move all affected bone surfaces in the concave-tending direction. The concave surface fills, the convex surface resorbs, and the flexure reduces. The bone straightens, and the tendency of the bone to buckle under compression or direct flexure strains is neutralized.
Creep	The progressive deformation, stretching, and adaptive shortening of soft tissue structures caused by constant aberrant loading over a prolonged period of time (Rodgers and Cavanagh 1984). Creep affects new tissue more significantly than old, and bone less than soft tissue.

References

Bleck, E. E. 1982. Developmental orthopedics III: Toddlers. *Developmental Medicine and Child Neurology* 24(4):533-35.

Bly, L. 1983. *Development of normal movement during the first year of life and abnormal development.* Monograph. Oak Park, IL: Neurodevelopmental Treatment Association, Inc.

Bly, L., and F. Sterne. 1980. *Baby treatment.* Lecture notes and instructional materials from neurodevelopmental treatment advanced course, New York, NY.

Brooks, S. 1985. *Mobilization applied to the neurologically involved child.* Lecture notes and instructional materials from advanced training course, Dallas, TX.

Crouch, J. E. 1985. *Functional human anatomy.* Philadelphia, PA: Lea and Febiger.

Franco, A. H. 1987. Pes cavus and pes planus: Analysis and treatment. *Physical Therapy* 87(5):888-893.

Frost, H. M. 1986. *Intermediary organization of the skeleton, vols. 1 and 2.* Boca Raton, FL: CRC Press.

Giallonardo, L. M. 1988. Clinical evaluation of foot and ankle dysfunction. *Physical Therapy* 68(12):1850-1856.

Gray, G. 1986. *Biomechanics of the foot.* Lecture notes and instructional materials from the South Carolina American Physical Therapy Association annual meeting, Charleston, SC.

Jordan, R. P., J. Cusack, and B. Rosseque. 1983. *Foot function and its relationship to posture in the pediatric patient with cerebral palsy and other neuromuscular disorders.* Lecture notes and instructional materials from Neurodevelopmental Treatment Association meeting, New York, NY.

Kapandji, I. A. 1970. *The physiology of the joints, vol. 2: Lower limb.* Second edition. Baltimore: Williams and Wilkins.

Mann, R. A. 1985. Biomechanics of the foot. In *Atlas of orthotics,* edited by W. H. Bunch et al., 112-125. 2d ed. Princeton, NJ: C. V. Mosby.

McCrea, J. D. 1985. *Pediatric orthopedics of the lower extremity: An instructional handbook.* Mount Kisco, NY: Futura.

McDonough, M. W. 1984. Angular and axial deformities of the legs of children. In *Symposium on podopediatrics—Clinics in podiatry,* edited by J. V. Ganley. Philadelphia, PA: W. B. Saunders Co.

Oatis, C. A. 1988. Biomechanics of the foot and ankle under static conditions. *Physical Therapy* 68(12):1815-21.

Pitkow, R. B. 1975. External rotation contracture of the extended hip. *Clinical Orthopaedics and Related Research* 110:135-139.

Riegger, C. L. 1988. Anatomy of the ankle and foot. *Physical Therapy* 68(12):1802-14.

Rodgers, M. M. 1988. Dynamic biomechanics of the normal foot and ankle during walking and running. *Physical Therapy* 68(12):1822-30.

Rodgers, M. M., and P. R. Cavanagh. 1984. Glossary of biomechanical terms, concepts, and units. *Physical Therapy* 84(12):1888-1902.

Root, M. L., W. P. Orien, and J. H. Weed. 1977. *Normal and abnormal function of the foot: Clinical biomechanics, vol. 2.* Los Angeles: Clinical Biomechanics Corporation.

Root, M. L., W. P. Orien, J. H. Weed, and R. J. Hughes. 1971. *Biomechanical examination of the foot, vol. 1.* Los Angeles, CA: Clinical Biomechanics Corporation.

Staheli, L. T., D. E. Chew, and M. Corbett. 1987. The longitudinal arch: A survey of 882 feet in normal children and adults. *Journal of Bone and Joint Surgery* 69-A(3):426-428.

Sutherland, D. H. 1978. The pathomechanics of progressive crouch gait in spastic diplegia. *Orthopedic Clinics of North America* 9(91):143-154.

Tachdjian, M. O. 1985. *The child's foot.* Philadelphia, PA; W. B. Saunders Co.

Tax, H. R. 1985. *Podopediatrics.* Baltimore, MD: Williams and Wilkins.

Tiberio, D. 1988. Pathomechanics of structural foot deformities. *Physical Therapy* 68(12):1840-49.

Valmassy, R. L. 1984. Biomechanical evaluation of the child. In *Symposium on podopediatrics—Clinics in podiatry,* edited by J. V. Ganley. Philadelphia, PA: W. B. Saunders Co.

Wilkins, K. E. 1986. Bowlegs. *Pediatric Clinics of North America* 33(6):1429-1438.

CHAPTER 2

Identifying Developmental Issues

Objectives for the Reader

- To describe the ways in which muscle action and weight-bearing influence the shape and size of developing skeletal structures, joint mobility, and alignment in the lower extremities.

- To identify the distinguishing features of skeletal structure and joint alignment in the trunk and lower extremities of the normal newborn infant.

- To describe the events that occur in normal sensorimotor development, particularly as they involve activity of the various muscle groups in the lower extremities.

- To identify the changes in alignment and mobility that occur with the combined processes of growth and modeling from birth through the age of 7 years.

- To apply the concepts of modeling and biomechanical factors to assessment of structural and functional deficits that commonly occur with neuromotor impairment in children.

Therapists who see normal gross motor development as a sculpting process can find valuable activities in the repertoire of movement skills achieved in infancy and early childhood. These can then be incorporated into therapeutic exercise programs.

Modeling of Young Bone— Influencing Forces

The infant skeleton is highly plastic and is composed primarily of cartilaginous tissue. The stresses applied over time to immature bone and supporting soft tissue structures can produce dramatic alterations. The tiny, conical "lotus foot," the result of years of painful nightly wrapping of the feet of Chinese girls in infancy and childhood, offers evidence of the plasticity of the developing skeletal system (Giannestras 1973; Hensinger et al. 1982; Matles 1965; LeVeau and Bernhardt 1984; Bernhardt 1988; Knight 1954; Frost 1986, Vols. 1, 2; Fabry et al. 1973; McCrea 1985; Tachdjian 1971). Intrauterine and sleeping postures and certain favored play positions have been cited as causative factors in certain pediatric deformities of the lower extremities (Giannestras 1973; Knight 1954; McCrea 1985; McDonough 1984).

Harold Frost (1986) has devoted more than 30 years to the study of bone modeling and remodeling. He reports that the subspecialty of orthopedic biomechanics began to develop in earnest in the 1940s with the work of such researchers as Venable, Stuck, Inman, and their colleagues and students. It is a new field and has developed by encompassing fads and changing emphases without a unified plan. Currently the field of biomechanics in medicine incorporates five major areas of investigation, each of which occupies a percentage of the available research and publications. The subdivisions are as follows (Frost 1986, Vol. 1):

1. Properties of materials both inside and outside the body—for example, bone, cartilage, plates, pins, acrylic implants, braces, casts (50 percent)
2. Kinematics—the dynamics of skeletal function (15 percent)
3. Pathophysiology of trauma and healing (25 percent)
4. Structural design of the adult skeleton (8 percent)
5. Design principles of the growing skeleton (2 percent)

The fifth subdivision, design principles of the growing skeleton, so far constitutes the least studied but perhaps the most basic subdivision of biomechanics. This area of study and its relevant concerns underlie and bear on all of the other subdivisions within the field of orthopedic biomechanics. Frost assembled the following account of the history of the development of the principles of modeling that are currently emerging (Frost 1986, Vol. 2).

Since people started contemplating the phenomenon of growth and aging, they have presumed that the developing skeleton faithfully followed some finished master blueprint, the details of which researchers have sought for at least the past hundred years. Wolff proposed in the 1890s that differences in mechanical usage could evoke changes in the internal architecture of bones, but he offered no mechanisms by which to quantify or predict those changes.

Prior to the 1950s, the capacity of the growing skeleton to respond to modeling influences was evident in the deformities that responded to procedures that were developed to manage anterior poliomyelitis in children. It became evident that many of the deformities could be prevented by using combinations of bracing, joint arthrodeses, physical therapy, and surgical transfers of muscle tendons of insertion. One of the reasons for the relative success of these procedures was the capability of these children to retrain their transferred muscles.

The waning of the polio epidemic left orthopedists with a repertoire of skills to aim at the population with cerebral palsy, even though the initial results were frustrating. Spastic limbs fought the braces, often worsening the deformities, and the lack of control over central sensorimotor processing impeded or nullified the potential effect of muscle transfers. Surgical outcomes for the spastic population were highly unpredictable (Frost 1986, Vol. 2).

Between 1958 and 1968, it was recognized that most osseous deformities of the older spastic child represent the effects of normal chondral modeling on hyaline cartilage and growing epiphyseal plates. These effects are dictated by the abnormal force environment of spastic contractual patterns, often combined with the effects of braces that might conceal spastic muscle dynamics but fail to correct them.

Children with spasticity and polio unknowingly carried out the natural experiments that overturned old ideas with newly perceived facts. These facts in their turn revealed at least some of the principles that govern the ways in which growing hyaline cartilage responds to mechanical usage.

In the 1960s some general principles of macromodeling were proposed by Frost (and Epker), under which certain predictions about the influences of various types of forces on skeletal architecture could be made. In the past 25 years, work in this area has continued, and several misconceptions about the fundamental design criteria of structural tissues have been challenged. For example, before 1960 orthopedic surgeons generally believed that mechanical compression stress somehow stimulated bone formation, and tension stress stimulated resorption, while dentists (particularly orthodontists) believed the opposite (Frost 1986, Vol. 1).

By 1966, Frost and Epker reached the following conclusions (Frost 1986, Vol. 1):

- The biological system "hears" strain rather than stress.
- This system fits its architecture to some average over time or to a history of its strains, rather than to single strains, even large ones.

- Dynamic rather than constant strains guide the system.
- A mechanism must exist that can transduce a flexural strain into a signal that cells can detect; in addition, this mechanism has the capacity to distinguish between the components of the flexural strain, recognizing bending that tends toward concave to be different from bending that tends toward convex.
- Articular cartilage on bone surfaces prevents modeling drifts on those surfaces.
- Widespread flexural neutralization occurs in vertebrate bony skeletons.
- Strains must exceed a minimum magnitude (the MES—minimum effective signal) before the biological system can perceive them.
- Modeling and remodeling are different processes.
- Modeling depends upon the growth process.
- Normal neuromotor function is somewhat stereotyped and controls bone and joint loading.

The next decade or two should see a growing body of research focus on the cellular, biochemical, and physical mechanisms that underlie the above events and concepts.

The Modeling Process—Current Perspectives

Frost wrote the following about the influence of outside forces on developing skeletal structures:

> A miniature model arises first in the uterus that does seem blindly and faithfully to follow a master genetic blueprint that distills the successful results from the innumerable evolutionary experiments performed since Precambrian times. The tissues of that model contain special principles of action that govern their growth and modeling responses to mechanical usage as well as to other factors.
>
> That model then enters the world as a growing passenger inside a newborn infant. As it grows, it experiences increasing vigor, frequency, and variety of usage by its owner . . . [Therefore] embryogenesis—ontogeny—creates the basic skeletal tissues and forms miniature models of the organs. The tissues of those miniatures then respond in special ways to their postnatal usage . . . Thus:

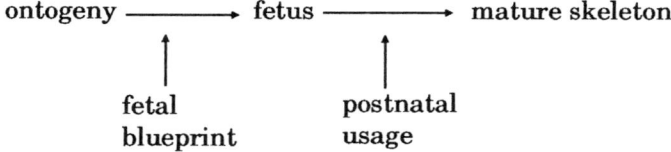

—Frost 1986, Vol. 1, p. 269

Chondral Modeling

The three types of cartilage include hyaline cartilage, fibrocartilage, and elastocartilage. Each is quite compliant compared to bone and is also strongly viscoelastic. In skeletal growth and development, both before and after birth, cartilage plays a dominant role. It determines the original number, location, and shape of the fetal models of most bones, as well as their orientations, alignment, and articulations.

> Postnatal functions of cartilage establish bone and limb length, body height and body proportions, facial and joint size and shape, the alignment of the segments of the spine and limbs, the locations, size and growth of tendon, ligament, and fascial attachments to bone, and the properties of growing and mature joints. Cartilage malfunctions of varied kinds cause most children's skeletal deformities, and many other skeletal diseases, as well as all joint disease.
>
> —Frost 1986, Vol. 2, p. 3

Cartilage is ultimately much weaker than bone under shear, tension, and compression loads. It is therefore capable of much greater unit creep than bone or mature tendon and ligament.

Hyaline cartilage forms articular cartilage, epiphyseal plates, and perichondral rings, and it lies at the bony attachments of tendons, ligaments, and fascia. Twenty percent of its volume is comprised of organic matrix, and extracellular water fills most of the remainder. Articular cartilage growth determines the shapes and thus the types of free motion of joints. Epiphyseal plate growth determines bone length as well as limb and joint alignment. Perichondral ring growth determines the diameters and cross-section areas of epiphyseal plates and joint surfaces (Frost 1986, Vol. 2).

Cartilage grows differently from bone: its precursor cells are located within rather than on the surface of the matrix. "Bone is shaped as a sculptor shapes plaster, by removing some at one surface and adding some at another. Cartilage models like a puff of smoke, by patterned and spatially oriented internal explosions" (Frost 1986, Vol. 2, p. 8).

During growth, bone replaces previously elaborated cartilage by the endochondral ossification mechanism. In doing this, it simply copies the configuration of the cartilage. Thus many skeletal disorders are actually disorders of chondrification in which normal bone modeling and ossification occur.

Bone Formation

Most bone forms by the process of endochondral ossification, which involves the destruction and replacement of hyaline cartilage that was originally shaped in the form of the (future) bone. Osteoblasts form spicules of osteoid material that accumulate, broaden, lengthen, and eventually join with adjacent spicules to form a meshwork of trabeculae (supporting bars or projections of connective tissue). Mineralization occurs in the matrix of trabeculae, which are laid down in response to forces applied to the cartilage model. For example, the bones of the foot reveal that tension forces of muscles and ligaments create loci of trabeculae in resistance to their pull (Bernhardt 1988). In more proximal bones, trabeculae are more concentrated in areas of greatest compression as well as tension (Frost 1986, Vol. 2).

In long bone, there are usually three ossification centers: one primary center in the middle of the shaft (future diaphysis) and two secondary centers—one at each end (epiphyseal plates). Most primary centers—except those of the small bones of the wrists and feet—appear shortly after the second month of fetal life. Most secondary centers in the epiphyses do not appear until after birth. Alternatively, the diameter of bone is increased by periosteal ossification and responds to externally applied forces of substantial magnitude.

The diaphysis (shaft) and epiphyses are separated by growth (epiphyseal) cartilages until ultimate length is achieved, at which time they close. The section of new bone tissue that lies between the epiphyseal plate and the diaphysis is the metaphysis. Mineral deposits begin to appear in newly formed bone matrix about one week after its formation and take six to twelve months or more to completely ossify the tissue. The mineralization process displaces water from the matrix in such a way that young bone has less mineral and more water than old bone, on a per unit volume basis. Thus it is less stiff and will therefore strain (deform under load) more significantly than older or mature bone. More rapid modeling occurs in the metaphysis than in the diaphysis, and in younger individuals compared with older ones (Frost 1986, Vol. 2).

Compact (cortical) bone is the dense, ivory-like outer layer. It is thickest around the hollow diaphysis (shaft) of long bones. Cancellous bone (spongiosa) is spongy, light-weight, elastic inner tissue. Cancellous tissue fills the epiphyses and collects at the enlarged ends of long bones.

Ossification and growth are complete by the 25th year.

Frost's Biomechanical Rules-of-Thumb for Normal Lamellar Bone

1. Strain rather than stress most directly controls modeling. The shape, stiffness, and the loads a tissue carries determine its strains.
2. Macromodeling determines the cross-section size and shape, the longitudinal shape, and the location (in tissue space) of growing bony diaphyses and metaphyses, except chondral effects.
3. The size and shape of a bone reflect the magnitudes and orientations of the typical larger dynamic loads it carried during its growth, and neuromotor factors control and pattern those loads.
4. Micromodeling aligns the preferred grain of lamellar bone during its deposition so it parallels the typical local tension and/or compression strains.
5. In order to occur in significant amounts, bone macromodeling requires concurrent general body growth. (Frost 1986, Vol. 1)

Frost's Chondral Modeling Axioms

These axioms pertain only to postnatal life. A different set of principles constructs the preformed models of bones and joints in the embryo and fetus.

- **Strain governs chondral modeling.** Load-induced dynamic strain probably most directly controls cartilage modeling.
- **The macromodeling system requires a minimum effective signal (MES).**
- **Chondral modeling features a dynamic strain-averaging property.** Like bone, cartilage adapts its structure to some history of mechanical usage, responding to an integration of many nontrivial dynamic loads averaged over some period of time. Unlike bone, however, constant loads may (and in fact probably do) have significant effects on chondral macromodeling, although some of those effects may relate to creep rather than to modeling. "For example, a constant valgus force of correct magnitude applied by a brace or cast across a growing knee or foot can change its alignment predictably by modifying the rates of longitudinal growth on opposite sides of those structures, thereby correcting a bow leg or a knock knee" (Frost 1986, Vol. 2, p. 10).
- **Chondral modeling occurs during growth.** Modeling ceases when growth stops. Like bone modeling, growth rate and bone age are directly related to potential effects of chondral modeling on skeletal architecture. Only that uncompleted fraction of growth can be modified or molded for therapeutic purposes.

Frost's Provisional Chondral Modeling Laws (postnatal only)

1. Modeling acts by modifying local growth speed.
2. Increasing the unit tension loads on a chondral plane increases its growth.
3. Increasing unit compression loads also increases growth up to a chondral growth/force response (CGFR) peak, beyond which it retards chondral growth. (Such excessive forces do not occur in normal movement or mechanical usage.)
4. Those growth responses apply only to time-averaged, dynamic (rather than static) unit loads.
5. Articular cartilage unit loading is normally high (except at the femoral condyles), so both increases and decreases in loading would retard its growth, with increases being more significant than decreases.
6. Epiphyseal and compression-loaded apophyseal plates normally take loads that fall under the CGFR peak; thus growth rate increases with normally increasing compression forces.

    Example: Resolution of genu varum/valgum—increased compression on the concave side of the knee joint increases growth rate, and reduced compression on the convex side of the knee joint reduces growth rate, until compression forces on both sides are equalized.

7. Tendon and ligament attachments to bone normally load in tension, which increases growth on the attachment site as tension increases. The result is formation of tuberosities, trochanters, the olecranon, the tibial tubercle, etc.

In reference to the magnitude and appropriateness of effective modeling forces, Frost explains:

> Even on weight-bearing joints, the major loads come from muscle forces rather than body weight, and they can readily exceed body weight by factors of two, five, or even to ten times . . . Furthermore, since the nervous system coordinates muscle contractual strengths and patterns, it follows that the chondral modeling contribution to joint configuration and limb alignment must reflect certain properties of that neurologic control as well . . . The realization that the postnatal skeleton is architecturally fluid to a significant degree, and that the stereotypism of the mature skeleton reflects the stereotypism of its mechanical usage during growth . . . is too new to have been digested by a majority of workers in the field.
>
> —Frost 1986, Vol. 2, p. 25

Clinical Examples of Chondral Modeling Errors

Epiphyseal Plate Errors (excluding diseases)

coxa valga

genu valgum

scoliosis

coxa vara

genu varum

spastic back-knee

tibial torsion

femoral torsion

Cartilage exhibits much larger amounts of creep than fibrous tissues, bone, and teeth. Total creep (rather than unit creep) adds up over the whole length and/or thickness of a structure. A form of creep in torque at epiphyseal plates underlies some limb torsions, as well as the effectiveness of certain orthotic and surgical muscle balancing methods of correcting the torsional deformities (Frost 1986, Vol. 2, p.13).

Fibrous Tissues

Fibrous tissues include those that assemble to form tendons, ligaments, and fascia. The matrix, comprised mostly of Type I collagen, consists of tropocollagen molecules with fixed lengths. However, the matrix assembles in variable quantity to alter length and weight. The tropocollagen fibers are bound together by chemical cross-links, which prevent them from sliding past each other and which provide the tensile strength and stiffness of the mature tissue (Frost 1986, Vol. 2).

As fibrous tissue is made, collagen fibers are laid down parallel to the tension loads and strains that were applied during their deposition. The fabric of fascial tissue might demonstrate two or three such preferred fiber orientations. Predetermined growth in length occurs at the ends of the tendons, ligaments, and fascia—as it does in bone—rather than in the middle. Repeated dynamic mechanical tension loads of sufficient magnitude to elicit activation of the modeling processes increase the diameter and cross-sectional area of the fibrous tissue structures (and thus their strength and stiffness) throughout the whole length of the structure (Frost 1986, Vol. 2).

With advancing age, fibrous tissues become stiffer and less compliant in tension. Under equal unit loads, young tissues strain more than old ones.

Developmental biomechanics is the study of the effects of externally applied forces on the musculoskeletal system during early life (Le-Veau and Bernhardt 1984; Bernhardt 1988). With increasing interest, medical professionals are investigating the influence of the forces of tension and loading on the shape and function of developing skeletal structures, both normal and abnormal. This field is, as Frost suggests, very new, but the information that is becoming available through these studies offers great possibilities for enhancing the effectiveness of intervention measures available to therapists, orthopedists, and orthotists, and for empirically evaluating the results of intervention.

It is known, for example, that the angle of femoral antetorsion (mistakenly referred to as "anteversion" in most related writings) is generally 20-35 degrees greater at birth than in adulthood, decreasing perhaps 5 degrees during the first postnatal year (Fabry et al. 1973; McCrea 1985; Engel and Staheli 1974; Bleck 1987; Staheli et al. 1968; Staheli 1977). Evaluation of the structure of the femur in children with hypertonic cerebral palsy, however, has revealed a significant persistence of, and in some cases an increase in, the degree of antetorsion that is normal at birth (Fabry et al. 1973; Bleck 1987; Beals 1969; Staheli et al. 1968). This phenomenon may become a focus of clinical research, perhaps using improved techniques such as computerized axial tomography to determine the angle of torsional declination of the femur (Murphy et al. 1987). Data gathered, using sophisticated radiographic technology, prior to and following various programs of therapeutic intervention, would contribute substantially to our understanding of the forces needed to reduce structural deformity. The following discussion concerns several aspects of structural development as a function of neuromotor activity as they are currently understood.

Features of Neonatal Structure and Joint Position

The Spine

The newborn's spine is kyphotic, and the thoracic area is rigid. The low back is flexed rather than extended; thus kyphosis is evident from the neck to the sacrum, as the entire spine forms a C-curve (Hensinger et al. 1982; LeVeau et al. 1984; Tax 1985; Asher 1975; Schafer 1987). The proportions of the segments of the newborn's spine differ greatly from those of an adult. The cervical and lumbar areas each comprise approximately 25 percent of the length of the spine (Tax 1985).

The Pelvis

At birth, the pelvis is small and tilted posteriorly relative to the frontal plane, more so in the prone than in the supine position. This alignment of the pelvis occurs in conjunction with the flexed attitude in the lumbar spine (Hensinger et al. 1982; Asher 1975; Schafer 1987; Bly 1983).

The acetabular roof of the hip joint is shallow at birth, and the acetabula is inclined downward 7 degrees from the sagittal plane. This acetabular inclination increases to a mature value of 17 degrees by the age of 3 years (Bernhardt 1988).

McCrea (1985) and Badgley (1949) suggest that the acetabulum is retroverted (directed posteriorly) in the neonate and gradually rotates to align on the frontal plane by the age of 3 years. The narrowness of the neonatal sacrum supports this suggestion. Bernhardt (1988) and Lloyd-Roberts et al. (1978), however, claim that the neonatal acetabulum is anteverted at birth.

The Hip

Newborn hips are maintained in a position of flexion and lateral rotation. Apparently they are held in that position by a combination of contracture of both the capsular structures and the muscles of flexion and lateral rotation, and perhaps a degree of structural retroversion of the acetabulum (Hensinger et al. 1982; LeVeau et al. 1984; Tax 1985; Bly 1983; Badgley 1949; Pitkow 1975; Haas et al. 1973; Phelps et al. 1985).

The anterior and inferior aspects of the hip joint are heavily endowed with ligamentous support structures, unlike the postero-lateral aspects (Kapandji 1970). By virtue of their spiral direction and attachments, the fibers of the iliofemoral and ischiofemoral ligaments that reinforce the hip joint capsule tend to recoil, pulling the femur into flexion and lateral rotation. They become taut when the hip is extended and rotated medially toward a close-packed (congruent) position (Kapandji 1970). In addition, there are nearly twice as many muscles of lateral hip rotation as there are of medial rotation (McCrea 1985; Kapandji 1970; Jordan et al. 1983).

Flexion contracture—The hip flexion contracture averages 30 degrees at birth (with a reported range of 30-120 degrees) when assessed by using the (highly variable) Thomas Test method (Hensinger et al. 1982; McCrea 1985; Haas et al. 1973; Sgarlato 1971; Hoffer 1980; Bleck 1982). Hip extension does not normally occur at any time during gestation. The study by Phelps et al. (1985) notes vast discrepancies in the findings by researchers relative to hip flexion contracture in infants. This study recommends using Staheli's Prone Hip Extension Test in order to determine the degree of existing contracture (See Staheli 1977, *Clinical Orthopaedics and Related Research.*) However, the study by Phelps excludes the neonatal population.

Rotation mobility—The range of hip rotation totals 120 degrees, with lateral rotation mobility exceeding that of medial rotation throughout the first 18 to 24 months of life (Tax 1985; Pitkow 1975; Haas et al. 1973, Phelps et al. 1985). In the position of flexion that prevails in the neonatal hip, the range of lateral rotation is highly variable, averaging 90 degrees at birth (range 45 to 110) (Hensinger et al. 1982; Haas et al. 1973). The average range of medial hip rotation is 60 degrees (with a range of -30 to 100 degrees) (Haas et al. 1973; Hoffer 1980).

Pitkow (1975) notes that with the hip extended (within its available limit), the range of lateral hip rotation exceeds the range of medial rotation by three times or more in children less than 6 months of age; this variance resolves before 3 years of age. Pitkow interprets his findings in terms of soft tissue contracture.

The lateral rotation contracture draws the greater trochanter posteriorly, anteverting the femoral neck 40-60 degrees relative to the frontal plane (Hensinger et al. 1982; McCrea 1985; Engel et al. 1974; Pitkow 1975; Beals 1969). This laterally rotated hip joint position is therefore synonymous with femoral anteversion (McCrea 1985). Acetabular retroversion, if present, would contribute to the maximum angle of 60 degrees of anteversion noted above, provided the measurement is taken relative to the frontal plane (McCrea 1985; Badgley 1949).

Most authors of orthopedic literature inaccurately describe "anteversion" as the angle of torsional declination of the shaft of the femur that results in a forward angulation of the femoral head and neck when the condyles are aligned on the frontal plane. The term "femoral anteversion," however, refers only to the "forward direction" of the femoral head and neck, relative to the frontal plane (McCrea 1985). The forward angle noted at the femoral head and neck when the femoral condyles are aligned on the frontal plane more accurately describes femoral torsion or, more specifically, "antetorsion." Antetorsion is discussed below (Fabry et al. 1973; Bleck 1987).

Abduction—Hip abduction mobility, measured in the neonate with the hips in 90 degrees of flexion, averages 76 degrees at each hip (with a range of 50-90 degrees) (Haas et al. 1973). By age 9 months, the average abduction range decreases to 59 degrees, where it remains through the age of 24 months (Phelps et al. 1985). Thereafter, 45 degrees of range at each extended hip is considered to be normal (Rang et al. 1986).

The Femur

The proximal femur, composed entirely of hyaline cartilage in the neonate, bears three growth plates: the longitudinal growth plate (LGP), the trochanteric growth plate (TGP), and the femoral neck isthmus (FNI). The LGP is located under the cap of the femoral head and is aligned on the transverse plane, partly because of the valgus orientation of the femoral neck and shaft (discussed below). The LGP contributes 30 percent of the growth of the length of the femur, assisted in small measure by the TGP (Siffert 1981). The proximal femoral shaft is therefore very pliable in infancy and childhood. The TGP and FNI primarily contribute to the modeling of the femoral neck and head, controlling thickness and reducing the valgus angle of the neck and shaft (Siffert 1981).

The newborn demonstrates a predominance of three structural features in the femur: coxa valga, antetorsion, and mild varus bowing (Hensinger et al. 1982; Matles 1965; Knight 1954; McCrea 1985; Tachdjian 1971; Bleck 1987; Tax 1985; Sgarlato 1971; Sutherland 1984; Siffert 1981). These deviations, plus occasional evidence of some anterior bowing, reflect early fetal skeletal design plus the position demanded by intrauterine confinement during the final two months of full-term gestation (Hensinger et al. 1982; Knight 1954; Tax 1985; Badgley 1949). They are indicators of skeletal immaturity.

Coxa valga—The angle of inclination between the neonatal femoral shaft and the neck is increased, compared to the mature value, up to a maximum of 150 degrees (Matles 1965; McCrea 1985; Tachdjian 1971; Tax 1985; Jordan et al. 1983; Cailliet 1983; Siffert 1981). This angle will reduce to 125-135 degrees by the age of 6 years (Jordan et al. 1983). Beals (1969), however, suggests that the angle of inclination between birth and 18 months reduces to 145 degrees, reduces again to 135 degrees by age 6 years, and by adulthood reduces another 10 degrees.

Antetorsion—Antetorsion is a medial twist of the femoral shaft, distal on proximal ends. At birth, the average declination angle of the femur (torsional twist) is 38-40 degrees (Hensinger et al. 1982; Matles 1965; Badgley 1949; Fabry et al. 1973; McCrea 1985; Tachdjian 1971; Tax 1985; Bleck 1982; Sutherland 1984; Beals 1969).

Despite the medial twist of the femoral shaft, the newborn femoral head and neck are anteverted by contracture of soft tissue and possibly by the posteriorly displaced acetabulum (Engel et al. 1974; Pitkow 1975; McCrea 1985; Badgley 1949; Jordan et al. 1983). The resultant resting angle—evident in the relationship of the patella to the sagittal plane and of the femoral condyles to the frontal plane—approaches 30 degrees of lateral rotation (Jordan et al. 1983; Tax 1985) (Figure 2.1).

Reduction of torsion in the femur appears to correspond with reduction of the hip flexion contracture, combined with activation of the hip extensors and lateral rotators (Bleck 1982). The rate of reduction of antetorsion is greatest during the first two years of life, during which antetorsion reduces from 40 to 30 degrees as can be shown by the radiographic assessment techniques that existed prior to the CT scan (Fabry et al. 1973; Engel et al. 1974; Bleck 1982; Sutherland 1984).

Figure 2.1 Neonatal femoral antetorsion and anteversion combine to leave the femoral condyles angled laterally relative to the frontal plane. Internal genicular position results in medial rotation of the lower leg on the femur.

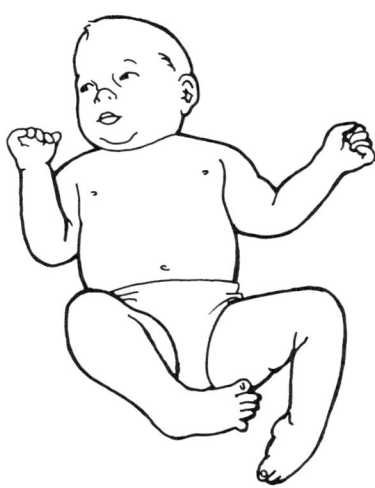

The Knee

Flexion contracture—The newborn demonstrates knee flexion contractures of up to 30 degrees with the hips maximally extended (Hoffer 1980). Two factors contribute to the formation of this contracture: maturation of the nervous system, which brings in flexor activity, and adaptive shortening of soft tissue structures secondary to positioning in utero (Hensinger et al. 1982; McCrea 1985; Tax 1985). Together, the two factors result in "physiologic flexion" that is observed in the full-term newborn at the elbows, hips, and ankles, as well as at the knees (Bly 1983; Sternat 1987).

Internal genicular position—The slightest degree of flexion at the knee permits the tibia to rotate on the femur (Schafer 1987). Uterine confinement forces the tibia and fibula to rotate medially on the femur. McCrea (1985) describes the medial rotation position of the lower leg under the femur as internal genicular position. When this deviation is great enough to prohibit rotary excursion laterally past 0 degrees or when it persists beyond early infancy, as often occurs in children with neuromotor disorders, "internal" (medial) genicular position should be distinguished from "internal" (medial) tibial torsion (McCrea 1985) (Figure 2.1). McDonough (1984) describes this deformity as a possible "component" of internal tibial torsion. In fact, they are separate features.

Genu varum—"Physiologic" genu varum is a feature of the newborn knee joint, although its presence is masked by flexion contracture (Hensinger et al. 1982; Bleck 1982; McDade 1977; Valmassy 1984). The combined features of femoral coxa valga (which, when the femoral head is seated in the acetabulum, displaces the distal femur laterally) plus lateral hip rotation, mild lateral femoral bowing, medial knee flexion contracture, and medial tibial rotation, result in a normal tibiofemoral varus angle of up to 17 degrees (McDade 1977; Hensinger et al. 1982; McDonough 1984). It should be noted that Bernhardt (1988) apparently disagrees with these studies.

The Lower Leg

Torsion—The newborn tibia and fibula are usually quite straight (that is, neither bowed nor twisted) in the newborn (Jordan et al. 1983). By clinical examination, the torsional declination of the lower leg bones is 0 degrees, with 5 to 10 degrees of either medial or lateral deviation (Hensinger et al. 1982; McCrea 1985; Tax 1985; Bleck 1982; Bernhardt 1988). The presence of flexion and rotary contracture can confound this measurement on clinical examination, because the flexed position of the knee joint permits the lower leg to rotate on the femur. This produces the appearance of medial tibial torsion in the shaft of the bone (McCrea 1985). Torsional status is best assessed radiologically using CT or MRI (Bleck 1982). The distal tibia and fibula are composed almost entirely of cartilage, rendering them pliable and highly responsive to applied torque forces (Tax 1985).

Apparent tibial varum (bowing)—The distal third of the lower leg appears to bow laterally approximately 15-20 degrees (Sgarlato 1971; Jordan et al. 1983). However, the long bones are in fact straight. The *bowing* is actually the result of lateral displacement of the posterior compartment muscles, which is caused by *medial rotation of the lower leg* combined with a medial deviation of the lower leg under the femur (genu varum). This deviation results from adaptive shortening of the medial knee joint musculature and connective tissues (McDonough 1984).

Retroversion of the proximal plateau—The tibial plateau aligns with the transverse plane at an angle of up to 27 degrees, positioning the anterior edge of the plateau more proximal than the posterior edge. This angle, masked in early infancy by knee flexion contracture, reduces to 5 degrees by the end of adolescence (Bernhardt 1988).

The Talocrural Joint

The tibia and fibula articulate with the talus at this joint. This is the place where the primary motions of ankle dorsiflexion and plantarflexion occur, within the context of concurrent pronation and supination, respectively.

Mobility—At birth, the ankle can be passively dorsiflexed up to 70 degrees, bringing the dorsum of the foot in contact with the tibia. Plantarflexion may be limited to 15-30 degrees (Hensinger et al. 1982; McCrea 1985; Hoffer 1980). The newborn ankle rests at approximately 15 degrees of dorsiflexion (Tax 1985). This hypermobility, which is evidently related to intrauterine positioning and to maternal hormonal relaxants excreted during birth, diminishes rapidly in the first weeks of life, resulting in a normal infant range of 45-50 degrees of passive dorsiflexion.

Alignment—The literature can be confusing regarding the structural rather than functional relationships between the newborn tibia, fibula, and talus at the ankle joint. On the issue of structure, some authors concur that the tibial plafond (its distal surface) is everted in such a way that the medial side is more distal then the lateral side (Bahler 1986; Tachdjian 1985). Tachdjian (1985) illustrates the talocrural joint in congruous articulation at birth, which results in a valgus deviation of the body of the talus under the tibia and in a valgus deviation of the calcaneus under the talus. Bernhardt (1988) agrees with this observation of hindfoot valgus deviation in the newborn.

However, Sgarlato (1971), Jordan et al. (1983), and Tax (1985) describe the open-chain alignment of the newborn hindfoot as one of predominant varus (inversion), which converts to valgus during infancy with the onset of weight-bearing. They describe a calcaneal valgus deviation at birth as an abnormality suggestive of intrauterine deformation and correctable within six weeks with gentle manipulations at diaper changes. If they are correct, does the inverted calcaneus at birth reveal evidence of an original lack of talocalcaneal congruity caused by shortening of the soft tissue structures—muscle, tendon, and ligament—that lie medial to the talocrural and subtalar joints? Is talocrural and subtalar joint congruity in eversion gained, then, in later infancy, when compression applied to the weight-bearing foot gradually lengthens the medial soft tissues to allow the calcaneus to evert?

Bahler (1986) suggests that the tibial plafond usually aligns on the transverse plane by the age of 12 years. (Is he referring to the full ossification of the distal tibial chondral model, or to the growth of cartilage that brings the plafond onto the transverse plane?) However, Bleck (1982) reports that arthrographic evaluation reveals that "even in toddlers, the superior articular surface of the talus is perpendicular to the distal tibial metaphysis" (p. 541). Does this finding indicate that the growing cartilage model of the tibial plafond reduces the effective distal plafond angle several years earlier than Bahler suggests? Or, does the talus alter its orientation to the tibia to align the trochlea on the transverse plane?

Another structural feature of the newborn talocrural joint is a relative shortness of the fibula in the area of the lateral malleolus (Jordan et al. 1983; Tachdijian 1985; Tax 1985). The longer, more distal lateral malleolus provides stabilization for the talus against eversion. Therefore, Tax (1985) reports, the newborn ankle joint (rather than the subtalar joint) allows slight frontal plane motion.

These questions remain to be answered satisfactorily by researchers. Further studies that include large populations of newborn infants and longitudinal studies of the same infants, perhaps using techniques other than arthrograms and roentgenograms, are needed to clear the confusion.

The Foot

The length of the neonatal foot averages 3-4 inches, which is long in proportion to the length of the leg (Tax 1985). The sole is triangular in shape. The first ray is pitched medially, abducting away from the second metatarsal by approximately 8-15 degrees (Tax 1985; Jordan et al. 1983; McCrea 1985). The talus, calcaneus, and cuboid bones reveal evidence of ossification at birth, as do the metatarsals (Giannestras 1973; Crouch 1970).

Hindfoot varus—The posterior calcaneus aligns in an average of 10 degrees (with a range of 8-22 degrees) of varus relative to the distal third of the lower leg when the subtalor joint is aligned in congruity (Tax 1985; Jordan et al. 1983). This deviation, together with forefoot varus (described below), is a function of the structure of the calcaneous (see *calcaneal torsion*, following).

Calcaneal torsion—The posterior segment of the calcaneus is inverted relative to the anterior portion at birth, by virtue of a medial twist in the body of the calcaneus. The degree of torsion gradually reduces with growth.

Forefoot varus—The newborn forefoot is inverted into varus position an additional 10-15 degrees on the hindfoot when the subtalar joint is aligned in congruity (Tax 1985; Jordan et al. 1983; Sgarlato 1971). The original embryonic "praying" apposition of the plantar surfaces of the feet is evident in this varus foot position, offering evidence of early intrauterine position (Bernhardt 1988; Jordan et al. 1983; Jaffe and Laitman 1982). Open-chain varus alignment that persists after birth appears to be maintained by both shortened medial soft tissue structures and talar torsion, as discussed below.

Talar torsion—Looking down on the newborn's foot from a superior (dorsal) perspective, the talar neck (the portion that extends forward toward the navicular) is elongated and deviates medially 30-37 degrees relative to the sagittal plane bisection of the talar trochlea (the superior surface of the talar body, or its posterior portion) (McCrea 1985; Bleck 1982; Tachdjian 1985). In the adult, the talar neck is proportionally shorter than in the newborn, and the adduction angle is 18-20 degrees (Bleck 1982; Tachdjian 1985).

The adducted position of the talar neck and head causes the remainder of the medial foot structures distal to the talus to angle medially (adduct) when the talonavicular joint is congruous (Jordan et al. 1983; Bleck 1982). The proximal navicular articulates with 80-90 percent of the talar head. The cuboid closely approximates and moves together with the navicular. The result is adduction of the foot, distal to the talocrural joint, of 0-10 degrees at birth (McCrea 1985). If this angle of adduction exceeds 10 degrees at birth, spontaneous resolution before the age of 3 years is unlikely; in-toe gait will probably persist (Bleck 1982).

Medial deviation of the talar neck is also accompanied by lateral torsion, which results in an inverted orientation of the talar head (Tachdjian 1985). The talus articulates with the navicular; thus the inverted talar head also supinates the medial forefoot via the talonavicular joint and the interosseus ligaments. This torsional angle appears to promote the forefoot varus deviation described above (Tiberio 1988).

Talar torsion refers, therefore, to the adduction and lateral torsion of the talar neck. It typically resolves with modeling, which responds to pronatory stresses on the forefoot in weight-bearing, combined with reduction in hindfoot pronation and with growth in size of the navicular (Bleck 1982; Tachdjian 1985).

Metatarsal alignment—The normality of evidence of metatarsus adductus, or a medial deviation of all of the metatarsals at the tarsometatarsal joints, is unclear. Hensinger et al. (1982) state that metatarsus adductus is a frequent finding that may be related to intrauterine positioning. It is often accompanied by "internal tibial torsion." They report, and McCrea (1985) concurs, that in the normal newborn foot, the lateral border of the foot is normally straight; in the case of adductus of the metatarsals, the lateral border of the foot is C-shaped. Therefore, by the process of deduction, it seems that the C-shaped foot is abnormal. Hensinger et al. (1982) also recommend that metatarsus adductus be treated early in case it does not resolve spontaneously.

Tax (1985) and McCrea (1985) also describe the normal newborn foot as triangular in shape. However, without explanation, Tax also reports that the normal newborn foot reveals 15-35 degrees of adductus of the lateral four metatarsals, with an additional 8-10 degrees of adductus of the first ray. Bernhardt (1988) seems to concur with this. This deviation into adductus would result (again) in a C-shaped foot, which is considered abnormal.

Agnew (1988) considers all metatarsus adductus (excluding that of the first ray) to be abnormal. He suggests that true correction of metatarsus adductus does not occur spontaneously in any case. Instead, the affected child typically rotates the hip laterally to clear the medially deviated toes out of the path of progression of the opposite foot, and a hindfoot pronation deformity evolves while the forefoot adductus persists. The result is "skewfoot," which is among the most difficult deformities to treat.

For the purposes of this text, we will presume the following:

- The normal newborn foot is triangular, and straight along its lateral border.
- Persistence of adductus of the metatarsals, with the exception of the first, is evidence of excessive constriction during the latter phase of uterine confinement. It is abnormal or at least undesirable.

Toes—The toes are hypermobile in infancy, although a lack of opportunity to hyperextend the metatarsophalangeal joints commonly results in some tightness in flexion.

Newborn Biomechanical and Structural Developmental Issues

To summarize the previous discussion, it appears that the newborn, while working to achieve motor control (and sculpting the underlying skeletal architecture into the appropriate adult configuration), is confronted with a variety of obstacles. These include the shape of the pelvis, long bones, and talus, and limitations of joint mobility in the spine and lower extremities. Thus we might compile the following list:

Neonatal Biomechanical Problem List

1. Rigid, kyphotic spine, including the lumbar area, in which the vertebrae are relatively short
2. Shallow acetabulae, inclined upward and possibly retroverted
3. Coxa valga
4. Antetorsion within the femoral shaft
5. Femoral lateral bowing
6. Hip flexion contracture involving muscle, ligaments, and joint capsule
7. Lateral hip rotation contracture involving muscle, ligaments, and capsule
8. Knee flexion (hamstrings) contracture, more medial than lateral
9. Physiologic genu varum
10. Internal (medial) genicular position—soft tissue contracture favoring medial rotation of the lower leg
11. Apparent lateral bowing of the distal lower leg (due to factors 9 and 10)
12. Straight (untwisted) shafts of the tibia and fibula
13. Short distal fibula, aligned anteriorly relative to the position at maturity
14. Everted tibial plafond
15. Excessive dorsiflexion and frontal-plane mobility in the talocrural joint
16. Hindfoot varus (in congruity)
17. Forefoot varus (in congruity)
18. Calcaneal torsion
19. Talar torsion
20. Metatarsophalangeal flexion contracture

The Sculptor's Tool Box

Within the infant's central nervous system there are built-in demands to achieve the upright position. As the infant responds to these demands, longitudinal growth and muscle action contribute to the revising of its skeletal design and arrangement (Asher 1975; Effgen 1987). The process is one of tireless weight lifting, first of the head and later of the limbs and trunk, as the trunk gains proximal antigravity control and strength in a cephalocaudal direction (Tax 1985; Asher 1975; Bly 1983; Sternat 1987; Effgen 1987; Scherzer et al. 1982; Salek 1977; Bobath 1967).

As the infant undertakes the strengthening and sculpting process, the postural arrangements of the spine, pelvis, and lower extremities are of particular interest to the developmental therapist. When forces are applied across joints that are malaligned (as occurs with ligamentous laxity) or when those forces are unbalanced (as in the case of hypertonus), the structural consequences typically become clinical concerns for the therapist, orthopedist, orthotist, and podiatrist (Hensinger et al. 1982; LeVeau et al. 1984; Fabry et al. 1973; McCrea 1985; Bleck 1987; Staheli et al. 1968; Staheli 1977; Bleck 1982; Tachdjian 1985; Root et al. 1977; Schafer 1987; Salek 1981; McDonough 1984; Valmassy 1984; Jordan et al. 1983).

As the events of normal sensorimotor development appear, they signal the achievement of several components of movement, including the following (Salek 1981; Scherzer et al. 1982; Bly 1983; Tachdjian 1985; Effgen 1987; Sternat 1987):

- Muscle strength and control against gravity in the neck, trunk, and extremities
- Muscle elongation through reciprocal innervation
- Joint capsule and ligament mobility within the spine and lower extremities
- Automatic postural reactions

The following discussion covers the apparent mechanisms by which the normal infant successfully resolves the structural problems observed at birth, particularly in the context of normal tonus, growth in size and length, and hereditary expectations.

Rigid, kyphotic spine—The component of proximal antigravity extension strength and control develops in a cephalocaudal direction. This is usually accomplished by the end of the fifth month (Bly 1983; Sternat 1987; Scherzer et al. 1982; Bobath 1967). By implementing this component repeatedly in antigravity righting reactions of the head and trunk (in prone and quadruped positions as well as sitting and standing positions), active and passive spinal mobilization into extension bring about a reduction in neonatal thoracic and lumbar kyphosis (LeVeau et al. 1984; Tax 1985; Asher 1975; Bly 1983; Sutherland 1984; Effgen 1987). The achievement of mature spinal alignment (particularly of lumbar extension) requires years of maintaining the upright position (Asher 1975).

Shallow acetabulum—The head of the femur and the socket of the acetabulum develop in relative congruity, guided by the loads that are applied to them (LeVeau et al. 1984; Bernhardt 1988; Siffert 1981). The most important of the loads that influence development of the hip joint are muscle tension and body weight applied in appropriate magnitude and direction (LeVeau et al. 1984; Frost 1986).

In hypertonic cerebral palsy, the prevailing hip joint position is one of flexion with adduction. (Evidence of medial rotation is exaggerated by distal torsional deformity.) This disrupts the application of appropriate muscle forces to the hip joint and frequently results in persistence of both coxa valga and a shallow acetabulum. It is worsened by resorption of the proximal shelf due to excessive, prolonged compression, with resulting subluxation or dislocation (Bleck 1987; Siffert 1981; Samilson et al. 1972). Contributing factors include the following:

- An imbalance of muscle power across the hip joint
- Hypertonus
- Muscle and connective tissue contractures
- Postponement of weight-bearing and of achievement of the upright posture
- Weight-bearing with the hips adducted
- Abnormal sitting and sleeping postures

Acetabular retroversion, if indeed it is a common newborn structural feature, resolves with growth and expansion of the sacrum, particularly at the sacral ala (Grant 1962). Acetabular migration to the frontal plane occurs in conjunction with the onset of upright weight-bearing between the ages of 18 and 30 months (McCrea 1985; Badgley 1949). Any measure of acetabular retroversion would increase the congruity between the acetabulum and the anteverted femoral head.

Coxa valga—The shape and angle of the proximal end of the femur is the product of modeling forces of sufficient magnitude to direct the process (Siffert 1981). The trabecular pattern reveals evidence of strong and repeated loading. Tension forces applied by the gluteus medius to the trochanteric growth plate (TGP) give rise to the enlarged greater trochanter. It is the enlargement and actual "raising" of the greater trochanter that accounts for much of the reduction in inclination angle between the femoral neck and shaft (Siffert 1981).

Compression applied to the head incites the TGP and the femoral neck isthmus (FNI) to produce stronger bone tissue along the uppermost border of the femoral neck. This lays the trabeculae parallel to the tensile strain that the upper border experiences. The longitudinal growth plate (LGP) gradually aligns perpendicular to the femoral neck as a result of this angular reorientation of the femoral neck. Vertical compression on the femoral head is evident in the density and arrangement of trabeculae along the medial border of the femoral neck. Here the periosteal layer thickens and strengthens the bony matrix by laying down trabeculae that are parallel with the compressive strains.

The greatest influence on the reduction of coxa valga is muscle action about the hip joint, which generates forces of far greater magnitude than static loading (Frost 1986, Vol. 2). These forces combine in co-activation to pull the femoral head into the acetabulum. As the upright position is achieved, at least 70 percent of the body weight is carried proximal to the hip joints (Perry 1975). The stabilizing demands on the gluteus medius muscle generate tensile forces that also greatly exceed body weight. These tensile forces applied to the cartilaginous proximal femur eventually produce and enlarge the greater trochanter (Siffert 1981). The angle of inclination is mature at approximately 125-135 degrees by the end of the sixth year (Jordan et al. 1983; Beals 1969).

Femoral antetorsion—The angle of femoral antetorsion will eventually be reduced from the newborn average of 40 degrees to the adult value of 5-15 degrees, which amounts to a total possible reduction of 25-35 degrees, by the age of 15 years (Hensinger et al. 1982; Fabry et al. 1973; McCrea 1985; Hoffer 1980; Bleck 1982). Radiographic methods used in 1973 showed that in the first year of life this measurement reduces to 31-35 degrees, which indicates that 5-10 degrees of reduction of torsion might be accomplished very early in life (Fabry et al. 1973).

The gluteus maximus and proximal segment of the adductor magnus attach to the proximal posterior femur along the linea aspera, which is a ridge formed by tensile forces. The line of pull of both muscles, plus the pull of the biceps femoris, from origin to insertion, favors lateral rotation and crosses the proximal femur, where the proportion of hyaline cartilage is greatest. Therefore, activation of these muscles applies a torque force to the proximal femur in the direction of lateral rotation.

The primary biomechanical requirements for reducing antetorsion within the shaft of the femur include the following:

- Reduction of hip flexion contracture, particularly that of the iliopsoas muscle, because it functions as an antagonist to the effective action of the hip extensors and lateral rotators (Jordan et al. 1983; Bleck 1982). The hip flexors become elongated primarily by reciprocal innervation (Sternat 1987; Lehmkuhl et al. 1983).

- Reduction of contracture in the anterior aspect of the hip joint capsule, which is necessary to allow the head of the femur to glide anteriorly as the hip extends (the rule of convex and concave) (Brooks 1985).

- Consistent tensile loading by the muscles that extend and laterally rotate the hip, of sufficient magnitude to apply lateral torque forces across the proximal femur (LeVeau et al. 1984; Frost 1986; Jordan et al. 1983; Bleck 1982).

- The application of these forces must occur in conjunction with longitudinal bone growth (LeVeau et al. 1984; Frost 1986; Kapandji 1970; Jordan et al. 1983; Lehmkuhl et al. 1983; Bleck 1987).

There is room for confusion here: Why must the child exert a force at the hip in the direction of lateral rotation, when the newborn hip is already positioned in anteversion? The difference lies in the action that occurs across the femoral growth plate.

A resting position, in which acetabular orientation and proximal soft tissue and capsular structures combine to maintain the proximal femur hip in an anteverted position relative to the frontal plane, is just that—a resting position that must be reduced to allow the normal range of medial hip rotation to occur. The torque force, however, which pulls in the direction of lateral rotation across the cartilaginous proximal femur, is a different factor. The proximal femur, which is maintained in lateral rotation, is presumably stabilized by the existing connective tissue so that actively applied lateral torque forces may be directed to the proximal diaphysis below the trochanters. The growing bone can thus alter in shape effectively, untwisting in response to the lateral torque forces.

Considering these anatomic, biomechanic, and kinesiologic findings, the following activities, as they develop spontaneously in the infant and preschooler, can be expected to apply the desired derotational shear forces across the proximal femur. These activities are repeated thousands of times in normal play. Strengthening occurs in the activating muscle groups as a result of the number of repetitions executed over the course of days, weeks, and years of a normal child's early life. Consider these activities as components of a daily therapeutic exercise program for the infant and young child with persistent femoral antetorsion.

Belly crawling: The pushing leg activates hip extensors with lateral rotators as the leg extends from a starting position of flexion, abduction, and lateral rotation (extreme frog-leg position).

Playing and creeping in all-fours (quadruped) position: Several activities that occur in quadruped require activation of the hip extensors, abductors, adductors, and lateral rotators. They include the following:

- Maintaining the quadruped position. Without adduction, the knees would slide apart.
- Rocking forward and backward (eccentric and concentric muscle action occurs at the postero-lateral hip).
- Diagonal loading on one knee and the contralateral hand during play.
- Reciprocal creeping, which demands stabilizing coactivation of the musculature about the loaded hip while it extends and laterally rotates.

Vaulting: Transitions between quadruped and sitting over one knee use eccentric and concentric proximal-on-distal muscle action of the hip extensors, abductors, adductors, and lateral rotators, together with the quadriceps and tensor fascia lata.

Other transitions:

- Between kneel-sitting and kneel-standing, with hips abducted and laterally rotated. Abdominal control of the pelvis is needed here to stabilize the pelvis against anterior tilt. Pelvic stabilization is needed to effectively activate hip extensors and to elongate anteriorly the hip joint capsule and ligaments.
- Between kneel-standing and half-kneeling positions. (In the half-kneel position, one knee supports the weight under an extended hip. The opposite hip and knee are flexed.) The transition from kneel-stand to half-kneel occurs as a result of a posterolateral shift of the center of gravity. The weight shift calls upon the hip lateral and posterior musculature to prevent a collapse into

sitting. As the infant plays in half-kneel position, the flexed anterior leg helps to stabilize the pelvis in a posterior tilt, which allows greater elongation of the hip flexors and anterior capsule proximal to the loaded knee. The hips are typically aligned in a small degree of lateral rotation.

- Between half-kneeling and standing positions, with the forward leg abducted. The hip and knee joints on the anterior leg extend with lateral rotation through the transition.
- Between squatting and standing positions, maintaining the hips in abduction and laterally rotated.

Climbing: Children begin to climb onto furniture and up staircases before the age of 12 months. Climbing offers loaded, proximal-on-distal activation of the desired muscle groups. Climbing also taxes all available joint mobility and strength in the pelvis and power extremities.

- In the all-fours position, with hips abducted and laterally rotated.
- In the upright position, with hips abducted and laterally rotated.

Walking: Lateral rotation occurs through most of the stance phase of gait, from the onset of independent walking (around 12 months) through maturity (Sutherland 1984; Rodgers 1988). The adductor magnus is also active from initial foot contact to mid-stance, while excessive electromyographic activity has been recorded in the gluteus maximus muscles in the beginning walker.

Running: Running exaggerates the rotary components of walking, applying greater torque force in the direction of lateral rotation on the stance leg at the end of the stance cycle (Rodgers 1988).

Femoral varus bowing—The reduction of varus bowing in the femur appears to demand the two components of longitudinal bone growth and the modeling effects of cantilever flexure drift. Cantilever flexure is imposed by weight-bearing in the upright position. Cantilever flexure drift occurs when compressive force of sufficient magnitude is applied to both ends of a bowed structure. The body's modeling system responds by forming new bone on the concave side and resorbing bone on the convex side. This results in what appears to be a drift, as Frost refers to it, of bone tissue toward the concavity (Frost 1986, Vols. 1 and 2).

Hip flexion contracture—Together with the fibers of the ligaments and capsule that cross anterior to the hip joint, the iliopsoas muscle maintains the hip in flexion throughout the first two to three years in most children (Pitkow 1975; Phelps et al. 1985; Hoffer 1980). The motion of hip extension is needed to actively and passively elongate the hip flexors and the anterior joint capsule. The iliopsoas flexes the hip. By its attachment to the lesser trochanter via the anterior aspect of the hip joint, the tendon of insertion can impede the distal and anterior glide of the femoral head, which is required for full hip abduction and extension. In this way, the contracted iliopsoas contributes to subluxation of the hip in children with neuromotor deficit.

The gluteus maximus functions as both an extensor and a lateral rotator at the hip (McCrea 1985; Kapandji 1970; Lehmkuhl et al.

1983). The lateral rotation component gains strength as the hip position gains extension (Lehmkuhl et al. 1983). In addition, the proximal component of the adductor magnus functions as a lateral rotator of the femur (McCrea 1985). It appears therefore that in early life, the gluteus maximus is the primary antagonist of the iliopsoas muscle, assisted by the proximal adductor magnus, and that activation of the gluteus maximus is a significant developmental event.

The motion of hip extension is also required to mobilize all of the hip joint ligaments and capsule, particularly the anterior aspect, because hip extension elongates most of the capsular tissue fibers (Kapandji 1970). With greater mobility in the noncontractile tissues at the hip, active extension and hyperextension can occur more effectively (Sternat 1987).

Lateral hip rotation contracture—The motion of medial hip rotation, both flexed and extended, is needed to reduce the newborn position of anteversion (rather than antetorsion) (Kapandji 1970). The close-packed position of the hip joint is one of hip extension, abduction, and medial rotation, which seats the femoral head in the acetabulum. Normal movement activities apparently operate to mobilize the tight soft tissues toward medial hip rotation by the age of 2 years, when the range of medial hip rotation is likely to be slightly greater than that of lateral hip rotation (Bleck 1982; Phelps et al. 1985). The discrepancy in the measures of medial as opposed to lateral rotation at the age of 2 years is minimal (averaging 7 degrees) and is influenced by existing femoral torsion.

Knee flexion contracture—By the age of 6 months, most infants engage in playing with and mouthing of the feet while lying in the supine and side-lying positions. With this activity, the hamstrings are elongated, both actively and passively. Soon after, babies continue to elongate the hamstrings through vaulting transitions and by assuming and locomoting in a bear-stand posture, quadruped on hands and feet, with both knees extended (Bly 1983).

Genu varum—By 2 years of age, physiologic genu varum resolves into genu valgum, which then increases, peaking at the age of 3 years at a maximum femoral-tibial angle of 12 degrees. After that, genu valgum resolves to the adult value of 5 degrees, usually by the age of 8 years (McDade 1977). The modeling forces at work in this process are those of variable compression on the medial and lateral condyles of the femur and tibia in standing and walking. Evidently these forces combine with cantilever flexure drift (described below), with reduction of coxa valga and medial genicular position, and with medial displacement of body weight associated with normal foot pronation in the young child in stance (Frost 1986, Vol. 2).

Compression within normal physiologic limits promotes growth of cartilage. In genu varum, the compressive forces on the medial condylar epiphyses are greater than those on the lateral condylar epiphyses. Therefore, the medial condyles increase their rate of growth while the lateral condyles, though they continue growing, do so more slowly by comparison. Consequently, varus resolves (Frost 1986, Vol. 2).

Cantilever flexure drift, in which bone forms on the concave side and resorbs on the convex side, evidently occurs simultaneously in the shaft of the femur. Meanwhile, the soft tissue contractures that hold the lower leg in medial rotation resolve. This action effectively aligns the lower leg parallel to the femur.

By the age of 12 months, the weight-bearing calcaneus assumes an everted position, probably to allow the varus forefoot to contact the ground. According to Root et al. (1971), calcaneal eversion in relaxed stance peaks at the age of 2 to 3 years, just prior to the peak of the valgus deviation in the knee joint. This suggests that the medial displacement of body weight over the foot in some way promotes a valgus orientation at the knee joint (McDade 1977). However, Valmassy (1984) suggests that the normal maximum relaxed calcaneal stance angle of eversion is greatest at 1 year (6 degrees) and diminishes each year by one degree.

The same variable compressive forces at the condylar epiphyses seem to operate to resolve genu valgum to 5-7 degrees by the age of 8 years. Meanwhile, the relaxed calcaneal stance angle also resolves to 0, with a maximum of 2 degrees, by the age of 5 years (McCrea 1985; Jordan et al. 1983; Root et al. 1971; Valmassy 1984).

Internal (medial) genicular position—More muscles cross the medial aspect of the knee joint than the lateral, and any degree of knee flexion allows the tibia to rotate on the distal femur. Thus the knee joint capsule and ligaments must be mobilized and lengthened to allow the tibia to rotate laterally during the final few degrees of knee extension. Efficient knee function requires outward rotation mobility of the lower leg on the femur, because complete knee extension is accompanied by a "corkscrew" motion of lateral rotation of the tibia on the femur (McCrea 1985; Schafer 1987).

Belly crawling is an excellent opportunity for reducing medial genicular knee position, because the entire lower extremity extends with lateral rotation on the propelling leg. Belly crawling typically occurs between the ages of 5 and 7 months. W-sitting (kneel-sitting between the feet) with the lower legs rotated outward applies a passive lateral rotation stretch to the ligaments in the flexed knee joint, and frequently occurs as a postural variation in normal infants. Later on, ambulation becomes the primary means of attaining needed mobility into lateral rotation of the tibia on the femur. The lower leg spins outward during most of the stance cycle, even in children of 1 year of age (Sutherland 1984; Root et al. 1977; Sutherland et al. 1980; Rodgers 1988).

Tibial and fibular torsion—In addition to the corkscrew phenomenon described above, the shafts of the tibia and fibula gradually twist laterally up to a combined average of 20-30 degrees, as measured at the TMA relative to the frontal plane. The change in the tibial and fibular alignments apparently occurs to move the inner vertical surfaces of the medial and lateral malleoli into position to stabilize the talus and to guide the angle of foot placement following swing, and to guide the angle of gait during stance. The fibular malleolus grows in length as well, providing adequate lateral support for the talus.

Staheli (1977, 1985) attributes the cause of certain in-toed gait deviations to failure to accomplish adequate lateral torsion of the tibia and fibula.

The normal factors of hereditary predisposition are evident in children who, with normal motor control and tone, reveal a familial inclination to demonstrate varying degrees of tibial torsion (Engel et al. 1974; Staheli 1977).

The same mechanism for modeling at the femur applies to the tibia and fibula. A torque force must be exerted in the direction of lateral rotation, across the growth plates and metaphyses of the tibia and fibula, during the time when longitudinal bone growth is occurring. Belly crawling and similar floor activities, which apply a lateral rotation force, seem to begin the process, while ambulation is the primary means by which lateral torque force is applied to the tibia and fibula. Additionally, standing on the toes in full plantarflexion applies a lateral torque to the tibia and fibula by reverse action of the triceps surae and the posterior tibialis as supinators (Lehmkuhl et al. 1983).

Apparent tibial varum—The lateral displacement of posterior compartment muscle bellies resolves as the knee joint gains lateral rotation mobility. The medial head of the gastrocnemius also hypertrophies as it gains strength. The distal varum in the lower leg usually resolves to 6 degrees by age 1 year, and to within 2 degrees by age 2 years (Engel et al. 1974; McDade 1977; Jordan et al. 1983).

Short distal fibula, displaced anteriorly—Simple bone growth accounts for the length of the fibular malleolus and its coverage of the lateral talus. However, proximal-on-distal activity in the triceps surae muscle group and the posterior tibialis (as occurs in toe-standing) seems to facilitate torsional modeling of the fibular malleolus to align it posterior to the frontal plane. With toe standing, the distal fibula is both twisted laterally and squeezed toward the midline of the leg. This offers the narrow posterior body of the talus secure housing when the weight-bearing ankle is plantarflexed.

Everted distal tibial plafond—The newborn foot is commonly aligned in varus in the open chain, but with the onset of weight-bearing on the feet, the varus forefoot seeks full contact with the ground and the hindfoot strains into valgus. Apparently this occurs to accommodate the lowering of the inverted medial forefoot. The stress of weight-bearing evidently works to elongate tight medial soft tissue structures at the foot. By 12 months of age, a normal calcaneal valgus deviation of up to 6 degrees relative to the sagittal plane appears in relaxed stance. Evidently, some measure of congruity is achieved among the everted tibial plafond, the talus, and the calcaneus. Weight-bearing on the everted calcaneus, combined with genu valgum in the preschooler, may apply a greater compressive force to the lateral plafond than to the distal, thus stimulating a greater rate of bone growth.

Excessive talocrural dorsiflexion mobility—Freedom from the uterine environment relieves the pressure on the feet that brought about dorsiflexion hypermobility. A drop occurs in the level of maternal hormones, released at the time of delivery to loosen pelvic support structures. The emergence of active ankle plantarflexion contributes to an eventual reduction in dorsiflexion contracture and hypermobility.

Hindfoot varus—The calcaneal-tibial angle is one of varus when the subtalar joint is aligned in congruity. Persistence of calcaneal torsion seems to account for this varus disposition of the neutral hindfoot (and the forefoot).

Everted calcaneal stance—By 12 months of age, the calcaneus deviates into eversion as the foot pronates in stance. The medial soft tissue structures, shortened during uterine confinement, evidently elongate under the stress of weight-bearing. Valmassy (1984) refers to this calcaneal deviation as the relaxed calcaneal stance angle and suggests that its normal value can be determined by subtracting the child's age from the number 7. This mild calcaneal valgus deviation in early childhood has been attributed to ligamentous laxity (McCrea 1985; Giannestras 1973).

Root et al. (1971) report that the calcaneal stance angle is between 5 and 10 degrees between the ages of 3 months and 3 years when the distal lower leg is aligned on the sagittal plane. However, the distal lower leg aligns in 6 degrees of varum at 12 months, gradually reducing to within 2 degrees of the sagittal plane by age 3 years. The calcaneal valgus angle then gradually resolves by 1 or 2 degrees per year to 0-2 degrees by the age of 7 years.

Agnew (1988) suggests that the prevalence of abnormalities of foot function and structure in the adult population indicates that the so-called norms that favor higher values of calcaneal valgus in stance in early life—such as 5-10 degrees between 3 months and 3 years—do not acknowledge the potential abnormality of those norms. In other words, "typical" does not equate with "optimal" for balance and function. This is the perspective presented in this book. It is preferable to err on the side of limitation of potentially excessive calcaneal valgus, although a little valgus is better than calcaneal varus (Rang et al. 1986).

Forefoot varus—The degree of forefoot varus reduces from 12-15 to 5-6 degrees in the first year, and to 0-2 degrees by the age of 5 to 7 years (Jordan et al. 1983). This reduction in varus occurs in conjunction with growth of the navicular, reduction in torsion in the talar neck, strengthening of the peroneus longus as a plantarflexor of the first ray, and reduction of the calcaneal stance angle of valgus.

Talar torsion—Bleck (1982) proposes that the force of correction of talar adduction and elongation is applied as the leg laterally rotates over the loaded foot in stance. He suggests that the lateral motion of the supinating navicular draws the talar head laterally through the latter portion of the stance cycle in gait. This book takes the point of view that the adducted talar neck might also respond to the application of supinatory forces that occur in walking on toes, and that feature plantarflexion of the medial rays.

Considering the torsional component in the talar neck (which results in inversion at the talar head), when the hindfoot gains stability against pronation, the varus-deviated forefoot and first ray seek full contact with the ground by plantarflexing and pronating in stance. The inverted talar head, which articulates with the navicular, endures corrective pronatory forces. More research is needed to verify or correct all of these presumptions.

Metatarsophalangeal (MTP) flexion contracture—The first evidence of self-imposed mobilization into hyperextension at the MTP joints occurs with belly crawling. The infant achieves a forward propulsion by pushing off with the plantar surface of the metatarsal heads and toes. Soon, bear-standing in quadruped applies more force into hyperextension at the toes. Shortly after achieving the upright position at 7 or 8 months, the infant rises onto toes, which also requires hyperextension at the MTP joints.

Toe hyperextension to between 56 and 90 degrees is a normal feature of gait, from midstance to terminal stance (Schafer 1987; Root et al. 1977). Most children with hypertonus lack this function in the foot. They retain toe flexion for grasp as a compensation for poor balance in stance and gait, and as a distal biomechanical consequence of abnormal alignment in the foot structures.

This part of the chapter has reviewed the kinesiological influences that contribute to the shape of the developing skeleton. Presented next is evidence of the application of these forces during the course of infant motor development.

Prone Position— Antigravity Extension Skills

The review of the course of normal motor development on the following pages emphasizes the kinesiological and biomechanical aspects of specific activities. The focus on the trunk and lower extremities is deliberate because upper extremity development, though no less important to the child's overall functional development, falls beyond the scope of this book.

The work of Bly (1983), unless otherwise indicated, serves as the primary resource for the following areas: the kinesiological aspects of development; the issues of identification of activating and elongating muscle groups; the progression of achievement of antigravity extension and flexion components; and changes in weight distribution. (For more global and detailed reviews of sensorimotor development, refer to the texts by Bly 1983; Scherzer and Tscharnuter 1982; and Connolly 1984.) Modeling influences that are not referenced are the author's own contribution.

The achievement of gross motor skills is viewed first in the infant under 12 months of age. The skills are further reduced to reveal cephalocaudal progressions of achievement of antigravity strength and accompanying joint mobility, beginning in the prone position.

These progressions begin again in supine, and again in sitting, quadruped, and standing positions. A sense of systematic progression emerges by examining the developmental course in this way. Postural and joint alignment changes in the child between the ages of 12 months and 7 years are then detailed, with associated distinguishing features of gait.

In prone, the gradual achievement of the first antigravity component of movement appears: extension strength and control in the neck, trunk, and hips. As extension activity and strength increase, the antagonistic flexors elongate by reciprocal innervation, and the anterior ligaments in joints of the spine and hips gain mobility into extension. Other features of movement reflect the added component of antigravity flexion in the neck and trunk. This is detailed more specifically in the supine progression below. All age-specific achievements are offered as guideposts to mark features in order of progression. They incline toward the higher end of the normal spectrum, rather than the lower, particularly for those skills that emerge in infancy.

Neonate—Flexion contracture at the hips, and kyphosis of the lumbar and thoracic spine, compel the newborn face and head to serve as the passive point of stability upon which active, random movement of the legs and pelvis occurs (Figure 2.2). Random kicking provides tactile sensory input to the legs and feet and begins the process of reduction of hip flexion contracture (Salek 1977; Salek 1981). (See the Neonatal Biomechanical Problem List earlier in this chapter.)

Abnormal

The child with neuromotor deficit who exhibits thoracic kyphosis and flattening (flexion) of the lumbar spine reveals persistence of the newborn spinal alignment and a lack of achievement of adequate extension strength and mobility early in life (Brooks 1985).

Figure 2.2
Birth to 1 month: kyphosis; posterior pelvic tilt; hip and knee flexion.

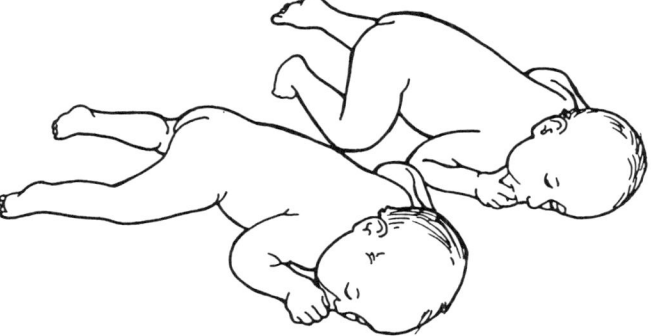

Two months—The trunk, neck, and extremities typically align asymmetrically (Figure 2.3). Abduction of the hips helps to lower the pelvis toward the supporting surface. This facilitates a shift of the point of stability from the face to the upper chest and forearms, which thus advances momentary head lifting. The movement of the hips toward abduction begins the process of mobilizing the medial/inferior aspect of the joint capsule, as the femoral head glides distally in the

Figure 2.3
2 months (child on the right): asymmetry.
3 months (child on the left): transition to symmetry; developing "frog-leg" posture.

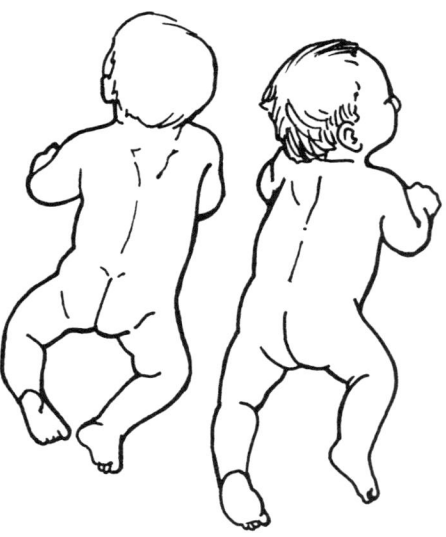

acetabulum. The tendon of insertion of the iliopsoas muscle endures tensile stress as well. The femoral head seats more deeply in the acetabulum.

Three months—During the third month the transition from the most asymmetrical to the most symmetrical periods in the developmental course occurs (Figure 2.3). Symmetrical antigravity extension of the neck and trunk is achieved through the thorax and appears in the low back area. This happens as the point of stability for head lifting and kicking shifts to the lower ribs. Symmetrical extension control is essential for lifting the head in midline; this skill is a major building block for further sensorimotor development. With increased antigravity trunk extension, spinal kyphosis diminishes at the thoracic and lumbar areas, and the pelvis begins to actively tilt anteriorly.

The hips become aligned symmetrically in a position of abduction, flexion, and lateral rotation. The knees remain in flexion and the feet contact each other. This configuration of the legs is the "frog-leg posture." It is the structural foundation for understanding the initial stages of the task of revising the design of the long bones. The frog-leg posture elongates the anterior and inferior aspects of the hip joint capsule. This is necessary to allow the femoral head to glide anteriorly and distally as the femoral shaft extends and abducts. The anterior hip capsule also endures pressure applied by the anteverted femoral head and neck (Brooks 1985).

Active kicking reveals activation of the gluteus maximus and implies that the work of reducing the iliopsoas contracture, the anterior hip capsule contracture, and (to a lesser extent) femoral antetorsion, has begun. The lack of hip extension diminishes the power of the gluteus maximus as a lateral rotator (Lehmkuhl et al. 1983). Furthermore, the gluteus medius activates and, because the small muscles of lateral hip rotation function as abductors when the hip is flexed, the muscle activity at the lateral hip joint draws the femoral head into the acetabulum. Forces of compression are applied to the femoral head and neck, tension is applied to the greater trochanter, and modeling to decrease coxa valga and to increase the depth of the acetabulum also begins.

Abnormal

Children with spastic cerebral palsy typically fail to exhibit a frog-leg posture in prone position at any time in their development. Instead they demonstrate "scissoring" (or tight adduction), which results in limited abduction range of motion and a lack of mobility in the anterior and inferior hip joint capsule (Brooks 1985). The potential modeling influences of kicking into extension from the frog-leg position are lost.

Many children with hypotonia, on the other hand, retain a frog-leg posture long after it is appropriate to do so. By relying on or enjoying the positional stability of this leg arrangement, they fail to gain adequate strength in the trunk and hips to move efficiently in lateral or rotary directions and to stabilize dynamically. These children often retain the newborn lateral rotation contracture long after it typically resolves. They generally exhibit accompanying increased angle of gait with pronation deformity.

Four months—Early in the fourth month the hallmark of achieving symmetrical antigravity control and bilateral extremity function occurs. The point of stability is at the belly and thigh. The pelvis is tilted anteriorly. The frog-leg posture prevails (Figure 2.4).

As the neck and spine extend with increasing strength and consistency, a corresponding increase in hip and knee extension with hip abduction is observed, and Landau swimming appears. Elongation of the iliopsoas presumably occurs by reciprocal innervation, and the anterior hip joint capsule is mobilized (Brooks 1985).

A synergistic pattern appears in the legs, as hip/knee/ankle extension (with adduction) occurs with a posterior tilt of the pelvis, and hip/knee/ankle flexion (with abduction) occurs with anterior tilting of the pelvis (Figure 2.5).

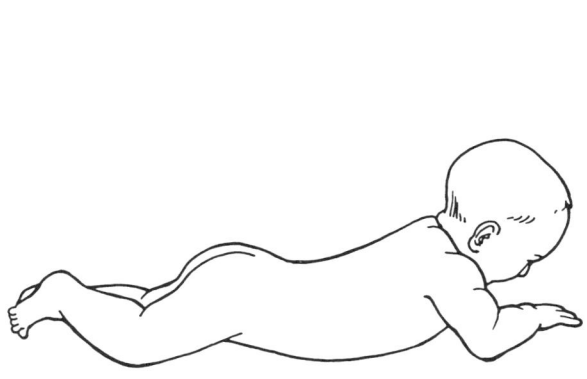

Figure 2.4 4 months: symmetry; chin tucked; "frog-leg" posture established

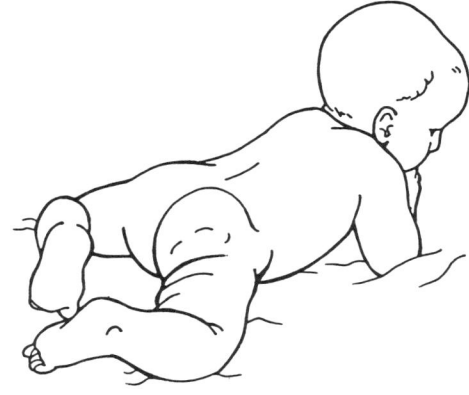

Figure 2.5 4 months: anterior pelvic tilt; bilateral kicking. Note activation of gluteus maximus muscle.

Five months—The weight-bearing point of stability for head and hand function and purposeful leg motions arrives at the pelvis; first the whole pelvis (Figure 2.6), then one side or the other (Figure 2.7), as the infant shifts into position for belly crawling. The frog-leg posture gives way to hip, knee, and ankle extension with hip adduction on the loaded side of the pelvis and trunk; pelvic rotation occurs. (See Figure 2.8, the infant on the right.) The result is disassociation of the lower extremities as the loaded side extends and the other flexes.

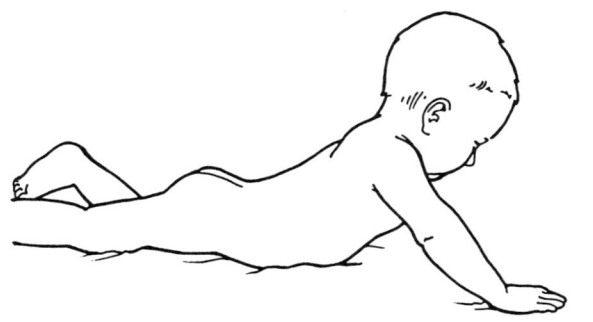

Figure 2.6 5 months: weight on the pelvis.

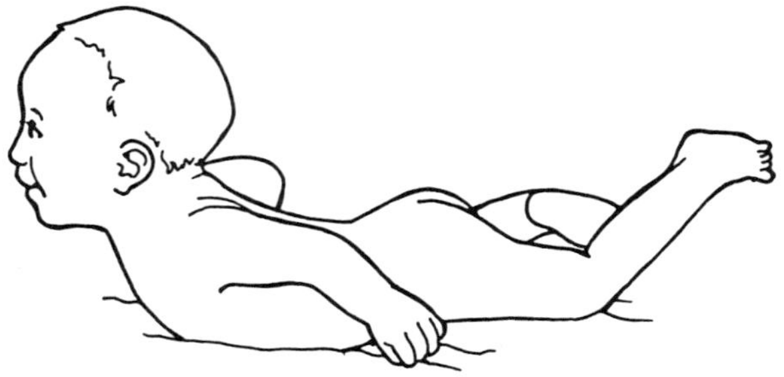

Figure 2.7 5 months: Landau "swimming"; antigravity extension complete; flexors are elongated.

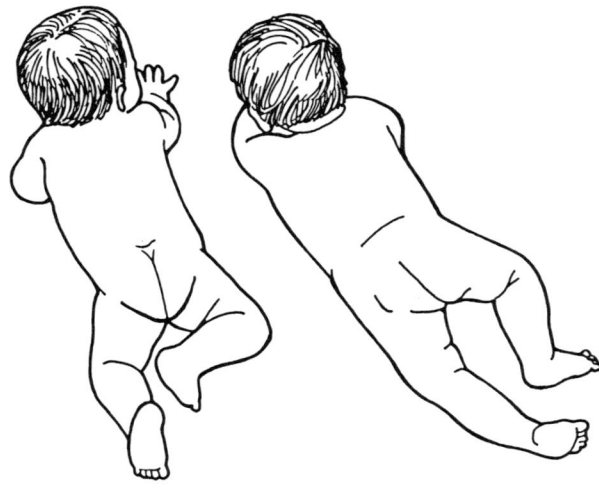

Figure 2.8 Weight shifts to one side of the pelvis; disassociation between the legs (Left: 5 months / Right: 6 months.). Belly crawling begins.

Six months—As the infant uses belly crawling to locomote, the propelling hip works against resistance in the direction of extension with lateral rotation and abduction while the infant pushes against the floor with the medial aspect of the ball of the foot. This event can presumably reduce antetorsion and coxa valga by applying torque and compression forces across the proximal femur. In addition, the metatarsophalangeal joints are first mobilized into hyperextension in the sixth month.

Abnormal Crawling

The child with hypertonus in the lower extremities commonly initiates forward progression by drag crawling (pulling along in prone while maintaining the legs in extension and adduction). This activity denies the opportunity for activating the lateral rotators and extensors of the hip and for mobilizing the toes into hyperextension. Disassociation of the legs from each other fails to occur.

Seven months—The baby achieves the hands-and-knees position, with all extremities abducted and symmetrically aligned (Figure 2.9). The hips remain abducted, and the knees are usually wider apart than the feet, although this becomes variable. The shallow acetabulae are (possibly) retroverted while the femoral neck and head remain anteverted. The position of hip abduction maintains congruity between the head of the femur and the acetabulum in the quadruped position (LeVeau et al. 1984). Rocking forward and back in this position activates the stabilizing musculature about the hip and applies a compressive loading force to the femoral head and neck and to the acetabulum. With rocking on hands and knees, the reduction of coxa valga continues in earnest.

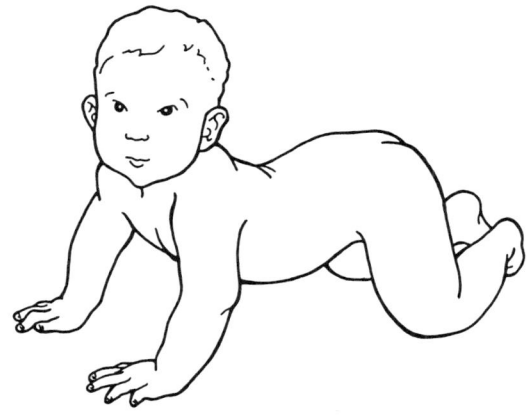

Figure 2.9   7 months: quadruped; symmetrical rocking occurs on the sagittal plane; hips rotated laterally, abducted.

Abnormal Quadruped

The child with a movement disorder (Figures 2.10 and 2.11) frequently exhibits an underdeveloped quality of symmetry, which is ordinarily achieved within four months in the prone and supine positions. Achieving symmetry requires antigravity strength into trunk extension and flexion (Bly 1983). The child in these illustrations is 26 months of age and reveals spastic diplegia. Here the lack of extension strength and mobility in the lower thoracic and lumbar spine is obvious. The pelvis does not tilt anteriorly. The hips are poorly aligned for seating the head of the femur in the acetabulum (Figure 2.10).

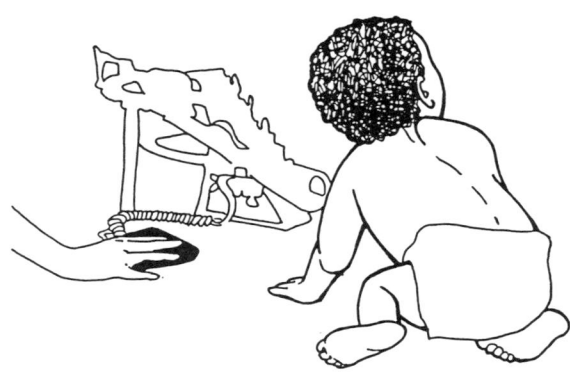

Figure 2.10 Spastic diplegia, age 26 months: asymmetrical quadruped; lumbar flexion; asymmetry.

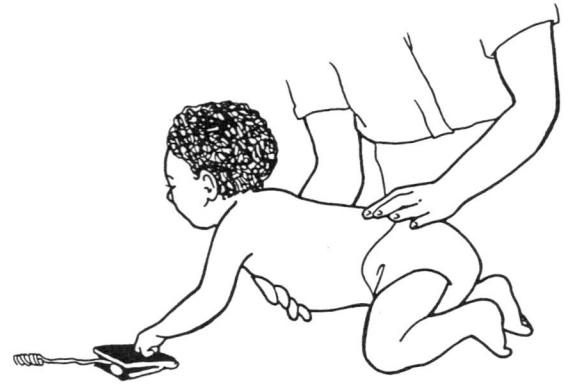

Figure 2.11 Spastic diplegia: simulating symmetry and normal leg alignment in therapeutic exercise and play.

Management Considerations

In movement training, the achievement of appropriate spinal extension and symmetrical arrangement of the supporting extremities requires close attention. Play facilitates active rocking in the normal hands-and-knees position (Figure 2.11).

Because of a typical persistence or worsening of antetorsion in children with hypertonus (Fabry et al. 1973; Beals 1969; Bleck 1987)—and considering the likelihood that the acetabulum has migrated to some degree toward the frontal plane with pelvic growth—the goals of management should be carefully considered. For example, in treating the child with developmental disability who is older than 30 months, full congruity of the hip joint surfaces must be maintained if the goal of therapeutic exercise is to attempt to improve hip joint congruity. The therapist should consider whether to abduct and rotate the TCA medially while activating the hip stabilizing musculature.

Also, as an alternative to prolonged sitting the therapist might position the child in a standing device that offers the following features: any necessary trunk and pelvic alignment; support in hip abduction and medial rotation; and maximum weight-bearing on the feet—rather than the chest and thighs—for a total of at least 2 to 3 hours per day, scheduled in sessions of 30 to 45 minutes each (LeVeau et al. 1984). Without promoting deformity, the less restrictive the device, the more the lower extremity musculature will be activated. The older the child, the less cartilaginous the proximal femur becomes, and the less likely it is that these simple loading forces will produce a significant change in the neck/shaft angle. Their consistent application might be worth the attempt, however, since surgical osteotomy is the remaining solution. As yet, researchers have not quantified any correlation between this type of static positioning and any changes in the angle of inclination of the proximal femur.

However, if the goal of therapeutic exercise is the reduction of femoral antetorsion, then the activation of lateral hip rotation and extension would be a more appropriate intervention. This is because of the direction of torque forces needed across the proximal femur. For example, from the beginning of independent ambulation, lateral torque force is applied to the femur as the hip extends after weight assumption (Sutherland et al. 1980). Timely and consistent facilitation during this pattern of the stance phase probably effects the desired therapeutic exercise goal, although more research is needed to gain objective measures of structural change.

The degree of ossification that has occurred in the femur dictates the potential influence of any vigorous exercise program on the angle of antetorsion. The younger the child the greater the modeling potential if one considers the plasticity of the skeletal structures in infancy. According to Bleck (1982), the age of 8 years is too late. —

The infant and young child normally engage in thousands of repetitions of movements that apply lateral torque forces to the femoral shaft. Considering this, exercise programs that take the form of a play activity or hobby—such as horseback riding (particularly developing the skill of "posting" in the saddle), adaptive gymnastics, play on climbing apparatus, and dance classes—could be important complements to individual therapeutic exercise. All of these activities require attention to activating the hip extensors and lateral rotators.

Orthopedic and radiologic assessment offer important information about these structures. The therapist should seek this type of assessment at the time of designing a therapeutic exercise program, particularly for the child who has bypassed the most impressionable period of infancy.

Supine Position— Antigravity Flexion Skills

The newborn's biomechanical status has been previously discussed. Next this chapter will consider the development of proximal flexion strength against gravity as a foundation for the achievement of control of the pelvis and of the hips.

The supine position is one of generous positional stability, offering support for the entire head and trunk. Antigravity flexion control and strength develop in a cephalocaudal direction and follow closely behind the countercomponent of extension. Flexion is usually established within one month after the achievement of antigravity extension strength and control in the neck and trunk. According to the progression illustrated here, antigravity extension is achieved in the fifth month and flexion is established during the sixth month. There is variation, of course, among different children.

One month—The newborn maintains the hips in flexion with lateral rotation and variable degrees of abduction (Figure 2.12). The presence of physiologic flexion appears in the elbows, hips, knees, and ankles. The primary feature of lower extremity function at this age is random kicking.

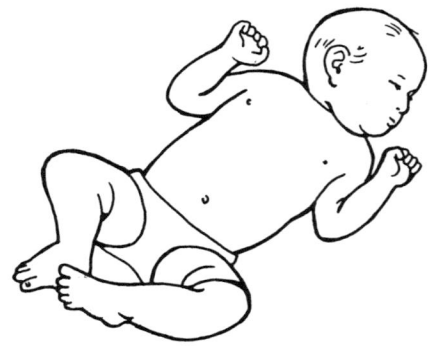

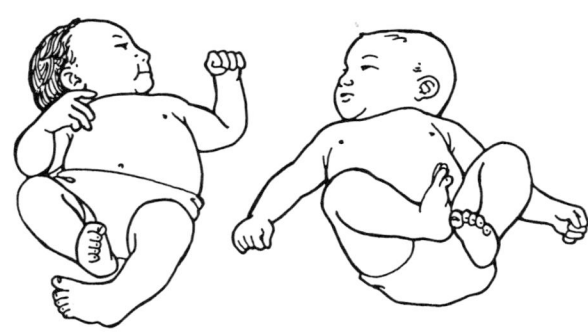

Figure 2.12   Birth to 1 month: "physiologic flexion" at hips, knees, ankles; femoral anteversion and antetorsion; "physiologic genu varum"; feet in varus; random kicking.

Figure 2.13   2 months (left): asymmetry. 3 months (right): transition toward symmetry.

Two months—The hallmark of asymmetry becomes evident as the asymmetric tonic neck reflex appears with a measure of consistency (Figure 2.13). This is also the child's "floppiest" period: a total head lag is evident during pull-to-sit. Gravitational forces and random kicking combine to reduce the hip flexion contracture.

Abnormal

Persistence of truncal asymmetry beyond 2 to 3 months indicates a lack of development of bilateral antigravity strength in the neck and trunk. This condition frequently leads to spinal scoliosis and hip dislocation.

Three months—Transition from asymmetry to symmetrical alignment occurs in this month. The emergence of symmetry offers evidence of increasing strength and control of bilateral flexors in the neck and trunk. This occurs on a base of some symmetrical stabilization by the extensors.

The legs are falling into a "frog-leg" posture, while foot-to-foot and foot-to-leg contact and self-exploration appear (Figure 2.13).

Four months—The hallmark of the fourth month is symmetry, as the baby achieves a midline orientation of the neck and trunk. The chin tucks into the neck, and both hands and feet come together (Figure 2.14). Bilateral kicking occurs in the legs; they move along the horizontal plane, away from and then toward the body. This kicking pattern repeatedly rolls the pelvis into anterior and posterior tilts and demands both eccentric and concentric activation of the abdominal muscles, respectively.

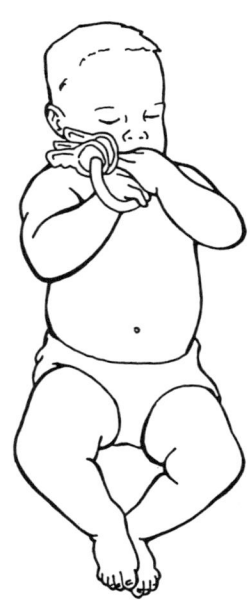

Figure 2.14
4 months: symmetry;
chin tuck;
frog-leg posture;
bilateral movements.

By this age, the child can often roll to the side-lying position, thus seeing and handling the feet and legs more conveniently than in the supine-lying position. Eye-foot and hand-to-foot contact appear. This sensory experience is lost to the child who is unable to use the muscles of antigravity flexion effectively (Bly 1983; Salek 1977).

Abnormal Posture

The child with hypertonus in the lower extremities (Figure 2.15) often does not demonstrate the frog-leg position. Instead, this child often seeks compensatory stability with the legs extended and crossed, thus allowing play with the arms extended away from the body.

Figure 2.15
Spastic diplegia, age 20 months: frog-leg posture never developed; hypertonus is evident in the legs.

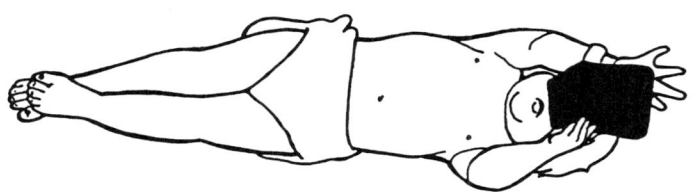

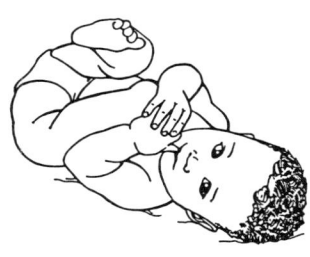

Figure 2.16
5 months: foot-to-mouth mobilizes posterior hip capsule and elongates proximal hamstrings.

Five months—The baby can grasp a foot and bring it to the mouth for exploration and play. Foot play and mouthing offer an avenue for enhancing awareness of one's own body and for developing a body image (Salek 1977) (Figure 2.16). While the child is mouthing a foot, the posterior hip joint capsule is mobilized by virtue of the position of extreme hip flexion. Passive and active elongation occur in the lumbar spine extensors, the proximal hamstrings, the hip extensors, and the hip medial rotators.

The bilateral leg movements of the previous period give way to individual leg movements. The foot-to-mouth position stabilizes the pelvis in a posterior tilt while the free leg engages in kicking away from the body. As the hip extensors and adductors are activated in kicking, the tensor fascia lata and iliopsoas muscles—together with the anterior hip joint capsule and ligaments—are elongated (Kapandji 1970; Brooks 1985).

Abnormal

The child who lacks this degree of antigravity flexion control loses the opportunity to handle and mouth the feet and legs while mobilizing the proximal joints.

Six months—The component of antigravity flexion control and strength is complete in supine at 6 months. The infant has achieved flexion control in supine when able to do the following:

- Maintain all extremities extended into space above the trunk (Figure 2.17). Preventing the limbs from toppling over places a significant demand for strength and control upon the abdominal muscles. The hamstrings are actively and successfully elongated by contraction of the quadriceps muscles while the hips are maintained in flexion.
- Lift the head off the support surface independently (Figure 2.18).

- Rotate and derotate the pelvis on the shoulders. The action of the oblique abdominals is evident in Figure 2.19, as play with the feet continues. The infant is now able to roll segmentally from the supine to the prone position, disassociating the pelvis from the shoulders. This activity in the oblique abdominals applies sculpting forces to the anterior and lower ribs.

Abnormal

It is reasonable to conclude that any limitation of hamstring mobility observed in the child with hypertonus began to develop at or before the age of 5 to 6 months (Figure 2.20).

Flaring of the anterior lower ribs and relative indentation of the sternum is a typical structural finding in children who lack control and strength in the oblique abdominals.

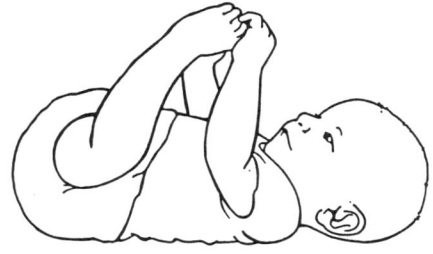

Figure 2.17 6 months: antigravity flexion control is achieved; knee extension elongates distal hamstrings.

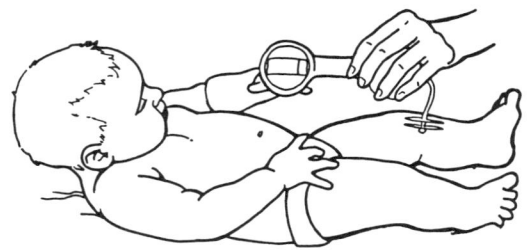

Figure 2.18 6 months: head lift against gravity reveals strength in neck flexors and trunk stabilizers.

Figure 2.19
Leg drops, side to side, strengthen oblique abdominals and hip abductors and adductors and build control of the pelvis by trunk musculature. The rib cage is sculpted by rotary tensile forces applied by oblique abdominals.

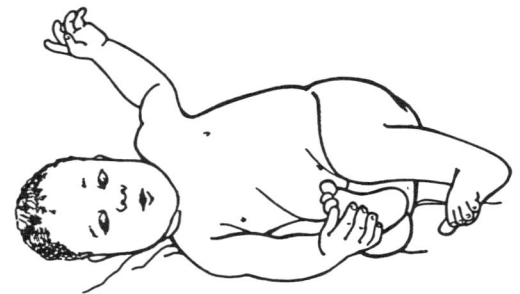

Figure 2.20
Lack of antigravity flexion control and strength for foot play promotes persistence of neonatal knee flexion contractures.

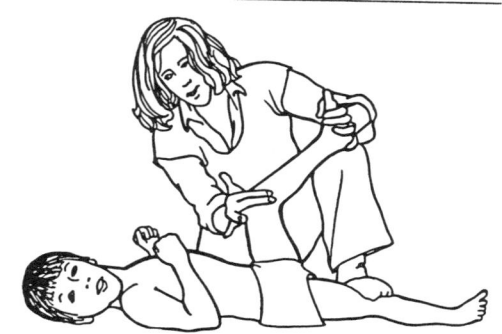

Implementing the Basic Antigravity Components

Sitting

Motor skills are not learned in isolation; they are grafted onto existing skills (Baddely 1984). For example, children who spend a significant amount of time in supine have been shown to advance more quickly to sitting than to crawling (Levitt 1984).

In the first six months, the infant gradually achieves the ability to maintain the sitting position when placed. From the first day of postnatal life, the pelvis aligns vertically in sitting, and the trunk falls forward of that (Bly 1983). Strength then develops in the neck, trunk, and hip extensors. The infant applies this strength to raise the trunk and head against gravity while maintaining the sitting position on a stable pelvis (Sternat 1987). Postural fixation, or the ability to stabilize the body against gravity, involves synergistic and balanced use of the antigravity musculature at the neck, trunk, and pelvic girdle (Sternat 1987).

During the same span of development, the neck and trunk gradually achieve verticality over the pelvis. At the same time, the hip joints loosen to allow an increasing degree of lateral rotation, abduction, and flexion. The knees remain in flexion. The result, usually established by the sixth month, is the achievement of "ring-sitting." In this position, the legs are arranged in a ring, with the soles of the feet directed toward each other and the flexed knees held in close proximity to the floor (Figure 2.21). This arrangement of the legs provides positional stability, which helps block a fall forward and laterally.

When the infant shifts weight laterally in ring-sitting, the hip on the loaded side abducts and laterally rotates, pressing the knee into the support surface. In this manner, the infant prevents a fall by counterpoising, making an adjustment in order to preserve upright equilibrium (Baddely 1984). This activation of the hip muscles applies a lateral torque force to the femur while preparing for the later execution of the same motions in vaulting transitions to the all-fours position.

In ring-sitting, the infant works to apply the component of flexion to the existing capacity for extension at the trunk, until a balance of the two opposing forces is accomplished. When the infant gains control of antigravity extension and flexion, the two components combine to produce lateral and rotary movements.

The quality of rotation within the trunk—that is, rotation of the shoulders on a fixed pelvis, or of the pelvis on fixed shoulders, or of both on the center of the body (as in creeping reciprocally or walking with arm swing)—is evidence of the sophisticated integration of extension and flexion capabilities (Bly 1983; Sternat 1987; Effgen 1987). The efficient control of the pelvis by the proximal trunk musculature, particularly by the oblique abdominals, facilitates the activation of the muscles of hip extension, lateral rotation, and abduction (Bly 1983; Lehmkuhl et al. 1983).

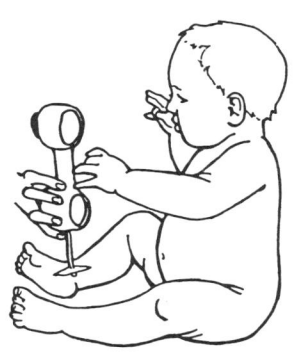

Figure 2.21
6 months: placed in sitting, the legs form a ring, requiring hip joint mobility and affording positional stability. The sacrum is vertical, the spine is erect, and extension predominates over flexion control as kicking occurs.

Abnormal Sitting

"Sacral-sitting" (Figure 2.22) suggests the lack of several essential components of movement, including the following:

- Antigravity extension mobility and strength.
- Joint capsule mobility, including the hips and spine.
- Muscle length, particularly in the shoulder protractors, rectus abdominous, hamstrings, and hip adductors.

Compensatory patterns occur in children with neuromotor impairment or delayed motor development, particularly if they must attempt a task that is beyond their capability (Baddely 1984). The child in Figure 2.22 demonstrates the following compensatory maneuvers in his effort to maintain the sitting position while sitting on his sacrum rather than on the ischial tuberosities:

- Trunk flexion into gravity.
- Head and shoulder protraction with shoulder elevation.
- Elbow flexion, as he hooks his hands under his thighs.
- Hip adduction and medial rotation.
- Knee flexion, apparently to press his heels to the floor.
- (And a mighty elevation of both eyebrows!)

Figure 2.22
Spastic diplegia, age 4 years: compensatory sitting on the sacrum; lack of trunk extension strength and hip joint mobility. Vaulting transitions and successful hand use are impeded.

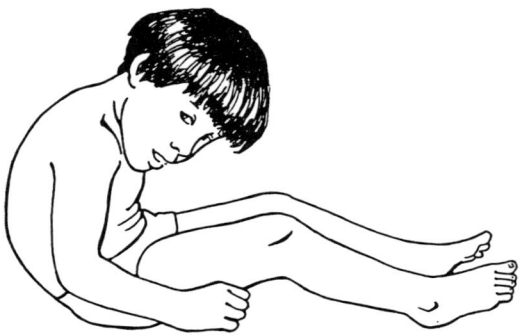

The child's hands are not available to him for dressing or play in this position. Clinical examination revealed the following:

- Weakness of the trunk extensors.
- Evidence of persistent femoral antetorsion.
- Contractures of the hip adductors, flexors, and extensors.
- Knee flexion contracture.
- Ankle plantarflexion contracture (equinus).
- Pronation deformity.

All of the compensations listed above appear in standing position also. Added to the child's structural deviations and contractures, they impose abnormal compressive and tensile forces on his foot structures.

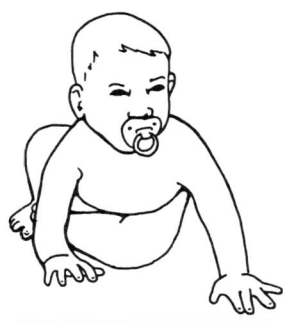

Figure 2.23
9 months: antigravity trunk control allows lateral and rotary movement. From ring-sit arrangement of legs, vaulting transitions occur between sitting and quadruped.

Movement is hardly possible without the capacity to maintain a posture against gravity, to rearrange body parts to move, and to continue to balance while moving (Baddely 1984). The limitations listed above deny the child in Figure 2.22 all of these requirements. He cannot apply the forces needed to activate the muscles of the hip effectively, nor to revise the structure of the femur.

In most normal vaulting transitions, the trunk is moved over the legs—first on the sagittal plane, and then in a rotary fashion (Figure 2.23). The ring arrangement of the legs is the base from which vaulting transitions to prone and all-fours will develop, with increasing evidence of rotary trunk control. The significance of the arrangement of the legs as these transitions are executed is discussed in the following section on vaulting.

Vaulting (Three-Point Kneel)

The vaulting transition occurs when the trunk is moved over the extremities between the positions of sitting and all-fours. The vault seems to be a significant feature of preambulatory movement and locomotion. This is because of its typical appearance in the latter months of the first year, and because of its countless repetitions in daily play. Vaulting is a common feature of floor play in children through early childhood (Figures 2.24 and 2.25). The components of strength, mobility, and stability are effectively implemented in the execution of the vault both as a transitional maneuver and as a play position.

Initially, the vault occurs on the sagittal plane with the pelvis positioned low to the floor and the hips in wide abduction. Thus movement of the pelvis and trunk applies mobilization forces to the hip joint capsule and to the ischiofemoral and pubofemoral ligaments (Kapandji 1970; Brooks 1985). This transition requires sagittal plane mobility of the pelvis and lumbar spine.

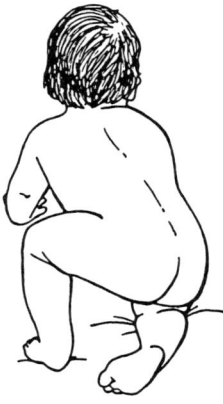

Figure 2.24   Vaulting between sitting and all-fours positions; hip joint mobilization and shear forces applied on the loaded (right) femur. Pelvic mobility is essential.

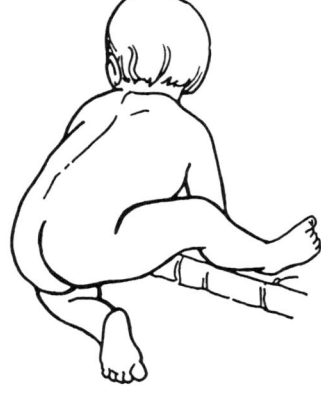

Figure 2.25   Concentric and eccentric activation occurs in the hip stabilizers and quadriceps. Hamstrings and adductors are elongated in the forward leg. Pelvis rotates.

As antigravity strength increases in the hip adductors, abductors, extensors, and rotators, as well as in the knee extensors (and as rotary control of the pelvis on the trunk improves), one knee bears an increasing proportion of the body weight as the vault is executed over it. Hip adduction, by reverse action, shifts the pelvis laterally over the stationary loaded knee.

Observation of normal infants has revealed that, proximal to the loaded knee, the hip is typically maintained in an abducted and laterally rotated position during the vault (see Figures 2.24 and 2.25). The hip and knee extensors work together while coactivation occurs in the remaining hip musculature to maintain the posture. Weight shifts, which lead to a change in posture between sitting and quadruped, occur by activating these muscle groups, both eccentrically and concentrically. The hip musculature, on the same leg as the weight-bearing knee, thus seems to be heavily engaged in the strengthening needed for dynamic stability and for reducing coxa valga and femoral antetorsion. These forces are apparent in the direction of the muscle fibers that attach to the posterior proximal femur during vaulting transitions.

As the vault is executed, the synergistic "total flexion" pattern in the legs gives way to more specific, disassociated joint motion. For example, consider the child in Figure 2.24. The right knee is loaded as the body moves forward over it. The right ankle and foot supinate to clear the foot out of the way of the passing pelvis, while the hip and knee extend above it. At the same time, the left leg, which is counterpoising, is positioned in hip flexion and abduction, knee flexion, and ankle dorsiflexion of varying degrees. The counterpoising foot is achieving contact with the floor as weight is displaced forward and backward, evidently gaining tactile and proprioceptive preparation for the eventual assumption of weight.

The infant in Figure 2.25 demonstrates that during a backward vaulting weight shift toward the sitting position, the hip flexion angle in the unloaded (right) leg increases as the knee extends and the ankle actively dorsiflexes. This combination of motions also brings about elongation of the hamstrings, hip adductors, and ankle plantarflexors by reciprocal innervation. This pattern of hip flexion with knee extension, ankle dorsiflexion, and loading on the heel is the one that appears in two future movement skills: 1) in the gait cycle, at the end of swing and the beginning of stance; and 2) in the equilibrium reaction to posterior weight shifts in the standing position (Gunsolus et al. 1975; Bobath et al. 1964). Because the right hip is rotated laterally, the primary contact area on the heel and foot is the lateral aspect. This is where heel strike will eventually occur in gait (Schafer 1987; Kapandji 1970; Salek 1977).

Management Considerations

Frequently in a program of therapeutic exercise and movement training there is indication to implement various features of vaulting transitions (Figures 2.26-2.28). Such intervention might include the repeated facilitation of those movements that occur in the context of vaulting transitions:

- Trunk rotation, pelvis on shoulders (Figure 2.28)

- Hip extension, eccentric and concentric, with lateral rotation: frontal-plane weight shifts initiated by active hip abduction and adduction on the loaded side

- Knee extension with hip flexion (unloaded)

- Ankle dorsiflexion with knee extension (loaded and unloaded: compression to the heel, lateral border, and forefoot)

If capsular limitation is interfering with joint mobility, active movement might be enhanced first by mobilizing the inferior and posterior aspects of the hip capsule and ligaments (Sternat 1987; Maitland 1977; Brooks 1985).

Figure 2.26
Simulation of the vaulting transitions in therapeutic exercise.

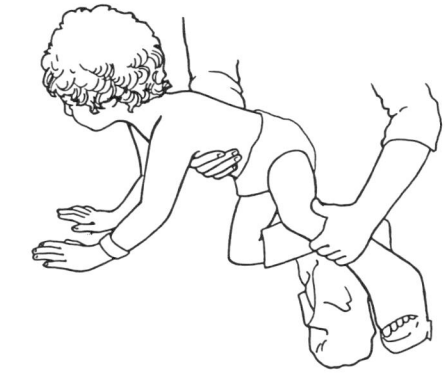

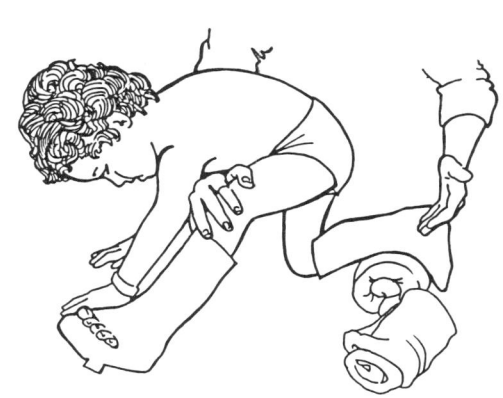

Figure 2.27 Proper weight shifts are facilitated to strengthen the loaded hip stabilizers and to elongate hamstrings actively on the forward leg.

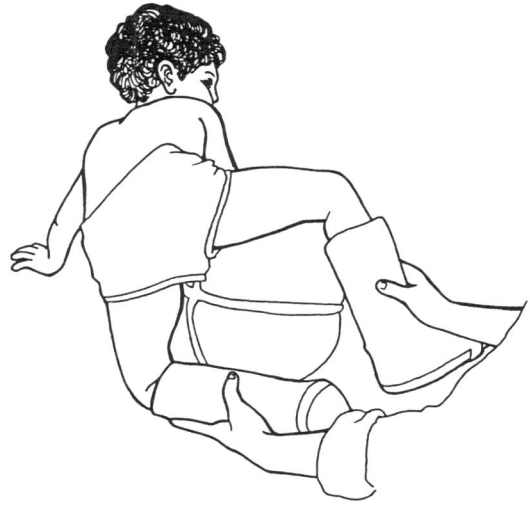

Figure 2.28 Components of vaulting are developed in therapeutic exercise, such as rotation of the trunk, distal-on-proximal segments.

Creeping (locomotion on hands and knees)

Active rocking forward, backward, and diagonally in quadruped elicits strengthening in the abdominals and in the muscles that stabilize the shoulders and hips. At the end of a forward shift, eccentric activation of the supporting shoulder flexors prevents the infant from plunging onto his face, and concentric activation of the same muscles—together with the hip flexors—initiates the shift backward. By associated reaction, this activity in the shoulder flexors facilitates activation in the abdominals; the lordotic sagging of the tummy that is typical of early quadruped position resolves. (See Figure 2.9.)

The significance of the support provided by the abdominals becomes evident in play in this position. When the abdominals anchor the pelvis, preventing it from deviating into a full anterior tilt, the adductors and the posterolateral hip musculature operate off of the stabilized pelvis. If the pelvis tilts forward and the infant reaches out to play, the hip stabilizers relinquish their support to the noncontractile soft tissues and the lumbar spine extensors, which then activate excessively to compensate for the lack of activity in the abdominals and hips.

The development of creeping usually begins with exploratory play on all fours, as the infant reaches out for a toy and leans forward and/or to the side. When the abdominals provide anterior support for the pelvis, this forward "reach and lean" results in diagonal loading simultaneously on the hand that is not reaching and on the opposite knee (Figure 2.29). The adductors contribute to unilateral hip stability in diagonal loading. The proximal band of the adductor magnus exerts a lateral torque force on the femoral shaft.

Reciprocal creeping applies this diagonal distribution of weight for the purpose of locomotion. The creeping matures in efficiency as the base of support narrows and counter-rotation occurs between the shoulders and the pelvis. In mature walking, the same counter-rotation occurs, and a reciprocal arm swing results (Sutherland 1984).

Reciprocal creeping also appears to apply lateral torque to the proximal femur as the hip above the propelling knee extends, usually in slight lateral rotation. In addition, the adductors, including the proximal adductor magnus, participate in stabilizing the upper leg

Figure 2.29
Reaching out to play on hands and knees prepares for reciprocal creeping.

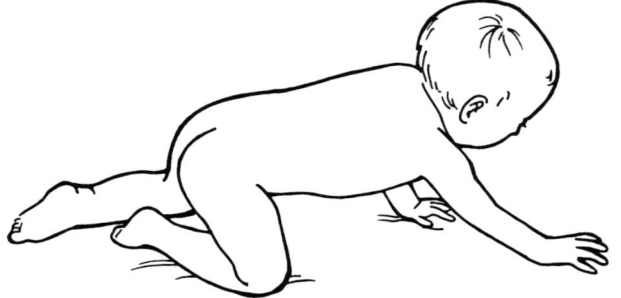

against sliding laterally. In a recent study of children with spastic diplegia, the achievement of reciprocal creeping in children between 1 and 2½ years correlated highly with independent ambulation skills (Badell-Ribera 1985).

Abnormal

Many children with hypertonus fail to creep reciprocally. Instead they "bunny hop," advancing both knees together after advancing both hands together. This sagittal-plane movement indicates an immature reliance on bilateral support and proximal muscle activation. Badell-Ribera (1985) found evidence of a high correlation between persistence of bunny hopping and low levels of ambulation skill—such as household and exercise ambulation—in children with spastic diplegia.

On the other hand, many children with hypotonia also fail to creep. They hitch in sitting position instead. Hitching suggests the presence of inadequate stabilizing control in the shoulders and pelvic girdle, including the hips, and perhaps a hypersensitivity to pressure sensation in the palms and knees.

Bear-Standing

Bear-standing (standing on hands and feet) can occur as early as six months, when the infant is developing extension at the knees (Figure 2.30). It is a more advanced skill than assumption of the quadruped position, because it places greater demands upon available shoulder stability and on control of the pelvis for successful execution. Three advances that are evident in the assumption of bear-standing:

- Elongation of hamstrings by the activating quadriceps—modified by the degree of flexion evident in the hips.
- Elongation of plantar fascia and plantar intrinsic musculature.
- Hyperextension of the toes by the application of pressure to the volar surface of the ball of the foot, modified by the degree of lateral rotation evident in the hips.

In normal walking in infancy, the stance phase of gait terminates over the first metatarsophalangeal (MTP) joint. This happens because of the increased angle of gait at this age (Sutherland 1984).

Figure 2.30
Bear-stand (on hands and feet).
Elongates hamstrings,
triceps surae muscles,
toe flexors, intrinsic muscles,
and plantar fascia.

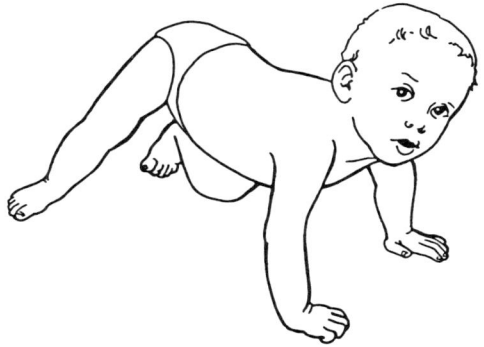

Management Considerations

In therapeutic exercise, bear-standing in varying degrees of hip flexion is often implemented to strengthen the quadriceps while actively elongating the hamstrings, with care to avoid applying deforming forces to the foot or toes (Figures 2.31 and 2.32).

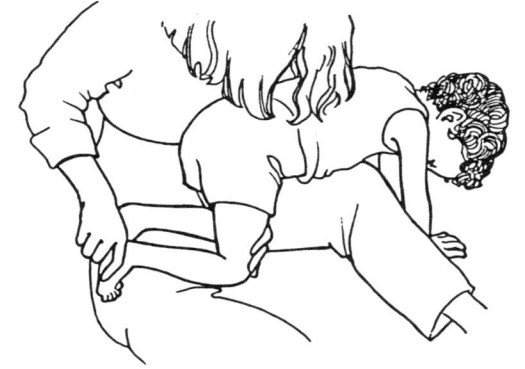

Figure 2.31 Simulate normal bear-standing in therapeutic exercise—maintain alignment of hindfoot and forefoot throughout.

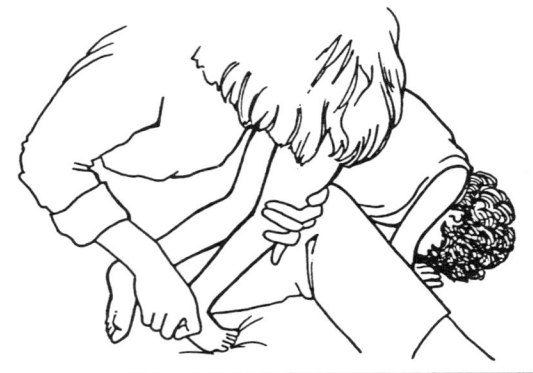

Figure 2.32 Include toe hyperextension to prepare for progression in gait from terminal stance to toe-off.

Kneeling Activities

As the infant continues on the course of neurologic maturation, the drive to gain the upright position becomes evident in the assumption of more vertical postures in play. Kneel-sitting occurs in the final three to four months of the first year as a logical progression from quadruped (Figure 2.33). During kneel-sitting, the knee joint is mobilized into flexion while the ankle and foot move into plantarflexion and supination. The feet and lower legs experience heavy tactile and deep pressure sensory input as the weight of the body is lowered onto them (Sternat 1987; Salek 1977).

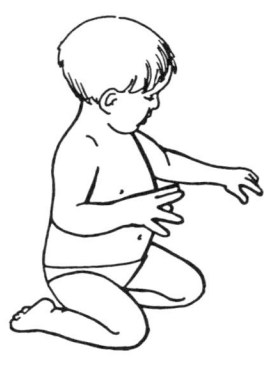

Figure 2.33 Kneel-sitting with hips abducted; trunk extension improved. Lateral shifts use trunk and hip control and lateral pelvic mobility.

Active rotation of both hips, in opposite directions simultaneously, brings about lateral and rotary transitions between the positions of kneeling, side-sitting, and sitting. Hip abduction and adduction occur simultaneously in opposite hips as well. To prevent landing too hard in side-sitting, an eccentric activation occurs in the hip abductors and medial rotators on the side that is closest to the floor. In hip flexion, concentric medial rotation of the uppermost hip occurs as a secondary function of several of the abductors, of the gluteus minimis, and of the proximal fibers of the gluteus maximus (Kapandji 1970; Lehmkuhl et al. 1983). Several hip abductors convert to rotators in full hip flexion and contribute to controlling these lateral weight shifts (Lehmkuhl et al. 1983). With these lateral/rotary transitions between kneel-sitting and side-sitting, the hip stabilizing and trunk musculature is elongated, activated, and strengthened. The hip lateral rotation contracture diminishes. Tensile forces are applied to the greater trochanter and proximal femur.

The transition from kneel-sitting to kneel-standing (on both knees, with the hips abducted and laterally rotated) initially evokes lumbar hyperextension with an anterior pelvic tilt and activation of the knee

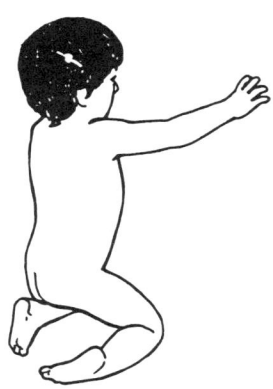

Figure 2.34
Kneel-sit to kneel-stand with hips abducted and laterally rotated.

extensors. The tight iliopsoas and anterior hip joint capsule resist the achievement of hip extension, and the child struggles for vertical alignment of the trunk (Figure 2.34). As the abdominal muscles become more effective in anchoring the anterior pelvis, the hip extensors and abductors increasingly participate in the rise to kneel-standing. Any activity in the hip extensors and lateral rotators elongates the hip flexors by reciprocal innervation and mobilizes the anterior hip capsule and ligaments. Reduction in femoral torsion is a likely structural consequence.

Kneel-sit to kneel-stand transitions can also help to address the problem of coxa valga by applying active (muscular) and passive (weight-bearing) compression to the head of the abducted femur as it is directed into the socket (LeVeau et al. 1984; Frost 1986, Vols. 1 and 2). Rang et al. (1986) state that in children with spastic diplegia, the ability to walk on the knees is evidence of potential for independent, unassisted ambulation in the upright position.

W-sitting (also known as the "reverse tailor" or the "TV squat"), in which the kneel-sit position is modified by lowering the pelvis to the floor between the legs, is seen consistently in some children with no neuromotor disability. These children often exhibit increased femoral antetorsion (mistakenly referred to as "anteversion"), usually of familial origin (Knight 1954; Staheli 1977; Bleck 1982; McDonough 1984). Studies have shown that in those children who do not demonstrate tonus abnormality, the existence of increased femoral torsion ("anteversion") imposes no significant limitation on athletic ability or functional skills (Staheli et al. 1985). Many individuals with normal tonus and increased antetorsion reveal a compensatory excess lateral rotation of the tibia (Fabry et al. 1973; Bleck 1987; Staheli 1977; Bleck 1982; Staheli et al. 1985; McCrea 1985).

Abnormal

The W-sitting position is commonly seen as a substitute for kneeling or sitting in children with neuromotor deficit, including both hypotonic and hypertonic types (Figure 2.35). After age 2 years, the W-sitting position reveals and promotes the exaggerated medial twist in the structure of the femurs. Considering the neonatal femoral configuration, it is not likely that the W-sitting position causes antetorsion, but rather that existing antetorsion fosters W-sitting, which then promotes persistence of excessive antetorsion by passive application of medial torque forces (McDonough 1984).

The selection of this position affords the child the greatest possible positional stability for sitting, because the pelvis is stabilized by the legs against toppling laterally. The legs function like outriggers on a canoe. Thus, consistent W-sitting in the child with few normal postural mechanisms usurps the potential femoral modeling influences of normal transitions between sit, kneel-sit, and kneel-stand. In this case, the transitions to kneel-stand and quadruped positions with the hips medially rotated call primarily upon activation of the hip flexors and adductors, quadriceps, and lumbar extensors. No forces of hip extension and lateral rotation are generated.

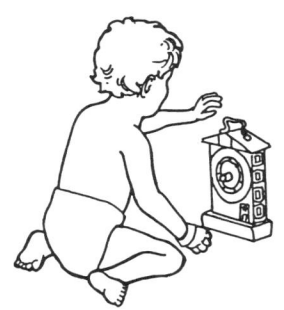

Figure 2.35
Compensatory "W-sitting" accommodates and promotes femoral antetorsion. This position prohibits hip extensors and lateral rotators from applying lateral torque forces.

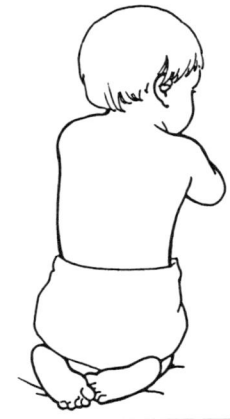

Figure 2.36
Hips abducted, feet together; elongates foot evertors and ankle dorsiflexors; reduces total flexion pattern. If overused, this arrangement of the lower leg can foster internal genicular position, medial torsional deformity in the tibia and fibula, and supination deformity in the foot.

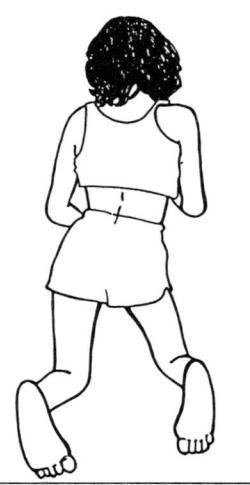

Figure 2.37
Asymmetry indicates lack of extension and flexion control in trunk; lumbosacral hyperextension occurs in lieu of hip extension; evidence of persistent femoral antetorsion is seen in the medially rotated hip position.

In addition, the lower leg is forced in W-sitting either into medial or lateral rotation on the femur—or sometimes both, as in windblown deformity (Figure 2.35). These deviations typically become chronic because the child uses only one sitting position in floor play. The result is adaptation of the soft tissues of the knee joint and torsional changes in the tibia and fibula. Abnormal torque forces at the knee joint are worsened if the ankle is fixed in dorsiflexion by a splint, orthosis, or cast while the child W-sits to play.

The child with spastic diplegia in Figure 2.36 demonstrates the long-term consequences of a lack of achievement of bilateral, symmetrical, antigravity strength and control within the trunk. This is evident by the deviation of her trunk from midline. She attempts to kneel-stand with the transcondylar axes rotated medially, which causes her feet to be placed farther apart than her knees. This configuration of her legs offers evidence of persistent femoral antetorsion as she attempts to seat the head of the femur in the acetabulum by reducing its anteverted position. She appears to rely heavily on her lumbar extensors and quadriceps to maintain kneeling. Likely causes of her postural malalignment may also include contracture of both the iliopsoas muscle and of the anterior hip joint ligaments and capsule (Bleck 1987; Bly 1983; Sternat 1987; Scherzer and Tscharnuter 1982; Root et al. 1971).

Management Considerations

In daily management, the W-sitting position can occasionally be adjusted to kneel-sitting on plantarflexed feet, with hips abducted to simulate the normal configuration (Figure 2.37). Once the base at the legs is revised, the child is given the opportunity to strengthen the femoral derotators and to develop transitions to other postures on the sagittal and frontal planes. Persistent positioning in this type of kneel-sit, however, has been identified as a contributing factor to such problems as in-toeing and medial rotation as well as torsional deformities in the lower leg and foot. Thus it is clear that the child should not use this play position exclusively (Knight 1954; McCrea 1985; Staheli 1977).

The child in Figure 2.37 evidently lacks essential basic antigravity components. At her age (11 years), it is highly unlikely that therapeutic exercise would reduce femoral antetorsion to any significant degree, so the biomechanical consequences at the feet and knees should be addressed with appropriate support systems to prevent progression of deformity. Conservative management includes the following:

- Therapeutic exercise, emphasizing mobilization of tight joint capsules.
- Elongation of tight muscles by reciprocal inhibition and strengthening of essential antigravity muscle groups.
- Serial casting as needed to reduce distal joint contracture.
- Adequate structural support for the feet.

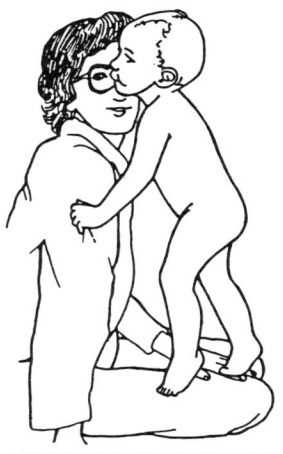

Figure 2.38
Scaling the parent:
another challenge to
strength, stability, and
mobility.

Cruising/Climbing/Preambulatory Skills

One of the natural developments of the ability to creep on hands and knees is that the infant commonly approaches the parents and attempts to creep up onto their bodies, pulling up to a standing position on a lap (Figure 2.38). Most parents seem to respond to the infant's apparent desire to stand by holding the child at the hands and helping in the effort if needed. In this fashion, the standing position is often introduced and experienced earlier than it would be without the parent's help—often in the sixth or seventh month. Later on, by the age of 10 to 11 months, the infant may climb on up the parent's body, scaling it like a monkey.

Management Considerations

The child with spastic diplegia in Figures 2.39, 2.40, and 2.41 has not had the chance to enjoy this experience, so "mother-climbing" was introduced in therapeutic exercise as a way to fulfill the child's apparently unmet need to thin his mother's hair while facilitating appropriate weight-bearing and strengthening.

The position of lateral hip rotation was maintained by his mother throughout this activity. She first facilitated numerous bilateral/symmetrical transitions between sitting and standing positions (Figure 2.39). Then she guided his weight shift onto one foot. This allowed his trunk to be aligned above that foot. He was then assisted as needed in placing his unloaded leg in proper position for the climb up onto mother's lap (Figure 2.40). He executed the elevation by activating his hip and knee extensors while his mother maintained his legs in a position of hip abduction. She then introduced lateral and rotary

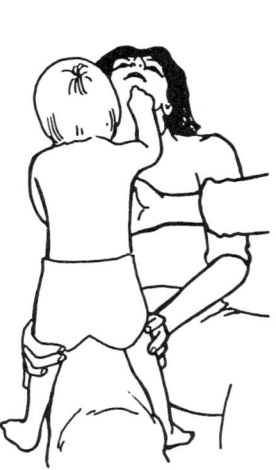

Figure 2.39
Simulating Figure
2.38 in therapeutic
exercise: beginning
with numerous repeti-
tions of bilateral/
symmetrical straddle-
sit to straddle-stand . . .

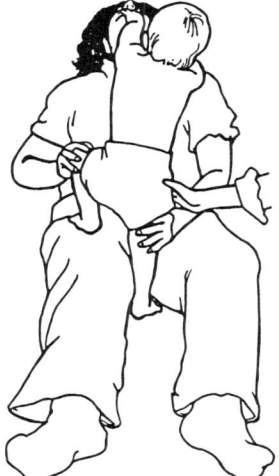

Figure 2.40
. . . facilitating a
weight shift to half-
stand for climbing—
mother maintains
normal leg alignment
with her hold on the
child's thighs . . .

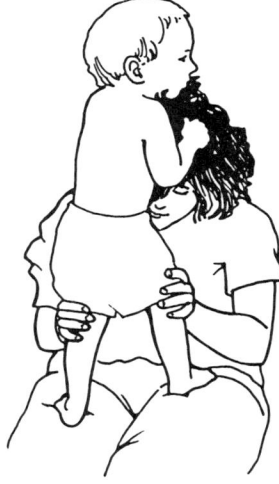

Figure 2.41
. . . and then offers
weight shifts by lifting
either of her support-
ing legs (while her
son successfully thins
her hair!).

shifts of his weight over each foot by raising first one of her supporting thighs and then the other (Figure 2.41). His attention to play rendered this therapeutic activity an enjoyable intervention for the two of them.

Pull to stand—The normal infant begins to pull-to-stand directly from the kneel-stand position by simultaneously extending both knees. This can occur as early as the seventh month. Soon after, the shift from kneel-stand to half-kneel position develops (Bly 1983; Scherzer et al. 1982) (Figure 2.42). A rotation of the upper trunk, such as occurs when an infant's attention is drawn over its own shoulder, often results in the initial assumption of half-kneel. This rotation of the trunk brings about a posterolateral transfer of the center of gravity, which elicits a flexion and abduction response in the opposite leg (Bly 1983; Effgen 1987). This diagonal transfer of the lower trunk is then applied to the transition between kneeling and half-kneeling, often without the component of trunk rotation.

From the half-kneeling position, the initial attempts to rise to standing will again involve simultaneous extension of the knees, with a central distribution of the center of gravity, until unilateral quadriceps strength improves (Figure 2.43). Because the typical half-kneel posture includes abduction of the flexed hip in front and lateral rotation of the supporting hip, a variation of the frog-leg configuration prevails. Loaded hip and knee extension occur on that base when the infant rises from half-kneel to standing. Soon after the gain in strength permits the rise to standing over the forward leg, the child can be expected to begin climbing in the upright position rather than on all fours.

It often happens that the infant who first learns to pull to stand using the rails of the crib or playpen cannot then sit back down without help. Extension skills in the legs continue to emerge in advance of

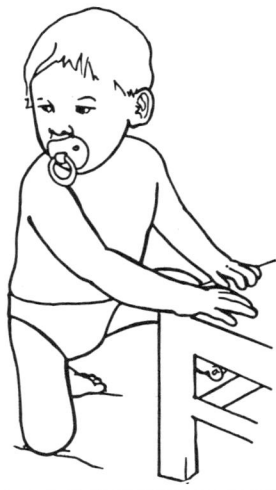

Figure 2.42
Transition from kneel-stand to half-kneel activates hip stabilizing muscles and elongates hip flexors.

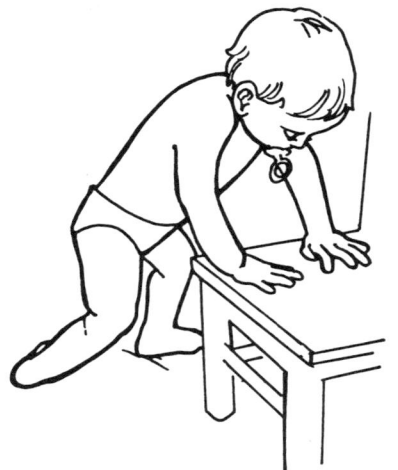

Figure 2.43 Initial pull to stand occurs with weight distributed over both feet, even from the half-kneel position.

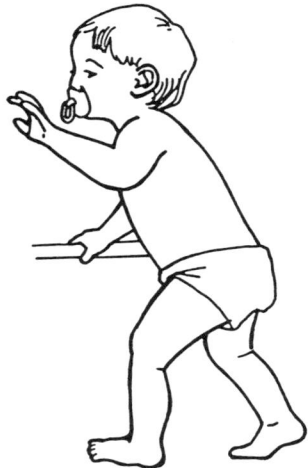

Figure 2.44
Cruising: closed-chain interactions in the legs and feet are explored; mature gait features of foot and ankle function are exhibited.

the flexion that is needed as a counterforce (Bly 1983; Scherzer et al. 1982). When the infant is able to overcome the extension and buckle at the hips to sit down, cruising (stepping while holding onto a support surface) typically begins in earnest (Scherzer et al. 1982) (Figure 2.44).

Abnormal

Many children with neuromotor impairment persist in pulling to stand over lower extremities that extend bilaterally, thus relying on primitive, sagittal plane weight transfer and function. These children miss the opportunity for disassociation, mobilization of the joints, strengthening, and modeling of the lower extremities that the transitions through half-kneeling provide. They also lack preparation for climbing, where further mobilizing, strengthening, and modeling can occur.

Cruising—It is while cruising that the infant begins to apply the strengths that were achieved on the floor to the challenge of maintaining—and continuously moving in—the upright position. As is evident in Figure 2.44, closed-chain motions appear in the legs and trunk as the infant, while stabilizing with the arms and hands, experiences rotational weight shifts and lateral movement. Cruising along furniture often begins as early as age 8 or 9 months and seems to be an important addition to the infant's growing repertoire of antigravity skills. Cruising provides opportunities for the infant to prepare for independent, unsupported standing and walking through strengthening, sensory input, and learning (Scherzer et al. 1982; Salek 1977).

Cruising usually begins with lateral movement, followed by rotary movement; side-stepping progresses to a forward rotation of the pelvis under the shoulders (Scherzer et al. 1982) (Figure 2.45). At this point in the infant's motor development, locomotion by creeping and stability in sitting are emerging and improving in efficiency.

Climbing—The achievements of disassociation between the lower extremities, and of antigravity power in the quadriceps and hip extensors, are expressed and enhanced in the skill of climbing both in quadruped (for example, up a staircase) and from a supported standing position (Figure 2.46). "High climbing" or "scaling" furniture of appropriate height applies and further develops the components of antigravity strength and joint mobility, particularly at the hips.

The child in Figure 2.46 achieves increased mobility into right hip extension by first flexing the left hip. This stabilizes her pelvis against tilting anteriorly. As the right hip extends, the right hip capsule and ligaments are drawn taut, and the flexors are both actively and passively elongated.

The work of reducing femoral antetorsion also appears to be underway in the weight-bearing hip during climbing activities. On ascending, the gluteus maximus is activated concentrically, as demonstrated by the right leg in Figure 2.46. It participates in raising the body over the uppermost leg and foot. On the return to the floor, eccentric activation occurs, as demonstrated by the right leg in Figure

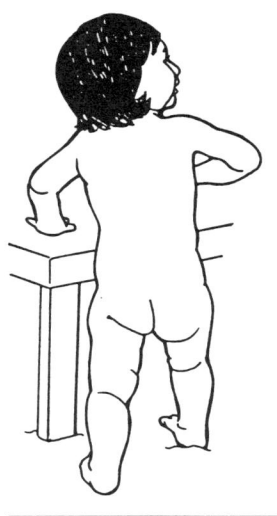

Figure 2.45
Cruising begins on the frontal plane and progresses to rotary motion.

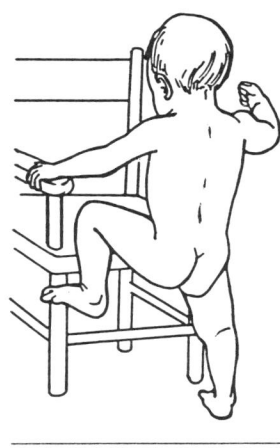

Figure 2.46
High climbing strengthens total body musculature through maximum ranges of motion, and applies lateral torque forces to long bones.

2.47. These movements are executed with the legs arranged in lateral hip rotation and abduction (Figures 2.46 and 2.47) and, once discovered, might be repeated hundreds or thousands of times.

Climbing also offers the infant the opportunity to learn about the dimensions of one's own legs and feet in relation to space (Salek 1977).

Squatting—When squatting appears, it is usually a transition from supported standing to sitting (or a stage in moving from half-kneel to standing) while the quadriceps are gaining strength. In a full squat position, the lateral hindfoot takes most of the body weight because the hips are abducted and laterally rotated (Figure 2.48). With each subtle backward shift of weight, the ankle dorsiflexors activate, apparently as a feature of the effort to regain balance (Salek 1977; Gunsolus et al. 1975; Bobath et al. 1964).

This is the first chance for the infant to strengthen the ankle dorsiflexors. They will eventually function to prevent the toe from dragging during swing and the foot from slapping to the ground after heel strike in mature gait (Sutherland 1984). Unlike the plantar flexors, the dorsiflexors do not require tremendous strength; they will not lift the body off the ground as the triceps surae do. However, they will be needed to aid in regaining balance if the trunk is displaced backward in standing (Scherzer et al. 1982; Salek 1977; Gunsolus et al. 1975; Bobath et al. 1964). The equilibrium function of the ankle dorsiflexors first appears in the squatting position.

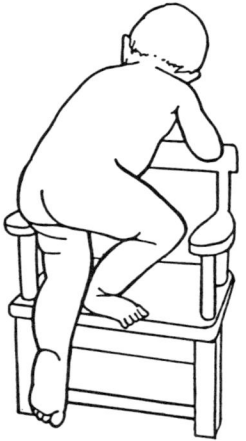

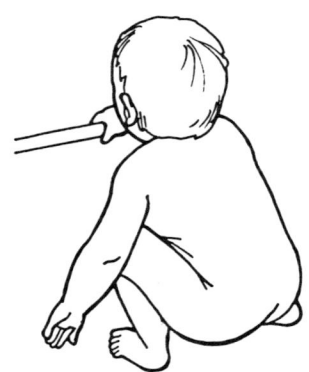

Figure 2.47 Climbing can enhance awareness both of body dimensions and of space.

Figure 2.48 Squatting with hips abducted: backward weight shifts activate ankle dorsiflexors and long toe extensors—preparing for balancing.

Standing—Postural Features of Progression

The newborn—The newborn infant placed in the standing position accepts part of its own weight, revealing evidence of "primary standing." This is also known as the neonatal positive support reflex (Figure 2.49). The trunk is kyphotic, the lumbar spine flat; thus the newborn cannot achieve upright extension in standing (Asher 1975).

The configuration of the legs in neonatal standing reveals the alignment features and joint limitations that were noted in prone and supine positions. The hips are flexed and laterally rotated, and the knees are flexed. The ankles are hypermobile into dorsiflexion. The consequence of these joint positions is that the heels align close together and contact the support surface. The newborn never normally stands on toes.

If the same infant is tipped forward, "newborn stepping" or "spontaneous stepping" appears, as the infant moves the legs in a stepping pattern (Figure 2.50).

Abnormal

With the exception of normal premature infants, newborns who toe-stand when placed upright are suspect for hypertonic neurologic deficit. Many children with neuromotor disorder never reveal newborn stepping, either because of hypertonus into extension, or because of a lack of tolerance for weight-bearing at all in standing (Salek 1977; Bly et al. 1980).

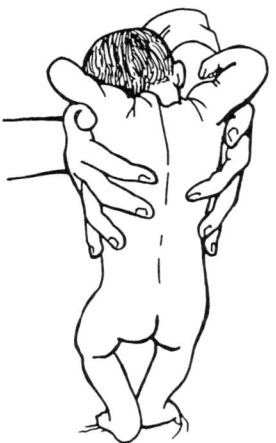

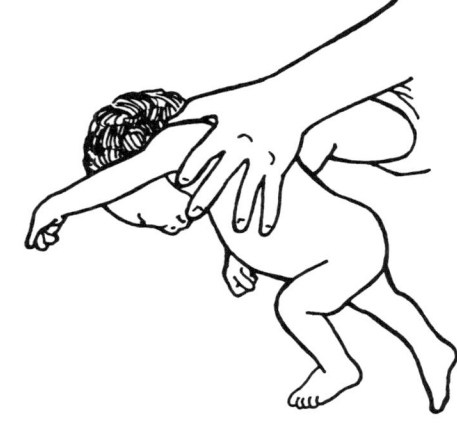

Figure 2.49
Newborn: primary standing with "physiologic flexion" at hips, knees, ankles; hips laterally rotated; knees apart; heels together and on the surface.

Figure 2.50   Newborn: "spontaneous stepping."

One month—Kinematic studies of 18 infants at 1 month reveal that normal early spontaneous stepping reveals tight synchronization of motions at the hip, knee, and ankle in patterns of flexion or extension. During the swing phase, the ankle plantarflexors exhibit little electrical activity on EMG; however, the tibialis anterior remains generally tonically active throughout the phase (Thelen et al. 1987).

Two months—The newborn stepping pattern begins to show variation in the second month, with the appearance of plantarflexion as an isolated motion at the ankle (Thelen et al. 1987).

Two to three months—In the second and third months, astasia (the refusal to participate in standing) occurs as a transient motor pattern in some children. By the end of the third month, weight is again accepted in supported standing.

Four months—The child in Figure 2.51 is 4 months of age. The trunk is flexed forward of the legs with less kyphosis than during the newborn period. No significant lower extremity strength or control has developed by this age, so the same alignment features are seen here as were observed in the newborn. The main difference is apparent in the activation of knee extensors. As the infant's knees extend, the features of genu varum and of lateral rotation at the femoral condyles (with medial rotation of the lower legs) become clearly visible. At this age, the feet are still close together in supported standing, with the heels on the surface.

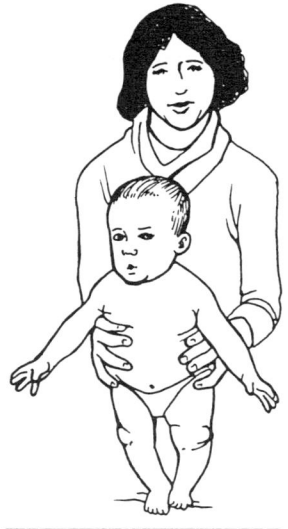

Figure 2.51
4 months: accepts weight with hips flexed and laterally rotated; knees extended; ankles flexed; heels close to each other; heels and forefeet contacting the surface.

There are several factors to consider in assessing the alignment of the hindfoot in the standing position in early infancy. First, the distal lower leg appears laterally bowed because of medial rotation of the lower leg. Second, the distal articulating surface of the tibia (the plafond) is everted (Bahler 1986). The trochlea (the uppermost surface of the talus) evidently articulates with the tibial plafond, resulting in eversion of the talar body. The off-weight-bearing calcaneus, however, is commonly held in varus at this age, apparently by shortened ligaments and muscle tissues on the medial side of the foot. (The newborn typically exhibits varus deviations of both the hindfoot and the forefoot.) The muscles of supination are more numerous and more powerful than those of pronation in the open chain.

Gradually, as the infant takes weight in the upright position, the foot passively pronates. The weak medial connective tissues evidently lengthen, and the weight-bearing calcaneus eventually aligns in valgus position, apparently along with the talus. Consequently, the weight-bearing bones of the infant's ankle and hindfoot align in pronation, which increases their flexibility.

Third, regardless of age, one of the basic functional features of the foot in the closed chain is that the forefoot (that is, the metatarsal heads) always seeks full contact with the ground (Gray 1986; Jordan et al. 1983; Root et al. 1977; Root et al. 1971). This is particularly true in the infant, because the center of gravity is displaced forward as the infant stands, forcing more weight to the forefoot by virtue of the line of gravitational loading (Figure 2.51).

Because the infant's hindfoot and forefoot are commonly at rest in a position of varus in the open chain, and the position of the forefoot when the subtalar joint is in neutral (congruent) alignment can approach 15 degrees, the very young infant stands on the outer borders of the feet. As weeks pass and upright standing increases in frequency, the entire plantar surface lowers to the floor with pronation. This happens because the varus forefoot, maintained by soft tissue contracture and lateral torsion of the talar neck, seeks contact with the ground and stresses the hindfoot into compensatory valgus to do so. Apparent tibial varum can thus exaggerate the appearance of hindfoot valgus as the forefoot lowers to the ground, particularly in early infancy (Jordan et al. 1983).

Six months—The distinguishing features of supported standing alignment and function include the following: a mild lordosis in the spine, which is becoming increasingly erect in standing; a widening of the base of support via reduction of medial genicular position (Figure 2.52); and a high level of activity, such as jumping, knee drops, stamping, and flip-flopping between the sole and the dorsum of the foot. The instability and poor control of the foot and ankle are most apparent at this age, because purposeful activity in the ankle plantar flexors and dorsiflexors has only recently appeared in prone and supine positions. The sensation of bearing weight on the feet can also be relatively unfamiliar at this age. The weight-bearing foot appears more pronated now than in previous months, evidently due to successful lateral rotation of the lower leg under the femur, which results in abduction of the foot.

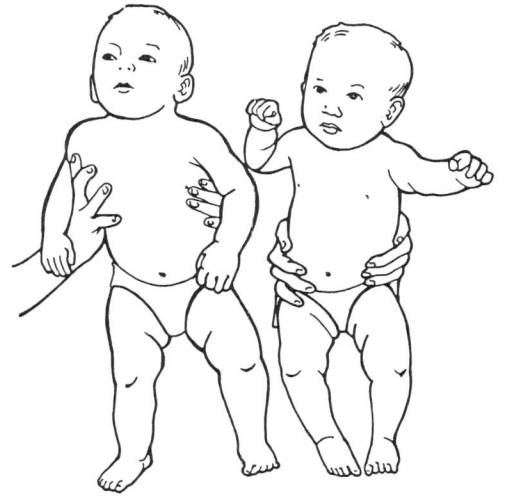

Figure 2.52
5 months (on the right): base of support widens. Medial lower leg rotation persists.
6 months (on the left): hips are abducted while knees are extended. Feet and ankles are very unstable on the frontal and sagittal planes. Heels are on the surface. Lower legs rotate laterally within the knee joints, promoting foot pronation in standing.

Seven to eight months—Standing on the toes emerges (Figure 2.53). The intrinsic toe flexors and the ankle dorsiflexors are elongated in toe-standing and the ball of the foot is mobilized as if to prepare for push-off later on (Sternat 1987; Salek 1981). Toe-standing appears before purposeful activity in the ankle dorsiflexors is evident in the standing position. This sequence of events is in keeping with the previous course of achieving antigravity extension control and strength before achieving those of antigravity flexion.

One might question the assignment of "positive support reflex" status to the appearance of toe-standing at the age of 7 months, since voluntary control is obviously well under way, as is the logical progression of control and strengthening from proximal to distal in the lower extremities. Because extension control has consistently emerged before flexion control more proximally, the emergence of ankle plantarflexion before dorsiflexion in standing follows suit, given the understanding that plantarflexion at the ankle is a distal function of extension. In the context of the extension synergy in the lower extremity (evident in decerebrate rigidity), extension at the ankle is synonymous with plantarflexion.

Furthermore, the musculature of the triceps surae group, particularly the soleus muscle, is intended for high endurance and high power work as a consistent stabilizer of the tibia on the talus in gait (Lehmkuhl et al. 1983; Soderberg 1986).

The calf musculature also needs power for successful climbing and running. The infant and preschooler will devote a considerable portion of time in the upright position to walking on toes rather than in the plantigrade position. However, if the child does not ever stand in plantigrade position, as the infant does in Figure 2.54, then hypertonus or motor dysfunction is suspected and should be investigated.

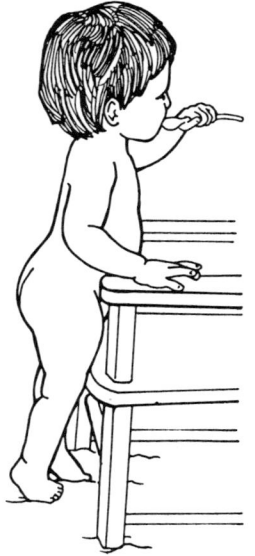

Figure 2.53
7 months: toe standing builds power in ankle plantar flexors for stability at the ankle and knee joints.

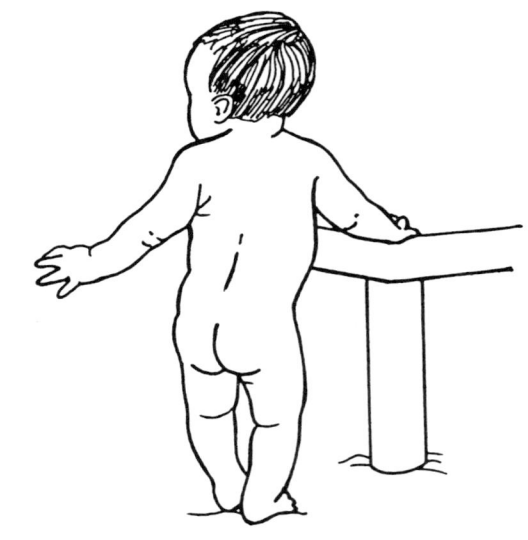

Figure 2.54 7 months: plantigrade standing also occurs. Trunk gains increased verticality.

12 Months to 7 Years— Postural and Gait Features

12 Months

Now that the infant has achieved independence in standing and is about to use ambulation as the primary means of locomotion, it is time to review the features of bone structure, joint mobility, and alignment of the lower limb segments to identify the changes that have occurred since birth. The arrangement of the lower extremities in standing influences current movement and stability skills. This arrangement also reveals the status of development of the supporting joints. This is particularly true at the feet and ankles, where appropriate distribution of weight is crucial to the establishment and maintenance of a stable structure (Salek 1977; Perry 1975).

The impact of improper weight distribution at the feet and ankles is readily apparent in the common deformities seen in the feet and ankles of children with cerebral palsy. This is more obvious after, rather than before, regular weight-bearing on the feet occurs (Scherzer et al. 1982; Gunsolus et al. 1975; Bobath et al. 1976; Baker et al. 1964). The difficulties are compounded when the child struggles to stabilize the trunk, head and arms—which together account for at least 70 percent of the total body weight on malaligned lower extremities (Perry 1975; Bobath et al. 1976; Baker et al. 1964). See Chapter 4 for a thorough discussion of these deformities and their functional influences.

Normal Values for Joint Mobility

The child at 1 year of age reveals the following evidence of progress in overcoming the joint mobility limitations of the newborn period (values are averaged):

- Hip rotation: With the hip extended, 58 degrees lateral/44 degrees medial (Phelps et al. 1985). With the hip flexed, total mobility increases to 120-130 degrees.
- Hip flexion contracture: The average limitation of hip extension is 9 degrees, using the Staheli Prone Extension Test. (The infant is placed in prone with hips flexed over the edge of a table. The hip is then passively extended until the pelvis begins to rotate.) (Phelps et al. 1985)
- Hip abduction: 54 degrees with hip flexed (Phelps et al. 1985).
- Knee flexion contracture: Resolved (Hoffer 1980).
- Ankle dorsiflexion: 25-45 degrees (passive) (Giannestras 1973; Jordan et al. 1983).
- Ankle plantarflexion: 45-50 degrees, minimum (McCrea 1985; Tax 1985).

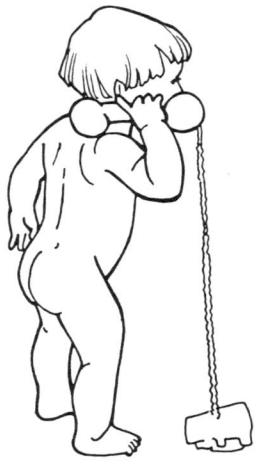

Figure 2.55
12 months: limited lumbar extension mobility. Hip flexion contracture draws stiff trunk into a forward lean. Effort to maintain vertical position requires upper back and shoulder extension.

Features of Structure, Alignment, and Posture

If one looks at the skeletal structure, joint alignment, and posture in the normal infant at 1 year of age, the following postural features can be identified when the infant stands erect:

- (Refer to Figure 2.55.) The pelvis tilts anteriorly approximately 16-20 degrees (Asher 1975; Sutherland 1984; Sutherland et al. 1980). Mobility into lumbar spine extension is limited (Asher 1975). Therefore, forward lean of the trunk is evident, with elevated and retracted arms (Asher 1975).

- (Refer to Figures 2.55, 2.56, 2.57, and 2.58.) Hip flexion is a consistent feature of postural alignment at this age (Hoffer 1980).

- Abduction is evident because the base of support averages 6 inches (Jordan et al. 1983; Sutherland 1984). Resolution of internal (medial) genicular position contributes to the wide base at the feet.

- Lateral hip rotation posture (that is, femoral head and neck anteversion), which is measured clinically by comparing the transcondylar axis of the femur to the frontal plane, averages 20 degrees (Jordan et al. 1983; Sutherland 1984).

- The entire foot is laterally rotated (abducted) approximately 20-30 degrees, in keeping with the position of lateral rotation at the hip joint and with weight-bearing pronation (McCrea 1985; Staheli 1977; Sutherland 1984) (Figure 2.58). At this age, the outwardly directed position of the hip and the foot favors frontal-plane positional stability by lengthening the lateral lever arms.

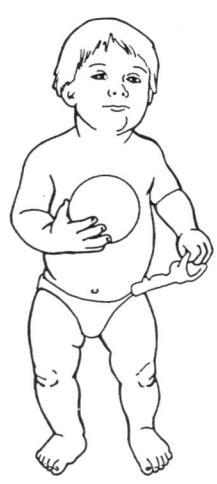

Figure 2.56
12 months: hip abduction, lateral rotation, and flexion persist.

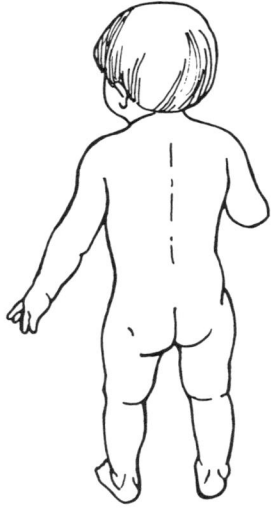

Figure 2.57
13 months: genu varum, antetorsion, and lateral hip rotation have partially resolved. Medial lower leg rotation is also reducing, which lessens apparent tibial varum.

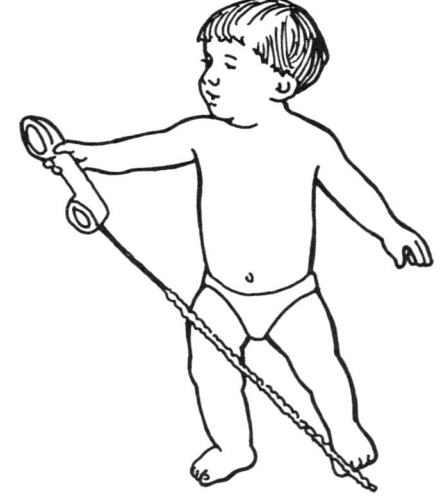

Figure 2.58 12 months: lateral shift of the center of gravity in play is not yet applied to gait.

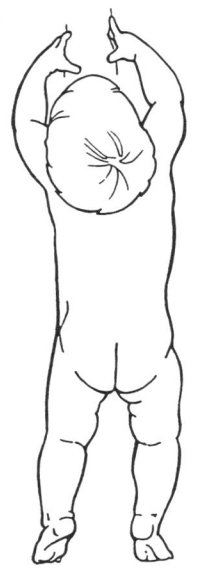

Figure 2.59
12 months: volitional toe-standing strengthens triceps surae and posterior tibialis muscles and reveals longitudinal arch formation. This muscle action serves to stabilize the ankle and foot and applies lateral torque force to the tibia and fibula.

Control of the triplanar motions of the talocrural, subtalar, and midtarsal joints is developing. With the feet aligned in abduction, lateral shift results in loading of the forefoot rather than the lateral border. This also elicits activation of the ankle plantar flexors for equilibrium, which helps to halt the lateral shift by stopping the fall of the tibia over the foot. The plantar flexors will soon be called upon to function similarly in gait (Sutherland 1984; Sutherland et al. 1980a; Sutherland et al. 1980b).

- Toe grasp is a common feature of stability-seeking in stance.

Skeletal structures in the lower extremities have altered as follows:

- Pelvis: Growth has occurred, particularly in the sacrum.
- Femur: Antetorsion averages 31-35 degrees (Fabry et al. 1973).
- Knee: Genu varum is reduced to 5-8 degrees (Hensinger et al. 1982; McDade 1977).
- Tibia: Mild apparent tibial varum of 6 degrees persists in the distal third of the lower leg (Jordan et al. 1983).
- Talocrural joint: The transmalleolar axis aligns at 6-10 degrees lateral rotation relative to the frontal plane (McCrea 1985; Jordan et al. 1983; Root et al. 1971). This measure should be taken with the femoral condyles aligned on the frontal plane.
- Foot: The longitudinal arch is observable in toe-standing at this age (Figure 2.59).
- Subtalar joint: The calcaneus aligns in 6 degrees of valgus in standing (calcaneal stance angle) (Valmassy 1984). Off weight-bearing, the STJ aligns in congruity in calcaneal varus, 5-10 degrees (Jordan et al. 1983).
- Midtarsal joint: 5-10 degrees of forefoot varus (open chain) with the foot neutrally aligned (locked). The entire area of the metatarsal heads contacts the floor in the closed chain.

Overcoming Pronation-Promoting Forces

As one considers the posture, alignment, and structural features of this age, it seems a wonder that the normal foot does not succumb to the multiple pronatory loads on it that originate both from the proximal and distal directions. In individuals who fail to resolve many of these biomechanical problems, compensatory pronation in the foot can be observed.

The factors that can cause the weight-bearing foot to pronate in the infant include any of the following: a wide-based, laterally rotated stance; femoral antetorsion; eversion of the tibial plafond and talar body; weak ligaments; and forefoot varus. How then does the infant escape severe pronatory consequences?

Postural features—One possibility may be by way of the existing genu varum in combination with a wide base of support and lateral rotation of the hip and foot. Through the first 18 months, this leg arrangement seems to displace a portion of body weight to the outer borders of the feet. Another is the mechanical support for the arches provided by any existing plantar fat pad (Figure 2.60). The fat pad (if present) will remain intact through the age of 2 years, after which

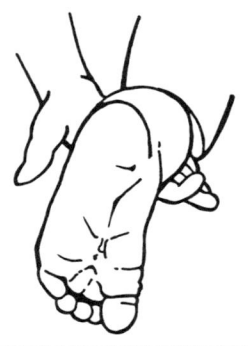

Figure 2.60
Normal, age 13 months: fat pad continues to mask and support the longitudinal arch while ossification and strengthening of the supporting ligaments continues. Forefoot varus diminishes to 5-6 degrees.

it will begin to "melt away," resorbing fully by the age of 4 years (Tax 1985; Valmassy 1984; Rodgers et al. 1984). Another protective factor is the modeling influence of normal "physiologic" pronation on strengthening the medial ligaments and fascia. The infant stands on a mildly pronated foot. The talus and navicular strain the medial connective tissue structures, which respond by thickening and gaining strength to resist pronation (Frost 1986, Vol. 2).

Squatting in abduction—Within the first month of walking, the infant finds numerous occasions to squat to varying degrees of knee flexion. The semi-squat is executed with a measure of lateral hip rotation and abduction (a recurrence of frog-leg alignment). The child in Figures 2.61 and 2.62 demonstrates a semi-squat posture. In this position, the quadriceps are strengthened together with the hip extensors, abductors, and ankle plantar flexors. All this muscle activity prevents the pelvis and knees from dropping to the floor (Lehmkuhl et al. 1983; Soderberg 1986). If this child did not use the lateral stabilizing musculature at the hips, the knees would contact each other in squatting, and the feet would pronate. (Refer to Figure 2.82 at the end of this chapter for an illustration of the consequences of chronic malalignment and muscle imbalance.)

An appropriate execution of squatting involves eccentric and concentric activation of the knee and hip extensors together with the hip abductors and lateral rotators. This applies loading forces to the lateral pillars of the feet and effectively protects the integrity of the medial supporting ligaments.

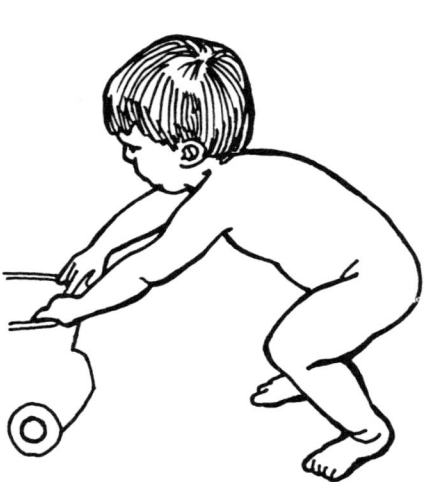

Figure 2.61   13 months: semi-squatting in abducted position builds strength and control in the quadriceps and triceps surae muscles.

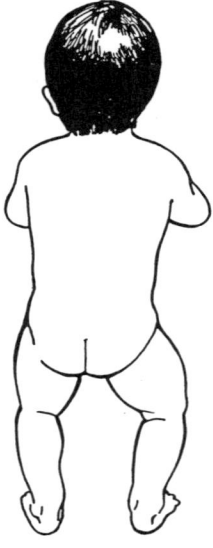

Figure 2.62
"Frog-leg" configuration persists in standing activities and facilitates activation of hip lateral rotators with abductors and extensors.

Equilibrium responses—In standing, equilibrium reactions are evident in the foot, though they are merely emerging. With lateral displacement of the center of gravity, supination occurs in the loaded foot. However, the degree is much less than in the more mature foot (Gunsolus et al. 1975). Active supinatory balancing responses of the medial pillar of the foot provide a means of strengthening the supinatory musculature needed to overcome pronation forces.

Toe-standing—Heel inversion occurs in toe-standing, which affects the windlass action of the medial aspect of the plantar aponeurosis (Figure 2.59). Concurrently, in toe-standing compared with plantigrade, the transmalleolar axis aligns more laterally relative to the frontal plane. According to some researchers, the plantar flexors are also supinators of the foot, increasing their power as invertors, as the angle between the TMA and the frontal plane increases (Lehmkuhl et al. 1983; Soderberg 1986). By reverse action, their activation can be expected to facilitate displacement of weight onto the lateral border of the foot as, over the next two or three years, the foot aligns closer to the sagittal plane, and the angle of the transmalleolar axis increases. This lateral displacement protects the foot structures from excessive medial weight-bearing forces that could lead to pronation deformity.

Walking—The most significant influence, however, seems to lie in the rotary components in the normal gait pattern. Even at this age, as the infant walks, the lower extremity medially rotates during the first 15 percent of the stance cycle, absorbing floor reaction forces at initial foot contact. Medial rotation of the leg combines with pronation of the foot through the mechanical links in the closed kinetic chain. Once weight is assumed, the rotation switches direction and lateral rotation occurs through the remaining 85 percent of the stance phase. Lateral rotation of the leg occurs with increasing supination of the foot, which converts the foot into an increasingly rigid lever for the carriage and forward propulsion of body weight (Sutherland 1984). Thus, if ligamentous integrity and bone structure in the foot are normal, the normal gait supports and protects the foot structures.

Figures 2.63 through 2.66 compare the feet of a child of 13 months with no neuromotor deficit to the feet of a preschooler of 30 months with spastic diplegia to identify normal and abnormal deviations in foot structure.

- The normal weight-bearing calcaneus at 13 months deviates into 6 degrees of valgus, measured relative to the sagittal plane (Valmassy 1984) (Figure 2.63). By comparison, the child with diplegia reveals the following:

- The calcaneae deviate into 15 and 25 degrees of valgus (Figure 2.64).

- The metatarsals normally align on a parallel with the sagittal bisection of the hindfoot (Figure 2.65).

- Active eversion and abduction are evident at the hindfoot and the forefoot of the child with diplegia (Figure 2.66).

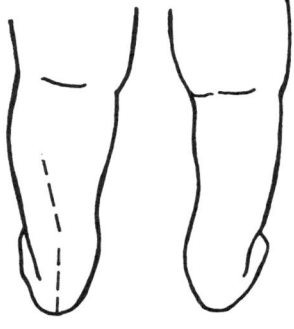

Figure 2.63
Normal, age 13 months: distal varum of 6 degrees; calcaneal stance is 6 degrees of valgus, relative to sagittal plane.

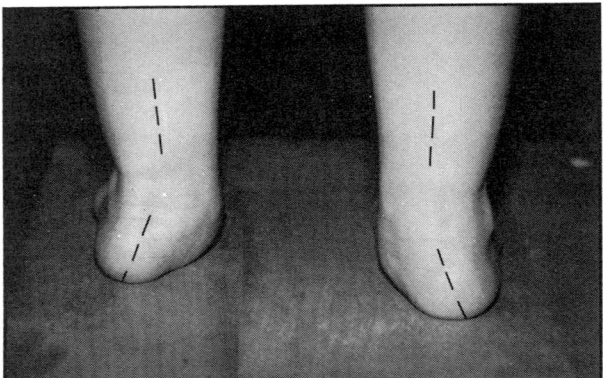

Figure 2.64 Spastic diplegia, age 30 months: Left: equinovalgus—heel elevation combined with 25 degrees of valgus. Right: pes planus—heel on the floor and 15 degrees of valgus.

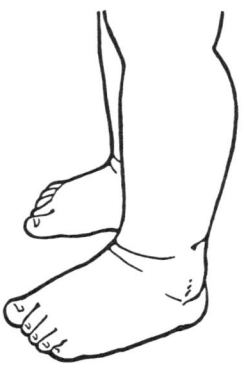

Figure 2.65 Normal, age 13 months: transmalleolar axis (TMA) at 6-10 degrees lateral, relative to the frontal plane. The forefoot is parallel to the hindfoot around the longitudinal axis.

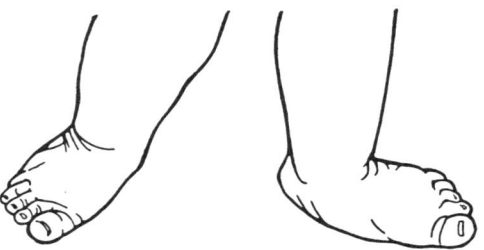

Figure 2.66
Spastic diplegia, age 30 months. Severe equinovalgus: TMA reduced to 0 degrees or less. The talus protrudes; the navicular head contacts the floor; the forefoot is abducted and everted; the first ray rotates medially; the toes deviate laterally.

With the resulting dorsiflexion and abduction of the forefoot and lateral deviation of the toes, the body weight is taken anteromedially from early stance through toe-off. The first metatarsal and its adjacent cuneiform (first ray) dorsiflex and invert, under the strain of loading, on the medial edge of the forefoot.

The medial supporting ligaments of the subtalar and midtarsal joints are severely strained and will gradually yield—by expanding and effectively lengthening—to the chronic abnormal tensile demand (Frost 1986, Vols. 1 and 2; Perry 1975; Baker et al. 1964). The lateral ligaments and muscle tendons will shorten accordingly, by physiologic adaptation mechanisms. This process is known as creep (LeVeau et al. 1984; Frost 1986; Rodgers et al. 1984).

- The lower leg segments in the child in Figure 2.66 rotate medially, bringing the right transmalleolar axis (TMA) to the frontal plane; the left TMA is aligned medial to the front plane. At 24 months, the normal pitch of this axis is 10-15 degrees lateral to the frontal plane (McCrea 1985). The congruity between the head of the talus and the navicular is disrupted, and the navicular dorsiflexes and abducts away from the medial aspect of the head of the talus.

- A high degree of integrity of the medial supporting ligaments for the subtalar joint (STJ) is evident in the respective 2:1 ratio of hindfoot inversion to eversion in the 13-month-old child in Figures 2.67 and 2.68. At birth, the same test might reveal a total range of 45-50 degrees, with generally equal distribution between inversion and eversion of the calcaneus, although the neutral (congruent) position is one of approximately 10 degrees of varus (Jordan et al. 1983).

- The 36-month-old child in Figures 2.69 and 2.70 has a diagnosis of asymmetric spastic diplegia. He demonstrates considerable instability of the subtalar joint: the range of eversion of the calcaneus is slightly greater than that of inversion. This excursion into eversion indicates laxity in the medial ligaments supporting the STJ, with concurrent adaptive shortening of the lateral soft tissues (Jordan et al. 1983; Root et al. 1971; Mann 1985).

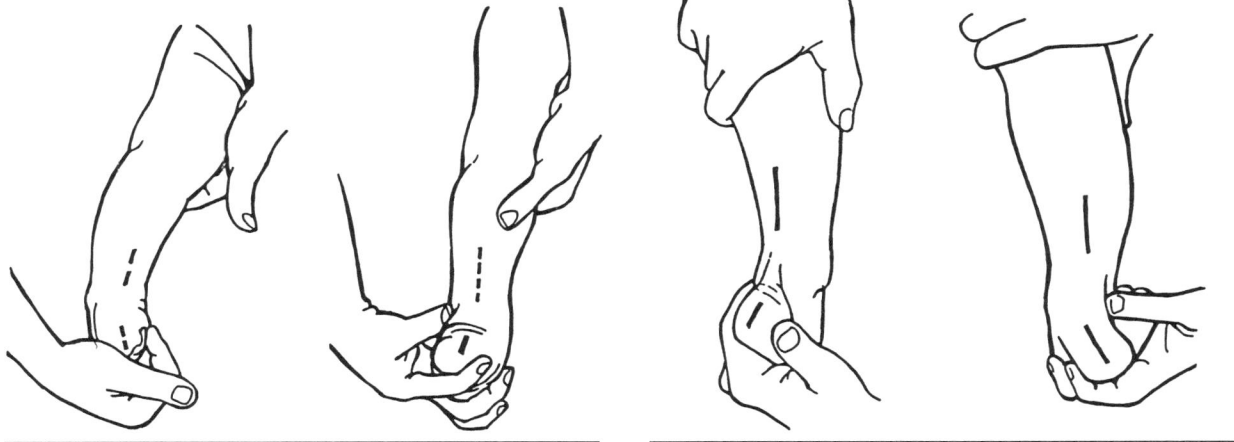

Figures 2.67 and 2.68
Normal, age 13 months: this STJ allows a minimum 2:1 ratio of calcaneal inversion to eversion respectively, indicating adequate integrity of medial ligaments that support the hindfoot and pronatory excursion for shock absorption.

Figures 2.69 and 2.70
Spastic diplegia, age 36 months: the STJ allows a 1:2 ratio of heel inversion to eversion respectively, indicating a lack of integrity of the medial support ligaments and a shortening in the lateral ligaments.

Stability Mechanisms

The beginning or "exploratory" walker of 11 to 16 months (who has walked less than six weeks) gains frontal-plane positional stability from the position of abduction and lateral rotation of the hips and feet, combined with a slight squat that lowers the center of gravity (Sutherland 1984; Sutherland et al. 1980a; Gunsolus et al. 1975; Okamoto et al. 1972).

Coactivation of the opposing (antagonist) muscle groups at the ankle joint has been documented both in standing and in gait (Okamoto et al. 1972; Sutherland et al. 1980a). The effect of this muscle activity is to diminish the hypermobility in the foot and ankle. Thus the muscle activity at least partially stabilizes those segments while the trunk and proximal joints gain stability. Toe grasping is a primary equilibrium response in the feet, whether the weight is displaced forward or backward. The typical response to a posterior shift of weight at this stage of development results in significantly more toe flexion than toe dorsiflexion (Gunsolus et al. 1975).

Gait Pattern and Determinants

Beginning walking—The average infant walks at the age of 12 months (Sutherland 1984; Scherzer et al. 1982). Learning, maturation, and bone configuration all contribute to the development of mature gait (Sutherland et al. 1980a). Significant differences are noted in timing and degree of sagittal plane gait components at the knee and ankle joints at 12 months when compared to those of an adult style of walking. Most of the rotational characteristics of pelvic and leg motion are exaggerations of those that occur in mature gait. Extensive studies have been undertaken by David Sutherland to distinguish normal gait patterns at various stages of early childhood. The results provide age-specific, objective data regarding transverse and sagittal plane rotations of the limb segments and the determinants of gait. (For those who need more detailed information than the scope of this text provides, Sutherland's publications are cited among the references.)

The 12-month-old child in Figure 2.71 achieved independent ambulation within 10 days of this photograph. She was a "beginning walker" and could be expected to (and did) reveal the following features of posture and equilibrium, gait, and muscle action in the lower extremities (McCrea 1985; Asher 1975; Sutherland 1984; Sutherland 1980a; Okamoto et al. 1972):

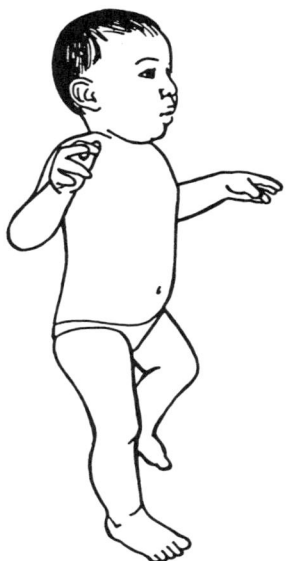

Figure 2.71
Normal, age 12 months: first steps are propulsive, while the pronated feet are apropulsive. Increased angle of gait, 25 degrees.

- Absent reciprocal arm swing.
- Persistent hip abduction throughout the stance and swing phases.
- Short step length, averaging 20 cm.
- Low duration of single-limb stance, averaging 32 percent of the gait cycle; this is an indication that the infant lacks hip stability.
- High cadence (step frequency), averaging 180 steps per minute, with a high degree of variability.
- Low walking velocity, averaging 60cm/sec.

The beginning walker typically exhibits the following gait-related events in the pelvis and joints of the lower extremities:

Pelvis—The total excursion in rotation on the transverse plane exceeds 20 degrees. Sagittal plane pelvic motion totals approximately 5 degrees around a median approximating 21 degrees at double stance (Sutherland 1984). The pelvis tilts posteriorly between foot contact and weight assumption, anteriorly through the full 5 degrees of motion during single-limb stance, and posteriorly from terminal stance to toe-off. The 1-year-old child shows a marked difference from the mature gait pattern in pelvic excursions on the frontal plane. At foot contact, the ipsilateral pelvis is aligned slightly below neutral position and rises perhaps 2 degrees until single-limb stance, when it lowers up to 5 degrees as the opposite side elevates during swing. This "hip-hiking" on the swing side diminishes considerably by the age of 2 years, when disassociation occurs between the pelvis and hip (Sutherland et al. 1980a).

Hip—Hip flexion is an active feature of forward progression at this age (Thelen et al. 1987; Okamoto et al. 1972). The rectus femoris has been shown on EMG to elicit hip flexion. Hip and knee flexion occur throughout the swing and stance phases. Hip flexion can approach 60 degrees at peak swing, lowering to slightly greater than 40 degrees at foot contact. The hips never fully extend after midstance but reach a maximum of minus 10 degrees in stance. The gluteus maximus remains active throughout the stance phase (Sutherland 1984; Sutherland et al. 1980a).

Femur—Postural lateral hip rotation is evident through both the swing and stance phases of gait. Immediately following foot contact, the femur rotates medially from a starting position of 20-25 degrees to 10-15 degrees of lateral rotation. It then rotates laterally to approximately 25 degrees at toe-off and essentially remains there until the next foot contact.

The moment of lateral rotation that occurs through the latter 85 percent of the stance phase is a consistent feature of gait throughout life (Rodgers 1988). It applies a torque force in the same direction across the proximal femur. Until ossification is complete, reduction of femoral antetorsion can be expected to continue with the combined components of an appropriate walking pattern and longitudinal bone growth.

Knee—The knee is flexed approximately 10 degrees at foot contact. This angle increases rapidly to 15-18 degrees, where it remains through midstance. After midstance, flexion increases dramatically to 60 degrees at toe-off and initial swing (McCrea 1985; Sutherland 1984; Sutherland et al. 1980a). The actions of knee flexion and extension occur in a different sequence throughout the gait cycle in early walking, compared with the mature pattern. Although EMG studies reveal that the rectus femoris and vastus lateralis are very active throughout both swing and stance phases in beginning walking, full knee extension is not usually demonstrated at any stage of the gait cycle at this age (Thelen et al. 1987; Okamoto et al. 1972). EMG analysis also reveals prolonged activity of the medial and lateral hamstrings during the stance phase (Sutherland et al. 1980a.) Thus the mature "knee-flexion wave," otherwise known as Inman's "double knee-lock mechanism," is not seen in gait. With the knee-flexion wave, knee extension occurs at heel strike, followed by flexion after heel strike, followed by extension in midstance, then flexion at heel-off (McCrea 1985; Sutherland et al. 1980a; Thelen et al. 1987).

The lack of knee extension in the stance phase is attributed to normal weakness in the ankle plantar flexors, rather than to underactivity in the quadriceps; the latter show prolonged stance phase activity (Sutherland et al. 1980b; Thelen et al. 1987). The ankle plantar flexors are the primary muscles that apply a stabilizing extension force to the knee joint in stance as they prohibit the ankle joint from falling into excessive dorsiflexion. As a contributor to knee flexion in stance, this factor of weakness in the plantar flexors in the infant becomes very important in assessing the motor-impaired child who exhibits crouch posture secondary to calcaneal deformity in stance and gait (Sutherland and Cooper 1978).

Tibia/fibula—Like the femur, the tibia rotates medially from a starting angle of approximately 20-25 degrees of lateral rotation at foot contact. This starting angle rapidly diminishes to 10 degrees by the assumption of weight on foot-flat contact. Thereafter, tibial lateral rotation occurs through stance until it exceeds 30 degrees at toe-off (Sutherland 1984). A lateral rotation force is applied, therefore, across the tibial and fibular growth plates and to the knee joint ligaments during most of the stance phase. This pattern of immediate medial followed by lateral rotation persists through maturity (Rodgers 1988; Sutherland 1984; Sutherland et al. 1980a).

When femoral antetorsion fails to reduce fully to 15 degrees or less, the lateral rotation movement at the lower leg can result in a compensatory external tibial torsion (Staheli 1977; Bleck 1982; Staheli et al. 1985).

The talocrural joint—The passive range of ankle dorsiflexion has diminished to 25-45 degrees, from 60-80 degrees in the newborn (Giannestras 1973; Jordan et al. 1983; Valmassy 1984; Tax 1985). The range remains exaggerated, however, over the mature value, and seems to contribute to the problems of stabilizing the knee and ankle in stance and gait (Sutherland 1984; Sutherland et al. 1980b). The existing coactivation of the dorsiflexors and plantarflexors seems to function to stabilize the ankle joint until proximal control is gained (Okamoto et al. 1972).

There is a relative foot drop in swing phase of gait, as the gastrocnemius fires along with the anterior tibialis (Sutherland et al. 1980a; Okamoto et al. 1972). Despite the evidence of coactivation in the anterior tibialis and gastrocnemius muscles, the ankle joint maintains 10 degrees of plantarflexion at the time of foot contact. Quickly the tibia falls forward over the loaded foot and the ankle achieves nearly 10 degrees of dorsiflexion, together with hip and knee flexion. The result is a slight squatting posture in gait (Okamoto et al. 1972). The dorsiflexed ankle position is maintained through most of the single limb support period of stance (Sutherland et al. 1980a).

Together with the posterior tibialis and the long toe flexors, the triceps surae muscle group performs four tasks in gait: (Sutherland et al. 1978; Sutherland et al. 1980b; Rodgers 1988).

- It contributes to stability at the knee joint by eccentric reverse action on the tibia.
- It halts the forward fall of the tibia (and thus of the body) over the talus from midstance to terminal stance phases.
- It supinates the ankle and hindfoot on the frontal plane through midstance to heel-off, thereby gaining maximum hindfoot stabilization and step length.
- It generates power prior to toe-off as a source of energy for forward acceleration of the same leg in its swing phase.

Weakness in the plantar flexors in infancy is cited as the primary reason for the delay in halting the fall of the tibia over the foot after contact (Sutherland et al. 1980a). The events of ankle dorsiflexion and plantarflexion are reversed, therefore, in the stance phase of the gait cycle in beginning walking. In this phase, ankle plantarflexion occurs at foot contact, and dorsiflexion follows with weight assumption (McCrea 1985).

The width of the weight-bearing foot in the area of the arch ranges from 70 percent to 135 percent of the width of the heel area, when measuring a chalk footprint of a child 1 year of age (Staheli et al. 1987). After the phase of beginning walking is completed, changes in gait pattern and related features continue to emerge.

15 Months

Features of Structure, Alignment, and Posture

The child in Figure 2.72 is 15 months of age. The main change in walking at this age, compared to an earlier age, is improved vertical alignment of the trunk and a slight reduction in coactivation at the distal lower extremities. Toddlers of this age seem to thrive on lifting and lugging large objects any possible distance. The demands on the stabilizing mechanisms increase with hauling heavy objects in play. The "volume" on proprioceptive input also increases, heightening the child's sensory awareness of joint position.

The child of 15 months normally reveals a mild genu varum, averaging 5 degrees. The varus-aligned knees begin to straighten immediately after birth and usually arrive on the sagittal plane during the latter part of the second year (age 18-24 months) (McDade 1977). There seems to be a relationship between walking and reduction in genu varum: varum is less often evident in children who have achieved ambulation than in those who have not (Engel and Staheli 1974). (The modeling influences at work are discussed previously, following the Neonatal Biomechanical Problem List.) If genu varum is not clearly resolving by 18 to 24 months and the tibiofemoral angle is 25 degrees or more, resolution will most likely require bracing (McDade 1977).

Stability mechanisms—Perham et al. (1987) found evidence of lateral equilibrium in stance on a tilt board in children age 15 months. However, only 50 percent of the children in this age group showed a functional response that involved extension of the lowermost leg and flexion of the uppermost leg to both right and left sides.

Features of Gait

The child who is walking at 15 months, after having walked independently for 3 months, demonstrates the emergence of reciprocal muscle action in the lower extremities. The base of support is narrowing while the hips remain in lateral rotation. The child squats less than during initial walking and thus stands more erect (Okamoto et al. 1972). Just prior to foot contact, the anterior tibialis activates, but foot-flat contact persists until late in this year (Schafer 1987; Thelen et al. 1987). A marked reduction in activity in the opposing muscle groups occurs at the knee and ankle joints during the swing and stance phases (Okamoto et al. 1972).

Once the infant achieves the upright position, and as the ala of the sacrum grow and expand, McCrea (1985) suggests that the

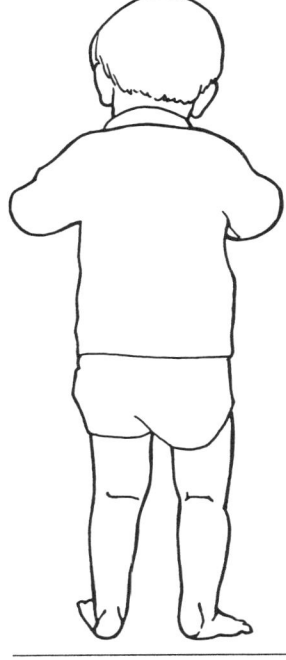

Figure 2.72
15 months: acetabulae have migrated closer to the frontal plane. Lateral hip rotation persists. Genu varum is diminishing. Feet remain pronated.

acetabulae begin to migrate to the frontal plane. A measure of lateral rotation position at the hips would resolve with that acetabular migration.

2 Years

Features of Structure, Alignment, and Posture

Spine and Pelvis—Pelvic tilting is an important mechanism in maintaining balance in the growing child. This tilting enables the body to adjust its weight distribution about the center of gravity as the body proportions alter.

The lumbar spine grows rapidly in the first two years of life. The intervertebral discs become wedge-shaped, allowing increasing degrees of hyperextension, and a pot-belly emerges in the second and third years. Most of the full range of anterior pelvic mobility is used in floor activities, such as moving forward from sitting to kneeling to standing and back. Lumbar hyperextension, rather than anterior pelvic tilt, is the primary influence on increasing lumbar lordosis at this age (Asher 1975; Sutherland 1984). The normal angle of anterior pelvic tilt ranges between 18 and 40 degrees, depending upon the authority cited (Asher 1975; Sutherland 1984).

Sagittal plane pelvic excursions remain generally the same as those at age 1 year, though the median angle is less than the 21 degrees of anterior tilt observed at age 1 (Sutherland et al. 1980a; Sutherland 1984).

Hip—By 24 months, hip flexion contracture has reduced to an average of 3 degrees, as determined by using Staheli's Prone Extension Test (Phelps et al. 1985). The gluteus maximus is active to a greater degree and for longer duration in stance than it will be in later childhood and adulthood (Sutherland 1980a). The gluteus maximus applies lateral torque to the femoral shaft.

The range of lateral rotation has been gradually diminishing since birth, while the range of hip medial rotation has been increasing. By 24 months, the two ranges can be expected to approximate each other. They may even reverse their relative status at this age (Engel and Staheli 1974). It has been suggested that at 24 months of age, many children reveal average ranges of hip medial and lateral rotation (with the hip maintained in extension) of 52 and 47 degrees respectively (Phelps et al. 1985).

Anteversion resolves to within 25 degrees after age 2 years (Jordan et al. 1983; Sutherland 1984; Phelps et al. 1985). In standing, the legs remain in lateral rotation between 10 and 15 degrees (Figure 2.73). In gait, the angle of lateral rotation of the foot reduces to 10 degrees or less and the base of support narrows (Staheli 1977; Staheli et al. 1985).

Femur—Antetorsion averages 28-30 degrees, indicating a 10-degree reduction in the angle of declination since birth (Fabry et al. 1973; McCrea 1985; Bleck 1982).

Knee—This year marks the beginning of "physiologic valgum" (less politely known as knock-knees) (McDade 1977) (Figure 2.73). The

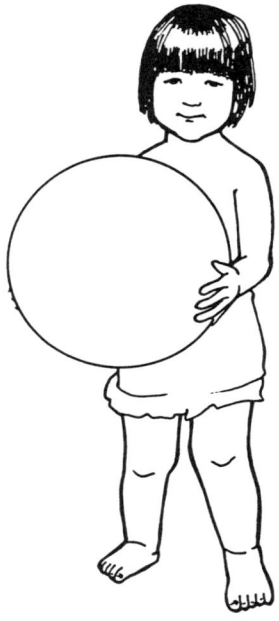

Figure 2.73
24 months: fat pad continues to mask most of the longitudinal arch. Genu valgum is evident. Pronation persists, with 5-degree calcaneal stance.

appearance of the normal 5 degrees of genu valgum might be exaggerated by the combined features of lateral tibial rotation and knee hyperextension (McDade 1977).

Tibia/fibula—The TMA (ankle joint axis) averages 10-15 degrees lateral, relative to the frontal plane (McCrea 1985). This new angle indicates that the tibia and fibula have twisted laterally in the past year. It also shows that ligaments of the knee joint have adjusted in length to allow lateral rotation of the tibia on the femur.

Foot—The neutral STJ manifests a varus deviation of the calcaneus, with a normal average range between 10 and 2 to 3 degrees. Forefoot varus, relative to the hindfoot, also persists—though to a lesser extent than during infancy—between 10 and 5 degrees. The relaxed calcaneal stance angle might measure 5 degrees of valgus relative to the sagittal plane (Valmassy 1984), or 5-8 degrees (Root et al. 1971). Valmassy (1984) suggests that the evaluating clinician subtract the child's age from the number 7 to obtain a normal maximum value for relaxed calcaneal stance. The relaxed calcaneal stance angle is not a position of neutrality of the subtalar and midtarsal joints; rather it is an angle of normal weight-bearing pronation in young children (Valmassy 1984).

The fat pad, if present, remains in place under the arch of the foot (Tax 1985; Schafer 1987; Jordan et al. 1983). The width of the weight-bearing arch drops to approximately 95 percent of the width of the heel area (Staheli et al. 1987).

Features of Gait

Stability mechanisms—In standing, equilibrium reactions in the feet reveal consistent toe-dorsiflexion in response to backward weight shift (compared to the toe-grasping seen in the beginning walker) (Gunsolus et al. 1975). Also, lateral displacement of the center of gravity (with the foot aligned close to the sagittal plane) elicits fully developed supination responses in the loaded foot. This in turn requires the activation of the medial foot and ankle musculature to control the medial pillar (Jordan et al. 1983; Salek 1977; Root et al. 1977; Gunsolus et al. 1975). Perham et al. (1987) discovered that children between ages 21 months and 24 months typically respond to lateral displacement on a tilt board by squatting and climbing down off of it.

Gait Pattern and Determinants

The latter half of this year between the ages of 2 and 3 marks the transition from immature to mature sagittal plane walking patterns as they are demonstrated in the various body segments. Mature timing of knee and ankle motions and reciprocal arm swing become established in walking by the end of this year. Rotary pelvic and leg motions diminish in degree (Sutherland 1984; Sutherland et al. 1980a).

Although the normal sagittal plane progression of joint action is important to the therapist as an instructor of movement, the determinants of gait are the significant features marking the onset of maturity. They include the following:

Velocity—A rapid increase in walking velocity, from 60 to nearly 85 cm/sec, occurs between 1 and 2½ years of age. The early gain in velocity is attributed to the achievement of longer step length. This is a function of improved stability in the supporting leg and foot rather than any significant change in hip and knee angles at heel strike. The reduced step length and velocity in immature gait seem most likely to be related to a lack of strength and control of the stabilizing musculature in the hips, knees, and ankles, and to the apropulsive nature of the pronated foot (Sutherland et al. 1980a; Thelen et al. 1987; Valmassy 1984).

Single limb support—The child of 2½ years shows a rapid rise in the percentage of the gait cycle devoted to single limb stance. This increases from approximately 32 percent at 1 year to over 35 percent at 2½ years (the adult value is 37-40 percent) (Sutherland et al. 1980a; Root et al. 1977).

Base of support and cadence—Both the base of support and cadence show a decrease between 1 and 2½ years (Sutherland 1984). The child at 2 years typically reveals patterns of motion in the lower extremities during walking, including rotations, knee flexion wave, and heel strike.

Rotations—Though evidence of the emergence of reciprocal arm swing might not be readily apparent (see Figure 2.74), its development can be detected by watching the trunk for counter-rotation between shoulders and pelvis, and by observing the forearm as the elbows flex and extend in keeping with the pattern of the arm swing (Sutherland 1984; Sutherland et al. 1980a).

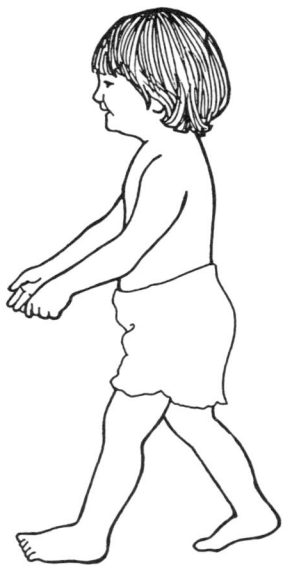

Figure 2.74
24 months: gait pattern often lacks full reciprocal arm swing and heel strike early in the second year. Hip extension is limited.

Lateral rotation of the femur and the tibia diminishes. This results in an average of 10 degrees of out-toeing by the age of 2 years (Staheli 1977; Staheli et al. 1985). Rotational asymmetry is common when comparing left and right sides, but it diminishes from an average of 7 degrees at age 1 year to 5 degrees at age 4 years (Scrutton 1969). During the stance phase, the femur bypasses the point of neutrality (or 0 degrees of rotation) into slight medial rotation (0-5 degrees) immediately after foot contact, which indicates that the lateral hip rotation contracture has reduced and that femoral antetorsion persists (Sutherland 1984; Sutherland et al. 1980a).

Once the weight is assumed by the stance foot (that is, after the initial 15-20 percent of stance is accomplished), closed-chain lateral rotation begins in both the upper and lower leg segments. This continues until toe-off, with greater excursion apparent in the tibia than in the femur. The same pattern occurs in mature gait (Sutherland 1984; Sutherland et al. 1980a).

Lateral torque forces are applied to the shaft of the femur upon lateral rotation at the hip (LeVeau and et al. 1984; Bleck 1982). When the lower leg is rotated laterally over the loaded foot, supination of the foot occurs. The plantar flexors of the ankle also supinate, or invert, the foot (Soderberg 1986). As the child approaches toe-off, the plantar flexors can be expected to apply a force of lateral torsion to the tibia by reverse action and their line of pull. The result is an increased resting angle of the transmalleolar axis relative to the frontal plane.

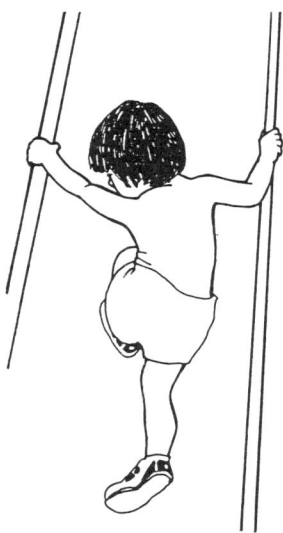

Figure 2.75
2 years: climbing quality is often influenced by available apparatus; it strengthens hip, knee, and ankle extensors.

Knee flexion wave—The angles of knee flexion and ankle dorsiflexion during both stance and swing cycles are greater at 2 years than at 1 year (Sutherland et al. 1980a). The "knee flexion wave" emerges in gait. Knee flexion after foot contact is followed by knee extension during single limb stance. Knee flexion recurs following terminal stance and heel-off, just prior to toe-off (Sutherland et al. 1980a; Thelen et al. 1987).

Heel strike—As early as 18 months, many children reveal heel strike, together with a resolution of foot drop in swing, as the triceps surae muscle group ceases to coactivate with the anterior tibialis at the end of the swing phase (Sutherland 1984; Okamoto et al. 1972). In the second year, therefore, the ankle dorsiflexes more adequately during swing than it did in the first year.

The preschooler continues the drive to achieve new motor skills and strengthens the lower limb musculature in the process (Figure 2.75). The application of lateral rotation and extension forces to the femoral shaft continues in play activities.

3 Years—The Onset of Mature Gait

Features of Structure, Alignment, and Posture

Spine and pelvis—The preschooler, age 2 to 3 years, reveals a characteristic pot-belly and lordosis, often with hyperextension at the knees. This indicates a need to distribute body weight over the feet on the sagittal plane while insuring balance (Asher 1975). The anterior pelvic tilt is variable, averaging between 28-40 degrees in stance. The main means of adjusting the degree of lordosis appears to continue to be flexion and hyperextension of the lumbar spine, rather than tilting the pelvis at the lumbosacral joint (Asher 1975).

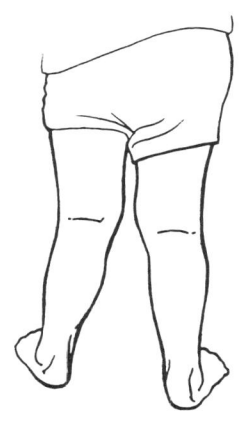

Figure 2.76
3 years: genu valgum is evident (condyles contact each other, medial malleoli do not) and can be exaggerated by normal knee hyperextension.

Hip—The limitation on hip extension can be expected to have resolved by now. Since birth, the total range of rotation has decreased to 95-110 degrees (Engel and Staheli 1974). The range of medial rotation is often slightly greater than that of lateral rotation at this age, indicating that the lateral hip rotation contracture of early infancy no longer imposes restriction on rotary mobility, although the femoral shaft remains medially twisted in excess of 25 degrees. This improved hip joint mobility is frequently evident in standing and supine positions in which the transcondylar axis of the femur aligns in mild medial rotation, relative to the frontal plane (Jordan et al. 1983).

Femur—The angle of antetorsion ranges between 26 and 28 degrees (Fabry et al. 1973; McCrea 1985; Bleck 1982).

Knee—Genu valgum generally peaks at 3 years, with the average tibiofibular angle approaching 12 degrees (Figure 2.76). A tibiofibular angle in excess of 15 degrees is considered abnormal (McDade 1977).

As mentioned above, hyperextension often occurs at the knees, apparently as a mechanism that collaborates with hyperextension in the spine, to maintain the center of gravity over the feet (Asher 1975). Knee hyperextension exaggerates the appearance of genu valgum when the hips are anteverted.

Tibia/fibula—The transmalleolar axis (TMA) remains at an average of 8-15 degrees of lateral rotation, relative to the frontal plane (McCrea 1985; Root et al. 1971).

Mild apparent tibial varum might persist, though it often resolves in the second year (Tax 1985; Jordan et al. 1983).

The fibular malleolus has grown longer. Radiographic evaluation reveals that its epiphysis is parallel with the talocrural joint on the transverse plane.

Talocrural joint—Dorsiflexion range of motion is diminishing as the plantar flexors gain strength and stabilize the ankle joint.

Foot—During this year, any existing fat pad under the longitudinal arch usually dissolves (Tax 1985; Asher 1975; Aharonson et al. 1980). The medial longitudinal arch, which has been evident in the open chain since birth, becomes increasingly apparent in standing. The width of the weight-bearing foot at the arch averages approximately 90 percent of the width of the heel area (Staheli et al. 1987). The calcaneus optimally aligns in up to 4 degrees of valgus in relaxed standing, relative to the sagittal plane (Valmassy 1984). Genu valgum can exaggerate the appearance of calcaneal valgus deviation if one were to measure the angle of the calcaneus without adjusting the tibial alignment onto the sagittal plane.

Stability mechanisms—The functional lower extremity equilibrium reaction to lateral tilt is described as *extension* in the lowermost extremity, and *flexion* in the uppermost extremity. Uphill trunk rotation does not occur, however, with consistency, and it may not be obligatory for functional equilibrium in response to lateral weight shift. Functional responses to lateral tilting were consistent for all children age 3 years and older (Perham et al. 1987).

Patterns of Normal, Mature Gait—a Review

Following is a brief review of the components of a normal gait pattern, covering the closed-chain motions that occur at the hip, knee, ankle, and foot during the stance phase. After the age of 3 years the gait pattern is nearly mature.

Pelvis: Sagittal plane motion—By age 7 years, the range of sagittal plane pelvic motion reduces to 2 to 3 degrees around a median angle approximating 17 degrees. At age 15 years, pelvic tilting is negligible around a median angle averaging 15 degrees. This indicates that sagittal plane motion of the hips has become fully disassociated from the pelvis.

Pelvis: Frontal plane motion—In mature gait, the side of the pelvis that is proximal to the advancing leg rises 5 degrees during weight assumption following foot contact. It then stabilizes in neutral position during single-limb stance and lowers 5 degrees between terminal stance and toe-off while the opposite leg is advancing. Thus, a total of 10 degrees of frontal plane pelvic excursion is needed for mature gait (Sutherland et al. 1980a).

Transverse plane motion—Approximately 20 degrees of rotation is needed for normal gait; 10 degrees on either side of the frontal plane. This range is limited, however, for such activities as segmental rolling and floor activities, in which the anterior superior iliac spines might form angles as great as 70 degrees to the frontal plane.

Hip—At the moment of foot contact, the hip flexes 25-40 degrees while rotating inward; the knee extends fully; and the ankle dorsiflexes to neutral (90 degrees). At contact, the entire leg continues to rotate medially, as the foot is lowered to the floor under the control of eccentric activation of the anterior tibialis and the long toe extensors (Schafer 1987; Sutherland et al. 1980a; Sutherland 1984; Rodgers 1988).

Closed chain in stance—Within the first 15 percent of the stance phase of the gait cycle, shock is absorbed by the entire lower extremity (Schafer 1987; Mann 1985; Root et al. 1977). The foot pronates, aided by proximal medial torque forces, causing the tibia and fibula—and therefore the knee—to pitch forward into flexion and medially into adduction with medial rotation (Mann 1985; Root et al. 1977). The resulting knee flexion further facilitates tibial medial rotation (Root et al. 1977) (Figure 2.77). The rotary forces travel both proximally and distally in adjustment to movement over the foot.

Following weight assumption (in which the foot is fixed against the floor under the load) the hip continues to extend and adduct, reversing its rotational direction from medial to lateral. By midstance, the center of gravity is aligned above the stance foot, and the calcaneus is optimally aligned in midposition (Figure 2.78). Children under 5 years of age might reveal more than 2 degrees of calcaneal valgus at midstance, though ideally no more than 6 degrees.

As the hip continues to extend and rotate outward, the knee joint—and therefore the tibia and fibula—rotates laterally as well. At terminal stance, prior to the stage between heel-off and toe-off, the following events occur:

- The hip achieves up to 15 degrees of passive extension beyond neutral.
- The knee extends fully, requiring 6 degrees of lateral rotation of the tibia on the femur.
- The ankle dorsiflexes up to 15 degrees over the supinating foot (Schafer 1987; Root et al. 1977).

If the foot did not supinate, it would have to spin outward with the hip and lower leg at this moment of gait, and motion into ankle dorsiflexion would be minimized (Sutherland et al. 1980a; Sutherland 1984; Perry 1974; Root et al. 1977). In midstance, the plantigrade foot is a stable base for forward movement of the body, enhancing the duration of single-limb stance. As stance progresses, continued supination converts the loaded foot into a rigid lever for transfer of body weight forward to the opposite foot. The forces of loading are therefore communicated efficiently through the extended knee and the rigid, supinated foot (Schafer 1987; Gray, 1986) (Figure 2.78).

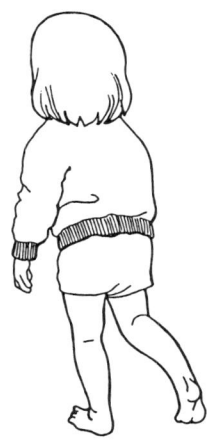

Figure 2.77
Normal gait, age 3 years: note lateral rotation at toe-off. Shock absorption occurs with medial rotation/pronation in early stance.

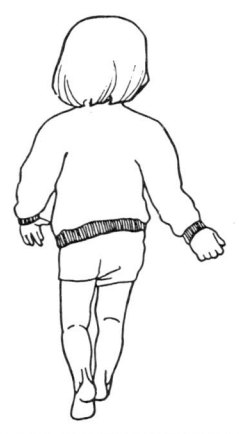

Figure 2.78
Normal gait, age 3 years: transition to adult style of walking occurs between 30 and 42 months of age. Knee flexion wave and heel strike with ankle dorsiflexion emerge. Angle of gait diminishes to average of 6 degrees.

Between terminal stance and toe-off, the ankle plantarflexes up to 20 degrees, as the plantar flexors activate to stabilize the ankle and foot for forward progression (Sutherland et al. 1980a and b; Sutherland 1984).

Swing—The femur and tibia rotate medially throughout the swing phase. The knee, which begins to flex after terminal stance and before toe-off, flexes up to 60 degrees following toe-off and extends through the swing phase, flexing slightly just prior to foot contact (Figure 2.77).

The Angle of Gait (or Angle of Progression)

Following foot contact, the moment of medial hip rotation reduces the average angle of gait to 25-30 degrees at age 1 year, 6-10 degrees in early childhood, and 0-6 degrees in school-aged children and adults (Sutherland et al. 1980a; Sutherland 1984; Bleck 1982; McCrea 1985; Engel and Staheli 1974; Root et al. 1977; Staheli et al. 1985; Schafer 1987) (Figure 2.78). Scrutton (1969) noted significantly lower values for angle of gait than other researchers, recording averages of between 2 and 3 degrees for children between ages 1 and 4 years.

The distinguishing features of gait at age 3 years are ranked by Sutherland et al. (1980a) in the following order of significance:

1. **Velocity**—Walking velocity rises sharply between the ages of 36 and 42 months, to nearly 105 cm/sec.

2. **Ratio of pelvic span to ankle spread**—This determinant is a proportional measurement in which the width of the pelvis is divided by the distance between the ankle joint centers at the time of double support. A rapid rise in this ratio occurs in the first 2½ years, increases more slowly until age 3½ years, then levels off until the age of 7 years (Sutherland 1984).

3. **Single limb support**—This determinant has increased to 35 percent of the cycle. The rise in percentage levels off significantly between 3 and 7 years, to slightly greater than 37 percent (Sutherland et al. 1980). The adult norm for single limb stance is between 37.5 percent and 40 percent (Root et al. 1977).

4. **Cadence**—This determinant tends to decrease steadily with age, with a possible sharp increase between ages 3 and 4 years, after which the decrease continues. Variability in cadence also decreases as stability improves (Sutherland 1984).

5. **Step length**—Because stride length is defined as the distance between the points of heel contact by the same foot, step length is roughly half of that distance, or the distance between consecutive points of heel contact by alternate feet. Step length, like single limb stance duration, is an indicator of dynamic stability in the stance leg and foot. It also shows the increase in hip extension at the end of the stance phase (with concurrent knee extension in the swing leg). This feature demonstrates a more rapid increase in the first 2½ years than thereafter, although the rise in step length, like that of limb length, is steady throughout the first 7 years (Sutherland 1984).

6. **Joint patterns**—The rotation patterns of the pelvis and lower extremities, the proportional base of support, and the patterns of knee motion and heel-strike are adult-like by this time, and gait is vigorous (Sutherland 1984).

7. **Toe-stepping**—Another significant feature of walking at age 3 is toe-stepping, rather than walking in a consistent plantigrade alignment of the foot (Figure 2.79). Both the soleus and the gastrocnemius are activated in toe-standing. The soleus is the long-distance, stabilizing muscle. The gastrocnemius activates phasically (although powerfully) in combination with the soleus, for such occasions as rising on toes, jumping, and running (Lehmkuhl and Smith 1983; Soderberg 1986). However, normally they never activate in isolation of each other in standing and walking activities (Perry et al. 1986).

Preschool age is a time of astounding achievements in all areas of development, a time in which the child applies automatic postural control and the components of joint mobility and antigravity strength to the mastery of new skills (Figure 2.80).

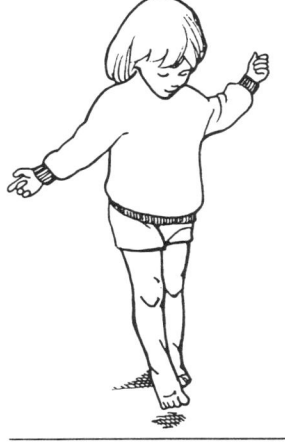

Figure 2.79
Toe-walking occurs in the second and third years, in combination with plantigrade walking; this builds power in the triceps surae muscle group and posterior tibialis.

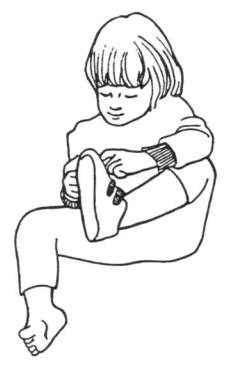

Figure 2.80
3 years: postural control and isolated lower extremity motions are well developed.

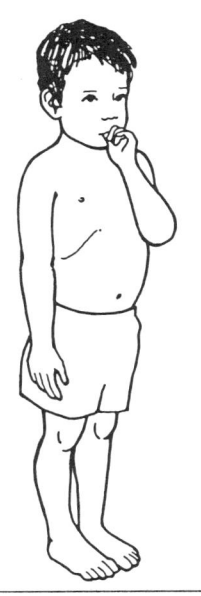

Figure 2.81
Normal, age 4 years: lordosis increases with lumbar extension mobility. Femoral condyles are aligned on, or are slightly medially rotated relative to, the frontal plane. Genu valgum is evident.

4 to 7 Years

Features of structure, alignment, and posture (normal and abnormal) are as follows:

Spine and Pelvis: Normal—The child of 4 years in Figure 2.81 exhibits typical features of posture and movement at this age. Lordosis increases through early school age; by the age of 7 years, the pelvis tilts anteriorly up to 30-40 degrees (Asher 1975). This resting angle normally falls under 30 degrees during the adolescent growth spurt and stabilizes at 15-20 degrees in adolescents and adults (Asher 1975; Sutherland 1984).

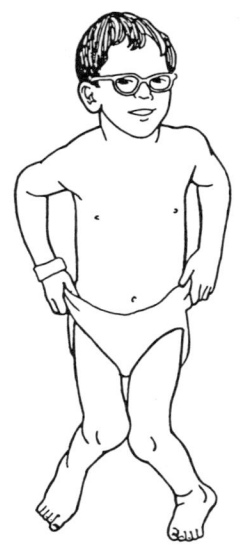

Figure 2.82
Spastic diplegia,
age 4 years: poor
antigravity strength
and control; apparent
femoral antetorsion;
hip and knee flexion
with concurrent
anteromedial weight
distribution over the
pronated feet; equinus.

Spine and Pelvis: Abnormal—By comparison, the child in Figure 2.82 reveals common compensatory patterns of postural adjustment in a diplegic child of 4 years of age. He demonstrates underdevelopment of antigravity extension strength and control in the upper trunk, hips, and knees. Note the shoulder girdle protraction and elevation, the forward lean in the trunk, the flexed hips, knees, and ankles, and the apparent medial hip rotation with adduction.

Hip—The total range of rotation remains at 95-110 degrees. The hip normally rotates medially an average of between 40 and 50 degrees (in a range of 25-65 degrees), and laterally an average of 45 degrees (in a range of 25-65 degrees) (Bleck 1982; Staheli et al. 1985).

Femur—The average angle of femoral antetorsion approaches 23-26 degrees between the ages of 4 and 7 years (Fabry et al. 1973; McCrea 1985; Bleck 1982; Sutherland et al. 1980a). Correction of antetorsion is complete between the ages of 8 and 16 years, when the value will fall to between 5 and 20 degrees (Fabry et al. 1973; McCrea 1985; Bleck 1982). Bleck suggests that no significant change in antetorsion angle occurs after the age of 8 years (Bleck 1982). However, Fabry and associates report that up to 10 degrees of reduction occurs, from an average angle of 24.40 degrees at 8 years to an angle of 15.35 at age 16 (Fabry et al. 1973). Beals (1969) reports higher values of 30 degrees at age 4 and 25 degrees at age 8, decreasing to 16 degrees in adolescence and 14 degrees in adulthood.

The angle of inclination of the head and neck of the femur is reduced to the adult value of 125-135 degrees by the age of 6 years (Beals 1969; Jordan et al. 1983). Coxa valga is resolved, though this angle continues to diminish into adulthood (Beals 1969).

Knee—Genu valgum resolves to a tibiofemoral angle of 7-10 degrees during this period (McDade 1977).

Tibia/fibula—The TMA angle has increased to the adult value of 15-30 degrees, indicating the full achievement of lateral torsion. The average angle is 22 degrees (McCrea 1985; Root et al. 1971; Staheli et al. 1985).

The fibular malleolus has grown and begun to ossify. This provides lateral support for the talus.

Apparent distal tibial varum is reduced to the adult norm of 0-2 degrees (Jordan et al. 1983).

Talocrural joint—The average range of talocrural dorsiflexion at age 4 to 5 years varies between 10 and 20 degrees when measured with the joints of the foot in neutral position (McCrea 1985; Jordan et al. 1983; Root et al. 1977). In the child of this age, the higher limits are more likely because years of wearing heeled shoes have not taken their toll on the available degree of flexibility. By the age of 7 years and into adulthood, normal dorsiflexion range with the knee extended is 8-15 degrees, with a minimum of 5-7 degrees (McCrea 1985).

The average range of 45 degrees of talocrural plantarflexion is evident from early infancy (McCrea 1985). Normal gait requires a minimum of 20 degrees of plantarflexion mobility (Root et al. 1971). Activities that involve climbing, kneeling, and toe-standing often require a degree of plantarflexion greater than 20 degrees.

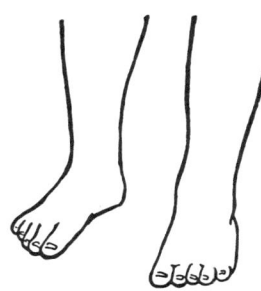

Figure 2.83
Normal, age 4 years:
feet are nearly mature
in alignment; axis of
mortice is aligned
more than 15 degrees
lateral to the frontal
plane; arch is low;
equilibrium reactions
are established.

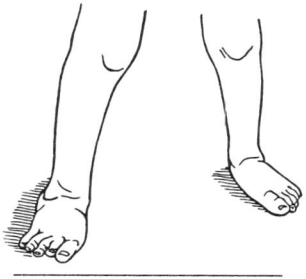

Figure 2.84
Spastic diplegia, age
4 years: pronation;
medial tibiofibular
rotation with knee
flexion; toe clawing.

Foot: Normal—At 4 years, open-chain assessment of neutral foot position reveals reduction in hindfoot and forefoot varus, toward a value of 4 to 5 degrees or less. Valgus deviation of the heel in relaxed calcaneal stance should not exceed 3 degrees according to Valmassy (1984). At 5 years and older, the normal calcaneal stance range is 0-2 degrees (Valmassy 1984; McCrea 1985; Jordan et al. 1983). Root et al. (1971) allow 6 degrees of calcaneus valgus at 5 years, and 5 degrees at age 6 years, but they presume that the distal lower leg is aligned on the sagittal plane. They also agree with a 2-degree maximum of valgus or varus at age 7 and above, in relaxed calcaneal stance. This value corresponds with the author's definition of calcaneal midposition.

The forefoot aligns within 2 to 3 degrees of perpendicular to the vertical bisection of the calcaneus in calcaneal midposition (Root et al. 1971; Aharonson et al. 1980) (Figure 2.83). The longitudinal arch is fully visible, though low. The average proportional arch-to-heel width of the weight-bearing foot continues to diminish steadily during these years from approximately 80 percent at age 4 years to approximately 70 percent at age 7 years. The decline in the width percentage continues into adolescence, after which it again increases gradually through later adulthood (Staheli et al. 1987).

In standing, body weight is carried by the heel (61 percent), the lateral border (4 percent), and the forefoot (35 percent) (Aharonson et al. 1980). Within the transverse plane, the forefoot is parallel to the sagittal-plane longitudinal bisection of the hindfoot; a line bisecting the hindfoot falls through the second toe or between the second and third toes. No forefoot adductus or abductus is evident. The toes are straight and parallel to the metatarsals (Figure 2.84) (Aharonson et al. 1980). All of these characteristics persist into adulthood in the balanced foot (Cavanagh et al. 1987; Root et al. 1971; Root et al. 1977).

Foot: Abnormal—The child in Figure 2.82 carries his weight on the anteromedial aspect of the forefoot. Dorsiflexion with abduction occurs at the midtarsal joint in weight-bearing.

Figure 2.84 more clearly illustrates the effects of creep on the alignment and structure of the foot within the first 4 years of the child's life. Pronation deformity is evident in both feet. There is related knee flexion and medial rotation of the lower leg, and reduction of the angle of the transmalleolar axis; valgus deviation of the calcaneus; abduction and dorsiflexion of the forefoot (note the curved configuration); dorsiflexion of the first ray; heavy loading on the medial first metatarsal head; and clawing of the toes with lateral deviation.

Features of Gait—Stability Mechanisms

The capacity for isolated function in the segments of the lower extremities is evident in the efficient execution of equilibrium reactions, play, and climbing activities (Gunsolus et al. 1975). (Figures 2.83 and 2.85) The ankle coactivation observed previously has resolved into reciprocal movements, and the motions of the subtalar and midtarsal joints have emerged. The result is a flexible and functional foot.

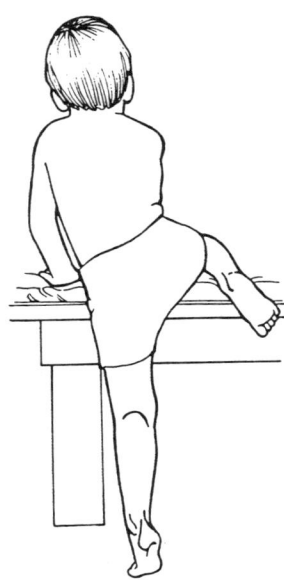

Figure 2.85
The components of movement combine to provide efficient control, joint mobility, and strength for isolated motions in the foot.

Current studies of equilibrium responses elicited by perturbations (rapid displacements of the support surface) demonstrate that no difference is evident in the sequence or timing of activation of muscle groups in the lower limbs when comparing school-age children to adults (Nashner et al. 1983). However, in evaluating the same responses in children at or under 6 or 7 years of age, differences were revealed in sensory organization capability: they were unable to balance under conditions in which there was a conflict between visual, vestibular, and proprioceptive inputs (Nashner et al. 1983).

Gait Pattern and Determinants

The four primary determinants that distinguish the gait in a child of 3 years from that of an adult include:

- Shortened step length
- High cadence
- Low walking velocity
- Limited duration of single-limb stance

The two primary requirements for resolution of these deficits and for achievement of a mature gait pattern are increased leg length and improved unilateral limb and foot stability. By the age of 8 years such resolution has occurred, and walking velocity and cadence are affected thereafter only by increasing leg length (Sutherland 1984; Sutherland et al. 1980a).

Summary

Developmental biomechanics offers a base of information upon which to make logical judgments about postural deviations and their functional implications in children with neuromotor disorders. The interrelationship between evolving antigravity strength and skills and the changes that occur in bone structure is fascinating, its significance made evident by the poverty of mature skeletal alterations and by the gradual development of deformity in children with cerebral palsy. It is no longer appropriate to assign these normal structural changes to "spontaneous" events related merely to longitudinal bone growth, because children with cerebral palsy also grow. In particular, the reduction of the newborn's hip flexion contracture, combined with the achievement of strength into hip extension and lateral rotation, appears to play a critical role in reducing femoral antetorsion. This information supports the longstanding concern of the proponents of neurodevelopmental treatment that these changes in mobility and strength be facilitated at the hip, and as early as possible. Clinical research is needed to draw conclusive evidence that might establish the validity of this concern.

Closed-chain biomechanics shows evidence of an interdependence between the alignment and structure of the leg and the foot. By reviewing the biomechanical consequences in the lower extremities during the course of motor development, it is possible to become familiar with the features of alignment and structure that distinguish the infant, toddler, and preschooler from the older child and adult.

The next chapter will pursue a more detailed understanding of the delicate balance of structure and function in the foot and leg. This will be done through a study of the structural anatomy and function of the foot, particularly of the joints within the foot. These principles will then be applied to the identification and management of the common problems of foot deformity in children with neuromotor disorder.

References

Agnew, P., DPM. December 8, 1988. Personal communication, Richmond, VA.

Aharonson, Z., A. Voloshin, T. V. Steinbach, M. A. Brull, and I. Farine. 1980. Normal foot-ground pressure pattern in children. *Clinical Orthopaedics and Related Research* 150:220-223.

Asher, C. 1975. *Postural variations in childhood.* Boston: Butterworths.

Baddely, H. 1984. Motor learning. In *Pediatric developmental therapy,* edited by S. Levitt, 34-43. Boston: Blackwell Scientific Publications.

Badell-Ribera, A. 1985. Cerebral palsy: Postural-locomotor prognosis in spastic diplegia. *Archives of Physical Medicine and Rehabilitation* 66:614-619.

Badgley, C. E. 1949. Etiology of congenital dislocation of the hip. *Journal of Bone and Joint Surgery* 31-A:341-356.

Bahler, A. 1986. The biomechanics of the foot. *Clinical Prosthetics and Orthotics* 10(1):8-14.

Baker, L. D., and M. H. Lowell. 1964. Foot alignment in the cerebral palsy patient. *Journal of Bone and Joint Surgery (Am)* 46-A(1):1-15.

Beals, R. K. 1969. Developmental changes in the femur and acetabulum in spastic paraplegia and diplegia. *Developmental Medicine and Child Neurology* 11:303-313.

Bernhardt, D. B. 1988. Prenatal and postnatal growth and development of the foot and ankle. *Physical Therapy* 68(12):1831-39.

Bleck, E. E. 1982. Developmental orthopedics, III: Toddlers. *Developmental Medicine and Child Neurology* 24(4):533-55.

Bleck, E. E. 1987. Orthopedic management of cerebral palsy. *Clinics in developmental medicine nos. 99 and 100.* Philadelphia: J. B. Lippincott.

Bly, L., and F. Sterne. 1980. *Baby treatment.* Lecture notes and instructional materials from neurodevelopmental treatment advanced course, New York, NY.

Bly, L. 1983. *Components of normal movement during the first year of life and abnormal development.* Monograph. Oak Park, IL: Neurodevelopmental Treatment Association.

Bobath, B. 1967. The very early treatment of cerebral palsy. *Developmental Medicine and Child Neurology* 9:373-390.

Bobath, B., and K. Bobath. 1976. *Motor development and the different types of cerebral palsy.* London: Heinemann Medical Books, Ltd.

Bobath, K., and B. Bobath. 1964. The facilitation of normal postural reactions and movements in the treatment of cerebral palsy. *Physiotherapy* 50:246-262.

Brooks, S. 1985. *Mobilization applied to the neurologically involved child—Advanced training.* Lecture notes and instructional materials. Dallas, TX: Sponsored by Curative Rehabilitation Center of Wauwatosa, WI.

Cailliet, R. 1983. *Foot and ankle pain, 2d ed.* Philadelphia, PA: F. A. Davis.

Cavanagh, P. R., M. M. Rodgers, and A. Iiboshi. 1987. Pressure distribution under symptom-free feet during barefoot standing. *Foot & Ankle* 7:262-276.

Connolly, B. H. 1984. Learning disabilities. In *Pediatric neurologic physical therapy,* edited by S. K. Campbell, 317-352. New York: Churchill Livingstone.

Crouch, J. E. 1970. *Functional human anatomy.* Philadelphia, PA: Lea and Febiger.

Effgen, S. K. 1987. Developing postural reactions. In *Therapeutic exercise in developmental disabilities,* edited by B. H. Connolly and P. C. Montgomery, 65-73. Chattanooga, TN: Chattanooga Corp.

Engel, G. M., and L. T. Staheli. 1974. The natural history of torsion and other factors influencing gait in childhood. A study of the angle of gait, tibial torsion, knee angle, hip rotation, and development of the arch in normal children. *Clinical Orthopaedics and Related Research* 99:12-17.

Fabry, G., G. D. McEwen, and A. R. Shands. 1973. Torsion of the femur. *Journal of Bone and Joint Surgery* 55-A(8):1726-1738.

Frost, H. M. 1986. *Intermediary organization of the skeleton, vols. 1 and 2.* Boca Raton, FL: CRC Press.

Giannestras, N. 1973. *Foot disorders: Medical and surgical management, II.* Philadelphia, PA: Lea and Febiger.

Grant, J. C. B. 1962. *Grant's atlas of anatomy, 6th ed.* Baltimore, MD: Williams and Wilkins.

Gray, G. 1986. *Biomechanics of the foot.* Lecture notes and instructional materials from the South Carolina American Physical Therapy Association annual meeting, Charleston, SC.

Gunsolus, P., C. Welsh, and C. Houser. 1975. Equilibrium reactions in the feet of children with spastic cerebral palsy and of normal children. *Developmental Medicine and Child Neurology* 17:580-591.

Haas, S. S., C. H. Epps, and J. P. Adams. 1973. Normal ranges of hip motion in the newborn. *Clinical Orthopaedics and Related Research* 91:114-118.

Harris, N. H. 1976. Acetabular growth potential in congenital dislocation of the hip and some factors upon which it may depend. *Clinical Orthopaedics and Related Research* 119:99-106.

Hensinger, R. N., and E. T. Jones. 1982. Developmental orthopedics I: The lower limb. *Developmental Medicine and Child Neurology* 24:95-116.

Hoffer, M. M. 1980. Joint motion limitation in newborns. *Clinical Orthopaedics and Related Research* 148:94-96.

Jaffe, W. L., and J. T. Laitman. 1982. The evolution and anatomy of the human foot. In *Disorders of the foot, vol. 1,* edited by M. H. Jahss, 1-35. Philadelphia, PA: W. B. Saunders.

Jordan, R. P., J. Cusack, and B. Resseque. 1983. *Foot function and its relationship to posture in the pediatric patient with cerebral palsy and other neuromotor disorders.* Lecture notes and instructional materials from symposium presented by Langer Biomechanics Group, Inc., sponsored by the Neurodevelopmental Treatment Association, New York, NY. (May 20-22).

Kapandji, I. A. 1970. *The physiology of the joints, vol. 2: Lower limb.* Baltimore, MD: Williams and Wilkins.

Knight, R. A. 1954. Developmental deformities of the lower extremities. *Journal of Bone and Joint Surgery* 36-A(3):521-527.

Lehmkuhl, L. D., and L. K. Smith. 1983. *Brunnstrom's clinical kinesiology (revised). 4th ed.* Philadelphia, PA: F. A. Davis.

LeVeau, B. F., and D. B. Bernhardt. 1984. Developmental biomechanics: Effects of forces on the growth, development, and maintenance of the human body. *Physical Therapy* 64(12):1886-1902.

Levitt, S. 1984. Motor development. In *Paediatric developmental therapy,* edited by S. Levitt. Boston, MA: Blackwell Scientific Publications.

Lloyd-Roberts, G. C., N. H. Harris, and A. R. Chrispin. 1978. Anteversion of the acetabulum in congenital dislocation of the hip: A preliminary report. *Orthopedic Clinics of North America* 9(1):89-95.

Maitland, G. D. 1977. *Peripheral manipulation, vol. 2.* Boston, MA: Butterworths.

Mann, R. A. 1985. Biomechanics of the foot. In *Atlas of orthotics, 2d ed.,* edited by Wilton H. Bunch and other members of the American Academy of Orthopedic Surgeons. St. Louis, MO: C. V. Mosby.

Matles, A. L. 1965. The newborn hip guide; technic of localizing head of newborn femur on roentgenograms. *New York State Journal of Medicine* 65:2345-2350.

McCrea, J. 1985. *Pediatric orthopedics of the lower extremity: An instructional handbook.* Mount Kisco, NY: Futura Publishing Co.

McDade, W. 1977. Bow legs and knock knees. *Pediatric Clinics of North America* 24(4):825-839.

McDonough, M. W. 1984. Angular and axial deformities of the legs of children. In *Symposium on podopediatrics—Clinics in podiatry,* edited by J. V. Ganley. Philadelphia, PA: W. B. Saunders Co.

Murphy, S. B., S. R. Simon, P. K. Kijewski, R. H. Wilkinson, and T. Griscom. 1987. Femoral anteversion. *Journal of Bone and Joint Surgery* 68-A(8):1169-1176.

Nashner, L. M., A. Shumway-Cook, and O. Marion. 1983. Stance posture control in select groups of children with cerebral palsy: Deficits in sensory organization and muscular coordination. *Experimental Brain Research* 49:393-409.

Okamoto, T., and M. Kumanoto. 1972. Electromyographic study of the learning process of walking in infants. *Electromyography* 12(2):149-158.

Perham, H., J. E. Smick, A. Hallum, and T. Nordstrom. 1987. Development of the lateral equilibrium reaction in stance. *Developmental Medicine and Child Neurology* 29:758-765.

Perry, J. 1974. Kinesiology of lower extremity bracing. *Clinical Orthopaedics and Related Research* 102:18-31.

Perry, J. 1975. Cerebral palsy gait. In *Orthopedic aspects of cerebral palsy: Clinics in developmental medicine nos. 52 and 53,* edited by R. L. Samilson. Philadelphia, PA: J. B. Lippincott.

Perry, J., M. L. Ireland, J. Gronley, and M. M. Hoffer. 1986. Predictive value of manual muscle testing and gait analysis in normal ankles by dynamic eletromyography. *Foot & Ankle* 6(5):254-259.

Phelps, E., L. J. Smith, and A. Hallum. 1985. Normal ranges of hip motion of infants between nine and 24 months of age. *Developmental Medicine and Child Neurology* 27:785-792.

Pitkow, R. B. 1975. External rotation contracture of the extended hip. *Clinical Orthopaedics and Related Research* 110:139-145.

Rang, M., R. Silver, and J. de la Garza. 1986. Cerebral palsy. In *Pediatric orthopaedics, 2d ed.,* edited by W. W. Lovell and R. B. Winter. Philadelphia, PA: J. B. Lippincott Co.

Rodgers, M. M. 1988. Dynamic biomechanics of the normal foot and ankle during walking and running. *Physical Therapy* 68(12):1822-29.

Rodgers, M. M., and P. R. Cavanagh. 1984. Glossary of biomechanical terms, concepts and units. *Physical Therapy* 64(12):1886-1902.

Root, M. L., J. H. Weed, and W. P. Orien. 1977. Normal and abnormal function of the foot. *Clinical biomechanics, vol. 2.* Los Angeles, CA: Clinical Biomechanics Corp.

Root, M. L., W. P. Orien, J. H. Weed, and R. J. Hughes. 1971. *Biomechanical examination of the foot, I.* Los Angeles, CA: Clinical Biomechanics Corp.

Salek, B. 1977. *The significance of structural and functional development in the normal foot and therapeutic implications thereof in the child with neuromotor disorder.* Unpublished article. Commack, NY: Suffolk Rehabilitation Center.

Salek, B. 1981. *Corrective footwear in young children with neuromuscular disorders.* Paper presented at the NDT Association Eastern Regional Conference, Philadelphia.

Samilson, R. L., G. Aamoth, and W. M. Green. 1972. Dislocation and subluxation of the hip in cerebral palsy. *Journal of Bone and Joint Surgery* 54-A:863-873.

Schafer, R. C. 1987. *Clinical biomechanics: Musculoskeletal actions and reactions, 2d ed.* Baltimore, MD: Williams and Wilkins.

Scherzer, A. L., and I. Tscharnuter. 1982. *Early diagnosis and therapy in cerebral palsy.* New York: Marcel Dekker, Inc.

Scrutton, D. R. 1969. Foot sequence of normal children under 5 years old. *Developmental Medicine and Child Neurology* 11:44-53.

Sgarlato, T. E. 1971. *A compendium of biomechanics.* San Francisco, CA: California College of Podiatric Medicine.

Siffert, R. S. 1981. Patterns of deformity in the developing hip. *Clinical Orthopaedics and Related Research* 160:14-29.

Soderberg, G. L. 1986. *Kinesiology—Application to pathological motion.* Baltimore, MD: Williams and Wilkins.

Staheli, L. T. 1977. The prone hip extension test. *Clinical Orthopaedics and Related Research* 123:12-15.

Staheli, L. T. 1977. Torsional deformity. *Pediatric Clinics of North America* 24(4):799-811.

Staheli, L. T., D. E. Chew, and M. Corbett, 1987. The longitudinal arch. *Journal of Bone and Joint Surgery* 69-A(3):426-428.

Staheli, L. T., M. Corbett, W. Craig, and H. King. 1985. Lower-extremity rotational problems in children. *Journal of Bone and Joint Surgery* 67-A:39-44.

Staheli, L. T., W. R. Duncan, and E. Schaefer. 1968. Growth alterations in the hemiplegic child. *Clinical Orthopaedics and Related Research* 60:205-212.

Sternat, J. 1987. Developing head and trunk control. In *Therapeutic exercise in developmental disabilities,* edited by B. H. Connolly and P. C. Montgomery, 55-64. Chattanooga, TN: Chattanooga Corp.

Sutherland, D. H. 1984. *Gait disorders in childhood and adolescence.* Baltimore, MD: Williams and Wilkins.

Sutherland, D. H., and L. Cooper. 1978. The pathomechanics of progressive crouch gait in spastic diplegia. *Orthopedic Clinics of North America* 9(1):143-154.

Sutherland, D. H., B. A. Cooper, and D. Dale. 1980b. The role of the ankle plantar flexors in normal standing and walking. *Journal of Bone and Joint Surgery* 62-A(3):354-363.

Sutherland, D. H., R. Olshen, L. Cooper, and S. L-Y. Woo. 1980a. The development of mature gait. *Journal of Bone and Joint Surgery* 62-A(3):336-353.

Tachdjian, M. O. 1971. *Pediatric orthopedics.* Philadelphia, PA: W. B. Saunders.

Tachdjian, M. O. 1985. *The child's foot.* Philadelphia, PA: W. B. Saunders.

Tax, H. R. 1985. *Podopediatrics, 2d ed.* Baltimore, MD: Williams and Wilkins.

Thelen, E., and D. W. Cooke. 1987. Relationship between newborn stepping and later walking: A new interpretation. *Developmental Medicine and Child Neurology* 29:380-393.

Tiberio, D. 1988. Pathomechanics of structural foot deformities. *Physical Therapy* 68(12):1840-1849.

Valmassy, R. L. 1984. Biomechanical evaluation of the child. In *Symposium on podopediatrics—Clinics in podiatry*, edited by J. V. Ganley, 563-579. Philadelphia, PA: W. B. Saunders.

CHAPTER 3

The Foot and Leg— Relating Function to Structure

Objectives for the Reader

- To distinguish between normal and abnormal alignment and mobility features at the pelvis, hip, knee, ankle, and foot at ages 1 through 7 years.
- To describe the motions that occur in the joints of the lower extremity as they operate in the open and closed kinetic chain.
- To identify the bones and joints of the ankle and foot, and to describe their axes and primary motions.
- To describe the following assessment procedures:
  - Staheli prone extension test
  - Knee tuck for hip flexion mobility
  - Hip rotation test for soft tissue status
  - Hip rotation test for femoral torsion
  - Ryder's test for femoral torsion
  - Genu varum and valgum
  - Popliteal angle test for knee flexion contracture
  - Thigh/foot angle
  - Genicular position
  - Tibial torsion
  - Subtalar joint (STJ) mobility
  - Neutral STJ position
  - Neutral foot position
  - Relaxed and neutral calcaneal stance
  - Relaxed and neutral tibial varum
  - Functional calcaneal midposition
  - Forefoot alignment (varus/valgus and abductus/adductus)
  - First ray mobility
  - Toe mobility and alignment
- To explain the purposes, normal findings, and limitations, if any, of these assessments as clinical tools.

Before explaining how to manage the structural and functional problems of the lower extremities commonly associated with neuromotor impairment in children, this chapter reviews the functions of the joints of the lower extremities in stance and gait. It also describes the associated clinical assessment procedures for the lower extremity joints and structures. The text of this chapter is organized to proceed in proximal-to-distal sequence. Because of the interrelated workings of the joints within the closed kinetic chain, certain joints and their functional participation are mentioned in advance of a direct discussion of their composition and motions. Problems of torsional and rotary deformity in the femur and lower leg are of particular importance in assessment, because they influence the structure and function of the foot and ankle (Regnauld 1986).

Issues related to sensory input as an influence on spasticity, withdrawal of the foot from contact, and vestibular organization fall beyond the scope of this text, although they must be considered in comprehensive therapeutic management.

The reader is encouraged to identify the features of structure and function that are discussed in this chapter. The assessment procedures can be conducted by first palpating bony landmarks on one's own leg and foot (Figures 3.1 to 3.4), then identifying them and conducting the tests on normal children. The resulting appreciation for normal alignment and function can then be readily applied to clinical assessment and intervention.

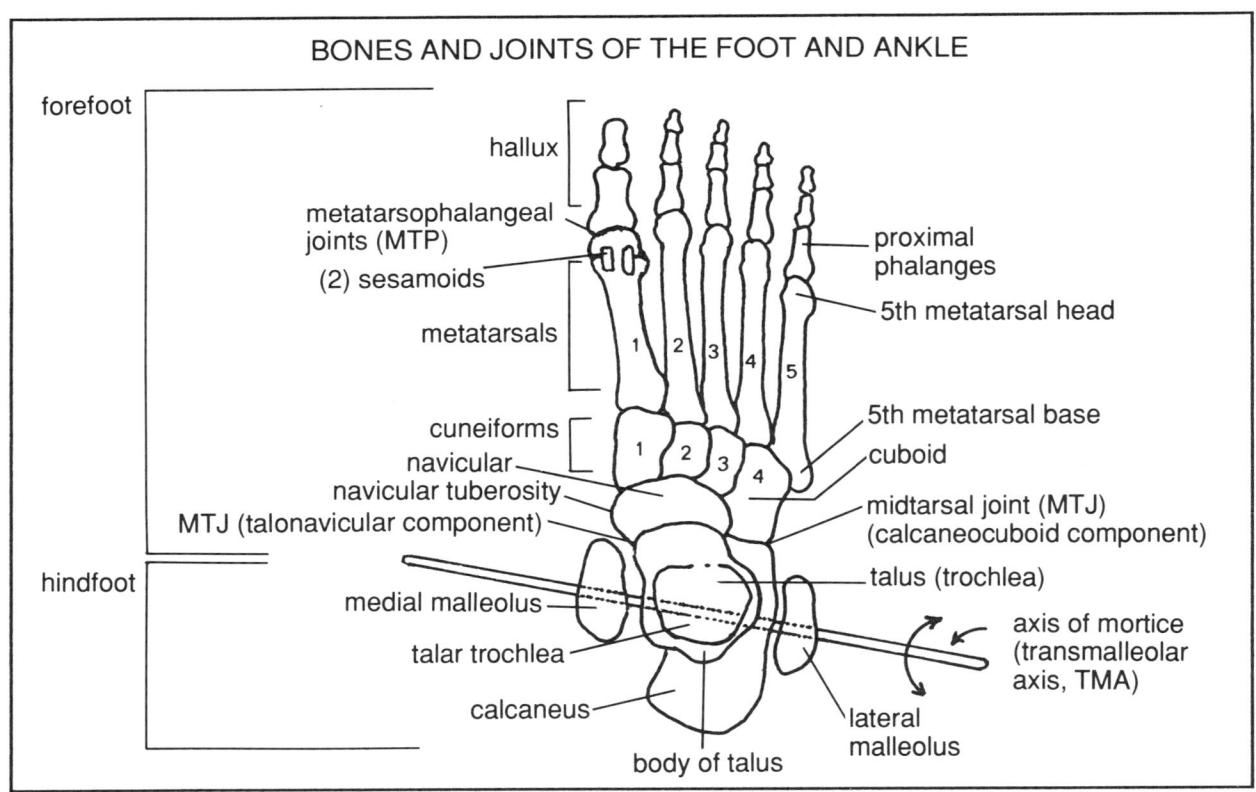

BONES AND JOINTS OF THE FOOT AND ANKLE

forefoot

hallux

metatarsophalangeal joints (MTP)

(2) sesamoids

metatarsals

proximal phalanges

5th metatarsal head

cuneiforms

navicular

navicular tuberosity

MTJ (talonavicular component)

5th metatarsal base

cuboid

midtarsal joint (MTJ) (calcaneocuboid component)

talus (trochlea)

hindfoot

medial malleolus

talar trochlea

calcaneus

axis of mortice (transmalleolar axis, TMA)

lateral malleolus

body of talus

Figure 3.1

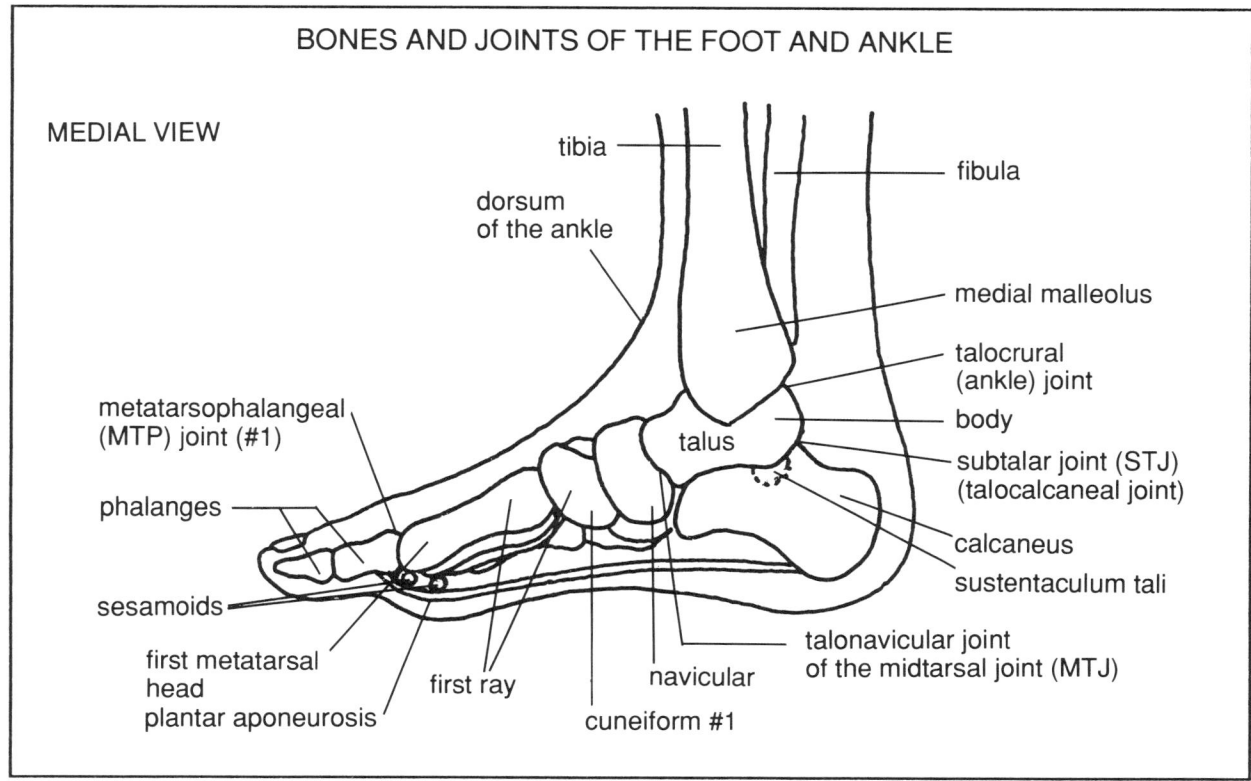

Figure 3.2

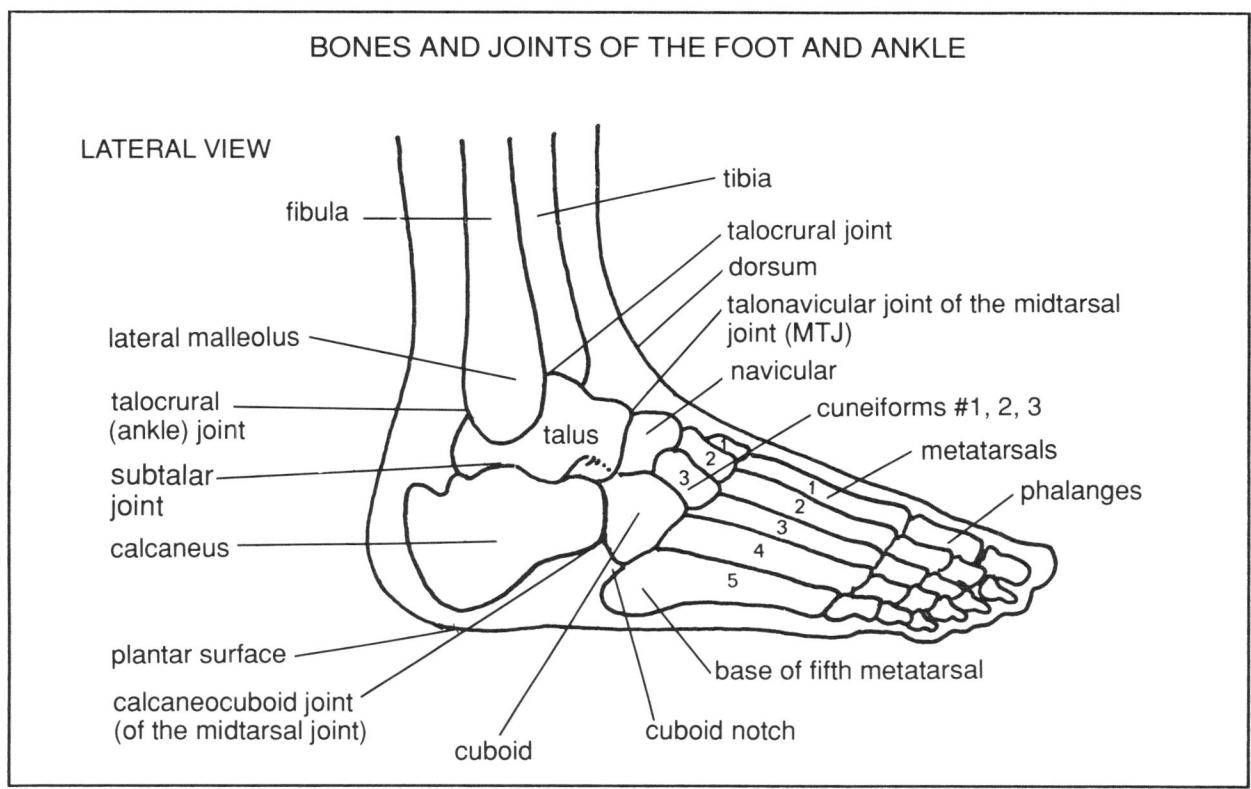

Figure 3.3

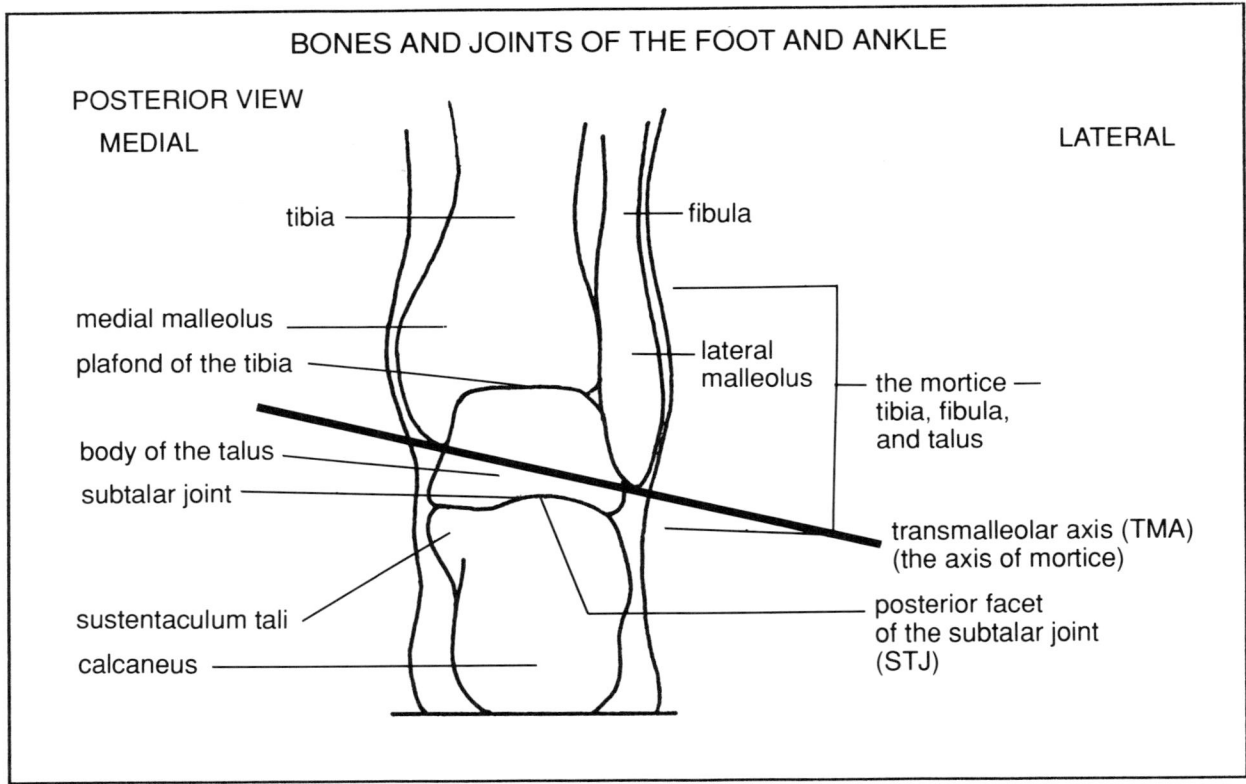

BONES AND JOINTS OF THE FOOT AND ANKLE

POSTERIOR VIEW
MEDIAL   LATERAL

tibia — ——————————— fibula

medial malleolus _____

plafond of the tibia —————

lateral
malleolus

— the mortice —
tibia, fibula,
and talus

body of the talus ———

subtalar joint —————

transmalleolar axis (TMA)
(the axis of mortice)

posterior facet
of the subtalar joint
(STJ)

sustentaculum tali ————

calcaneus ——————

Figure. 3.4

The Hip Joint

Sagittal Plane Motions

Mature walking on a level surface requires a maximum total of 55 degrees of combined hip flexion and extension (Sutherland et al. 1980a; Sutherland 1984; Schafer 1987). Limitation on hip extension shortens stride length and increases the anterior tilt of the pelvis.

Full hip flexion mobility is also needed for supple movements of the pelvis over the proximal femurs, as in sitting and in floor activities involving vaulting forward from sitting to quadruped.

If the posterior aspect of the hip joint capsule or the proximal extensors of the hip are contracted, anterior pelvifemoral mobility is restricted. The pelvis aligns posteriorly in sitting, and possibly in standing, in accordance with the degree of limitation (Brooks 1985; Bleck 1987).

Assessment for Evidence of Hip Flexion and Extension Contracture

Perry et al. (1976) evaluated the electrical activity emanating from specific muscles during the performance of eight of the well-known stretch tests commonly used to detect tight muscles (these tests help in making surgical decisions). They compared EMG recordings of the muscles tested with those of surrounding musculature and with EMG recordings of the same muscles in gait.

The stretch tests that were evaluated included:

- Straight leg raising
- Hip flexion with knees flexed
- Adductor stretch with hips and knees flexed
- "Thomas test"
- Lateral rotation of the extended hip
- Lateral rotation of the flexed hip
- Phelps-Baker "gracilis" test
- Prone rectus test of Duncan or Ely

In this Perry study, the researchers evidently did not evaluate Staheli's prone extension test, the popliteal angle test, or tests of the distal lower extremity musculature.

The EMG results indicated a margin for error in presuming that the mobility limitation that may be encountered in any of these stretch tests indicates functional influences of the specific muscle or muscle group being tested. None of these stretch tests was specific to any one muscle, though the straight leg raise correlated highly with increased activity in the hamstrings muscles. The other tests showed activity in more muscles than the one (or group) being tested. For example, hamstrings activity increased during the "gracilis" test and the iliopsoas was active during the prone rectus test and during other tests.

Rang et al. (1986) advise using these stretch tests to determine evidence of fixed contracture, but they support Perry and others in seeking to determine functional influences of specific muscles on the gait pattern by other, more sophisticated means. Dynamic EMG serves that purpose.

After age 3 years, the newborn hip flexion contracture is normally resolved when evaluated using Staheli's Prone Hip Extension Test (Staheli 1977, CORR; Phelps et al. 1985). This evaluation tool is simple to use and seems to offer greater precision and reliable measurement of the status of flexion contracture than does the Thomas test. The reason for the difference is stabilization of the pelvis and lumbar spine (Bleck 1987).

Staheli's Prone Hip Extension Test

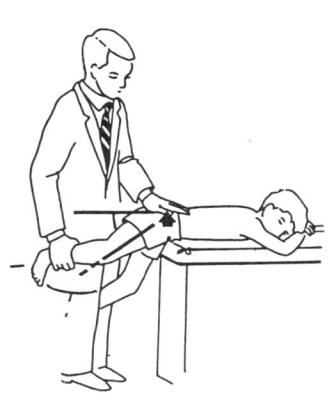

Place the child in prone with legs hanging over the edge of the examining table. Allow the untested leg to dangle or rest on a stool, or clasp it between your knees.

1. Lift the leg to be tested on the sagittal plane until the distal pelvis just begins to rise. Rest one hand on the sacrum to detect pelvic motion.

2. At that point, measure the angle formed by the femur and the surface of the table. (The femur is located between the greater trochanter and the lateral femoral condyle.) Normal hip extension = 0 (or 180) degrees.

Bleck (1987) uses a hip flexion contracture of 15-20 degrees as indication for surgical reduction. In mature gait, if the normal hip extends 15 degrees past neutral, a finding of 15-20 degrees of contracture represents a functional contracture of 30-35 degrees.

Knee Tuck Test for Hip Flexion Mobility

Use this test to assess for hip extension contracture of the proximal muscle tissue and/or capsular structures.

Place the child in supine. Maintain the sacrum on the table and flex the hips and knees fully, bringing the knees toward the chest. Normally, most of the length of the thighs contacts the torso without lifting the pelvis from the surface.

Rotary Hip Motions

As noted in Chapter 2, children as young as 24 months are likely to exhibit a mild excess of medial hip rotation range of motion compared to lateral rotation; they can average 52 degrees medial rotation and 47 degrees lateral rotation with the hip extended (Phelps et al. 1985; Bleck 1982). This discrepancy seems to be caused by the persistence of approximately 30 degrees of antetorsion in the femur, combined with reduction of the neonatal hip lateral rotation contracture (Phelps et al. 1985; McCrea 1985).

After the age of 2 years, full rotary mobility in the soft tissues of the hip joint is available for gait. When the hip is extended, a minimum total of 15-20 degrees of rotary motion is required for mature walking, although we use a greater range of motion for many other activities of daily living (Sutherland 1984; Root et al. 1971).

The purposes of measuring the rotary mobility in the hip joint in childhood are to determine the following by clinical examination:

- The status of reduction of the normal lateral rotation contracture.
- The status of the hip joint ligaments in general (whether lax or taut).
- The likelihood that excessive antetorsion persists in the femur.

Assessing Hip Rotation Mobility

The lateral rotation contracture of infancy precludes the use of this evaluative technique to determine evidence of antetorsion for a child under 2 years of age (Sutherland 1984; Pitkow 1975; Phelps et al. 1985).

The test positions used to evaluate hip rotation mobility include the following:

- Prone with the hips extended and the knees flexed
- Supine with the hips and knees extended
- Sitting with the knees flexed (short-sitting)
- Sitting with the knees extended (long-sitting)

Each of these positions alters the tensile forces on the femoral head. The tensile forces are applied either by the capsular structures, which tighten in either extension or flexion, or by the two-joint muscles of the hip and knee (Brooks 1985; Soderberg 1986; Maitland 1977;

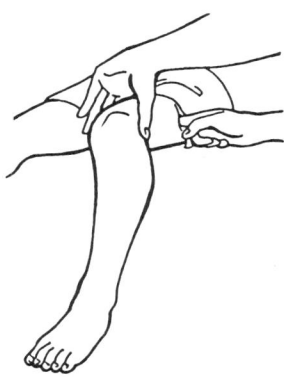

Figure 3.5
Ryder's test for femoral torsion: Place the patient supine, with the knees flexed over the edge of the table. Align the greater trochanter on the mid-frontal plane (at the center of the proximal thigh) to determine neutral position. Note the angle between the tibia and the sagittal plane with the trochanter centered. This is the neutral hip position.

Grant 1962). The position of hip flexion is "loose-packed," which means that tension on the ischiofemoral and pubofemoral ligaments is relieved. Because the hip is extended in the upright position and extension is the "close-packed" (stable) position of the hip joint, the values obtained in measuring hip rotation in extension are pertinent to the functional skills observed in stance and gait (Brooks 1985; Soderberg 1986; Gross 1987).

By comparing the rotary motion findings with the hip flexed with the findings obtained with the hip extended, the examiner might discover that a limitation on mobility that was noted with the hip extended is no longer apparent with the hip flexed. This indicates a limitation of extensibility in one or more of the hip ligaments, and perhaps in the rectus femoris or tensor fascia femoris muscles (Ryder et al. 1953; Root et al. 1971; McCrea 1985). If rotary hip motion is more limited in long-sitting (with the hips flexed and knees extended) than in supine (with both hips and knees extended), hamstrings tightness is the probable contributor to the discrepancy (McCrea 1985; Jordan et al. 1983).

When testing hip rotations with the knees flexed, the range of hip rotation mobility is determined by measuring the angle that the tibial crest forms with the sagittal plane as it is moved through an arc of motion on the frontal plane. When the knees are extended, the position of the femoral transcondylar axis (TCA) is compared to the frontal plane (the table surface).

Determining Hip Rotation Excursions from Neutral Hip Position

McCrea (1985) suggests testing soft tissue extensibility after first finding the neutral position of the hip joint, which is the center of the arc of motion.

1. Palpate and center the greater trochanter on the frontal plane of the hip joint (Figure 3.5) by rolling the upper leg as needed. Having thereby established neutral hip position, support the lateral or medial proximal thigh on a folded towel to maintain the central position of the greater trochanter. Proceed to evaluate the range of rotary mobility.

2. Move the lower leg in an arc on the frontal plane to measure the ranges of hip medial and lateral rotation relative to the neutral position (Figure 3.6).

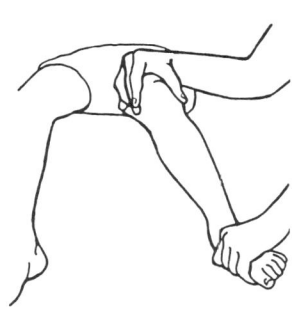

Figure 3.6
To assess soft tissue extensibility around the neutral hip position, place the greater trochanter on the frontal plane and measure the range of rotation in both directions. Repeat in sitting and long-sitting to detect differences in range.

For example, if the angle of the TCA is 10 degrees of medial rotation when the greater trochanter is centered, the measurement of rotation begins at 10 degrees of medial hip rotation rather than with the TCA aligned on the frontal plane. (This discrepancy also indicates existing medial torsion of the femoral shaft.)

If the soft tissue structures are normal, the available total range of hip rotation is equally divided around the established neutral position in all patient positions (supine and sitting).

If the child lacks a well-defined greater trochanter, which often occurs in severe cerebral palsy, this test is less precise.

The Femur

Torsional Status

As discussed in Chapter 2, a high incidence of increased femoral antetorsion occurs in children with cerebral palsy (Bleck 1987; Staheli et al. 1968; Fabry et al. 1973). Increased antetorsion has been identified as a possible cause of in-toed gait, foot pronation deformities, and compensatory lateral rotation and/or torsion of the lower leg (Staheli 1977, PCNA; Engel et al. 1974; Root et al. 1977; McDonough 1984).

These problems are magnified in children with neuromotor disorder, primarily because they lack postural control and the variable compensatory mechanisms needed to diminish the biomechanical consequences of this proximal torsional deformity.

Two clinical tests for antetorsion are discussed next.

Hip Rotation Test for Evidence of Femoral Torsion

A determination of the actual angle of femoral torsion, which compares the axis of the femoral neck to the transcondylar axis (TCA), requires elaborate radiologic assessment, such as computerized axial tomography (CT scan). This test requires the use of sophisticated techniques of identifying bony landmarks (Murphy et al. 1987). A high correlation has been found, however, between clinical findings for hip rotation mobility in extension and the existence of torsional deformity in the femur in children older than 2 to 3 years (Sutherland 1984; Staheli 1977, PCNA; Bleck 1982; Engel et al. 1974; McDonough 1984). The assessment method used in studies that confirmed this correlation was originally described by Phelps of the Dupont Institute in 1961, and has since been advocated by Staheli and Bleck (Staheli 1977, PCNA; Bleck 1982; Bleck 1987). In this book, the test will be referred to as the *Rotation Test for Femoral Torsion.*

Begin by placing the child in prone or supine. In the test position, the hips are extended and the knees are flexed 90 degrees.

1. Align the thighs and both tibial crests on the sagittal plane (Figure 3.7). The femoral condyles (TCA) are thus aligned on the frontal plane.
2. Move the feet along the frontal plane, first outward simultaneously to determine the range of medial rotation, then inward one at a time, to assess lateral rotation range.
3. Compare the angle that the tibial crest forms with the sagittal plane. Take care to prohibit the pelvis from rotating with these maneuvers, because this can distort the finding (Figures 3.8 and 3.9).

After the age of 4 or 5 years, when the range of hip medial rotation exceeds 60 degrees and lateral rotation is limited to 25 degrees or less, clinically significant femoral antetorsion is evident for the population that is not neuromotor-impaired, and often results in compensatory excess tibiofibular lateral torsion (Bleck 1982)

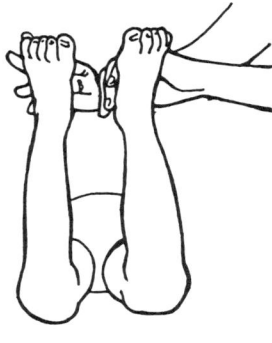

Figure 3.7
Hip rotation test for evidence of femoral antetorsion: Patient is prone with the knees flexed and the lower legs aligned on the sagittal plane . . .

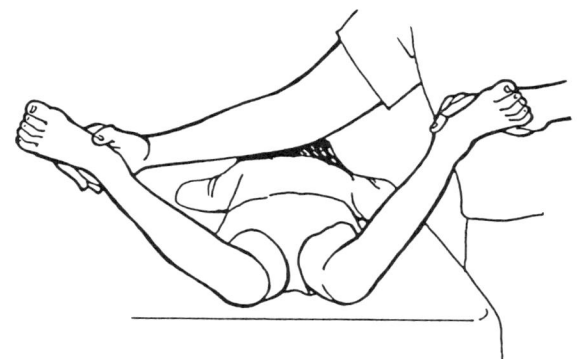

Figure 3.8 . . . Let both lower legs fall outward, away from each other. Do not force motion beyond the end point. Measure the excursion of each leg into medial rotation relative to the sagittal plane (average range = 45 degrees).

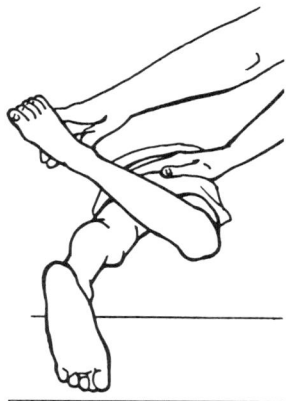

Figure 3.9
. . . Then gently stabilize the pelvis and flex the knee on the side to be tested. Assess lateral hip rotation, one leg at a time, with the opposite knee extended (average range = 45-50 degrees).

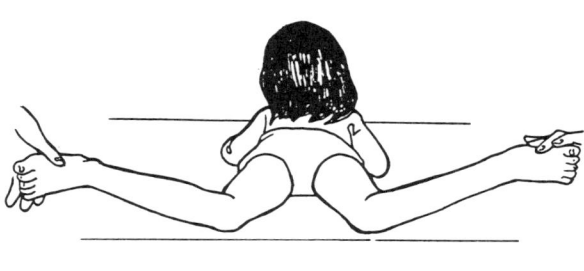

Figure 3.10 Evidence of abnormal femoral antetorsion: hip medial rotation exceeds 60 degrees (illustration shows 75 degrees) . . .

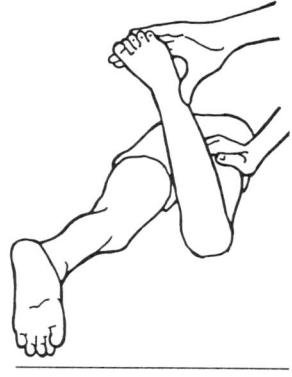

Figure 3.11
. . . Lateral rotation is less than 30 degrees (illustration shows less than 25 degrees).

(Figures 3.10 and 3.11). For the same population, antetorsion is considered to be <u>severe</u> when the value for medial rotation is equal to or greater than 90 degrees; 80 to 90 degrees is considered moderate; and 70 to 80 degrees is considered mild (Staheli 1977, PCNA). However, in my experience with children with neuromotor dysfunction who lack effective compensatory mechanisms, even the mild range of 60-70 degrees of medial rotation imposes significant functional impairment at the pelvis, hips, and distal structures.

Ryder's Test for Femoral Torsion

Ryder's test can reveal evidence of femoral torsion in the presence of hypermobility or laxity of the hip joint structures and adds another dimension to the findings discussed above. However, Ryder's test presumes that the greater trochanter has been formed by tensile modeling forces imposed on it by the gluteus medius. Many children with hypertonus fail to develop the greater trochanter, retaining coxa valga. The value of Ryder's test is limited in examining for evidence of femoral torsion in these children.

Begin to conduct Ryder's test by placing the child in supine with hips extended and knees flexed 90 degrees over the edge of the table.

1. Palpate the position of the greater trochanter of the femur to determine its proximity to the frontal plane, which is located at the center of the proximal thigh on its lateral aspect (Figure 3.5). This same maneuver is described previously for finding neutral hip position. In the mature hip in which the femur exhibits 5-15 degrees of antetorsion, the lower leg aligns on or very near the sagittal plane with the trochanter centered in the hip.

2. If rotation of the hip to align the trochanter on the frontal plane results in an angle greater than 10 degrees between the tibial crest and the sagittal plane, measure the angle.

As the angle of medial torsional declination of the femoral shaft increases in severity, the resting position of the trochanter can be palpated closer to the table surface (or more posteriorly) both in supine and sitting positions. Placing the TCA on the frontal plane forces the femoral neck into anteversion because of the femur's twisted shaft. As the trochanter is palpated and moved up to the center of the hip joint by medially rotating the hip, the lower leg aligns at increasing angles to the sagittal plane. If the angle of medial rotation is increased beyond 10 degrees with the trochanter centered, suspect torsional deformity.

Neither of these two tests gives the clinician a value that reveals the angle of torsional declination of the femur. However, they both offer evidence to suggest that structural deformity of the femur is a factor to be considered in management. Radiographic studies to determine the degree of torsion are indicated only when surgery is being considered or planned, to serve as a baseline for post-operative evaluation of results. These studies would also provide data for clinical research that is intended to reveal objective evidence of the influence of therapeutic exercise and/or other conservative intervention measures on the torsional status of the femur.

The problem of excessive femoral torsion is more significant in the management of cerebral palsy than in the management of head injury in the older child and adult. By age 5 years, the newborn value of 40 degrees of antetorsion is reduced to 23-26 degrees. By 8 years, this value decreases to 20 degrees. By age 15, the adult value of 5-15 degrees is achieved (McCrea 1985; Engel et al. 1974). Therefore, if a significant degree of structural maturity in the femur is achieved prior to the injury to the central nervous system, the closed-chain consequences of femoral antetorsion are of no major concern in rehabilitation.

The Knee

Sagittal Plane Motion—Flexion/Extension

Full mobility is available into both flexion and extension between the ages of 6 and 12 months. In gait, the knee extends fully as the same hip flexes 40 degrees prior to foot contact. It flexes up to 60 degrees after terminal stance (Root et al. 1977; Schafer 1987; Bleck 1987). In floor activities and self-dressing, greater degrees of motion are often used.

Functional position of the knee joint in standing is one of slight flexion, between 5 and 10 degrees (Perry 1974). Hyperextension beyond 0 degrees (on the sagittal plane) is a transient phenomenon in many children between the ages of 2 and 4 years. It offers evidence of the fairly steep, greater than 20 degree retroversion of the proximal tibial plateau (Bernhardt 1988). The inclined plateau favors mechanical knee extension. The task of achieving active control of the quadriceps and hamstrings in the context of this structural deviation is evidently arduous, requiring years of strengthening as the plateau models into the mature angle of 5 degrees. True genu recurvatum that approaches 20 degrees is abnormal and is usually associated with ligament laxity (Tax 1985).

The presence of knee flexion contracture can interfere significantly in floor play, self-help skills, and posture in stance. Knee flexion contracture can contribute to persistence of medial genicular deformity, patella alta, and reduction in step length and energy efficiency in gait (Mann 1985; Waters et al. 1985). Hamstrings contracture is also among the factors known to contribute to hip subluxation in children with cerebral palsy.

Using EMG analysis, stretch tests have been shown to lack specificity to isolated muscles, with the exception of standard straight leg raising for detecting hamstrings tightness (Perry et al. 1976). However, Rang et al. (1986) note that a contracture of the iliopsoas muscle can diminish the value measured in the straight leg raise. While the examiner lifts one leg into hip flexion with knee extension, the hip flexion contracture imposes an anterior pelvic tilt via the opposite, extended hip. Rang et al. (1986) uses the popliteal angle test, which is described below, to obtain a measure of knee flexion contracture.

Bleck (1987) allows no more than 20 degrees of flexion contracture as a criterion for optimum function when lengthening hamstrings. He arrives at this measurement by using the popliteal angle assessment procedure described below. Other authors consider a popliteal angle of 20-40 degrees as an indication for surgical intervention (Ray et al. 1979). It appears that they arrive at this measurement by extending the knee joint to its maximum end point, which reveals the maximum extensibility of the tendons and fascia, rather than that of the muscle fibers. The extensibility of the muscle fibers is evident at the initial point of resistance (Tardieu et al. 1982; Tardieu et al. 1987).

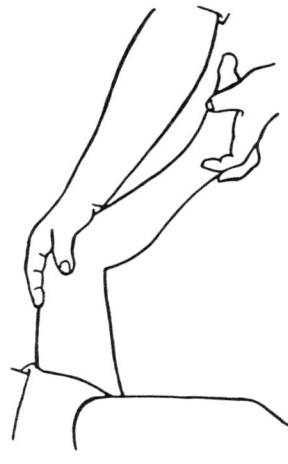

Assessing Knee Flexion Contracture— The Popliteal Angle

Knee flexion contractures can have three components: shortened hamstrings, shortened proximal gastrocnemius, and shortened posterior joint capsule and related ligaments. Capsular contracture is usually suspected if knee flexion contracture is evident when the same hip is fully extended (Rang et al. 1986, Bleck 1987). When ankle dorsiflexion is added to the popliteal angle test, some evidence of the possible contribution of the gastrocnemius muscle to the prevailing knee flexion contracture might be derived. If the popliteal angle of limitation is significantly greater with the ankle dorsiflexed than without dorsiflexion, the origin of the gastrocnemius is probably a contributing factor, and taking measures to try to lengthen the hamstrings would not adequately relieve the contracture. To perform the test:

Place the child in supine on the table or mat.

1. Extend the hips and knees fully. Note the presence of knee flexion contracture with hips extended. This would indicate capsular shortening.
2. Extend the opposite hip fully without tilting the pelvis anteriorly, and hold it down.
3. Flex the hip on the test leg 90 degrees to the frontal plane and maintain the thigh on the sagittal plane. (I use a gravity driven angle finder to ascertain the perpendicular relationship of the femur to the table.)
4. Extend the knee to the end of the free or comfortable range, and take a measurement of the angle between the longitudinal bisections of the thigh (the femur) and the tibial crest. The resulting measure is the knee extension deficit, or the number of degrees required to achieve full knee extension with the hip flexed 90 degrees (Reimers 1974). (I use an angle finder to measure the position of the tibial crest relative to the perpendicular upper leg.) Take two readings: initial endpoint (connective tissue and resting muscle tissue) and final endpoint (passive tissue extensibility). The finding pertaining to the initial endpoint of resistance is more significant to functional ability than the final endpoint.
5. Have an assistant maintain the position of the hips as you dorsiflex the ankle joint while protecting the foot from pronating.
6. Repeat the popliteal angle test with the ankle dorsiflexed initial and final endpoints.

Frontal Plane Deviation—Genu Varum and Valgum

By the age of 7 to 9 years and on through adulthood, the condyles of the tibia and femur—and thus the axis of the knee joint—should align on the transverse and frontal planes in the standing position. Knee joint motions of flexion and extension occur, therefore, on the sagittal plane (Wright et al. 1964; McCrea 1985).

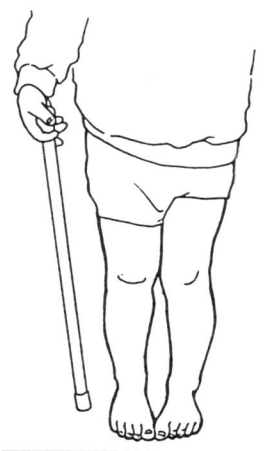

Figure 3.12
Normal neuromotor
status, age 3 years:
Genu valgum is
evident. With the
femoral condyles in
contact with each
other, the malleoli
are separated less
than 6 cm.

Between birth and 7 years, epiphyseal stimulation in weight-bearing results in unequal growth plate activity. Frontal plane deviations into genu varum and genu valgum may be seen in the same child at different ages, although via rotational changes in the femur and lower leg, the condyles within the knee joint remain in close proximity to the transverse plane. By the age of 2 years, neonatal physiologic genu varum has converted to valgum, which continues to develop until it peaks at 12-15 degrees at the age of 3 years (McDade 1977; Griffin 1986) (Figure 3.12). A gradual reduction in valgum then proceeds through the age of 7 years, after which the normal adult value of 5-7 degrees of valgum is attained and maintained (Staheli 1977, CORR; McDade 1977). These tibiofemoral values are obtained on radiographic examination.

Two clinical tests for evidence of genu varum and valgum follow.

Assessing for Evidence of Genu Valgum and Varum

The simplest method of determining the existence of genu varum or valgum is to align the legs in extension and place each TCA on the frontal plane, with either the malleoli or the medial femoral condyles in light contact with each other. This can be done in supine or standing position. The knees should not be hyperextended.

Genu varum—Because physiologic genu varum resolves by the age of 2 years and normally never recurs, any space between the femoral condyles, with the TCA aligned on the frontal plane and the medial malleoli contacting each other, is abnormal after age 2.

Genu valgum—In the preschool-aged child, if the space between the medial malleoli exceeds 2 inches (5 cm) while the femoral condyles are in contact with each other, the soft tissues that support the medial ankle and foot are at risk for pronation deformity. Persistence of genu valgum that features a tibiofemoral angle greater than 15 degrees after the age of 3 years places excessive pronatory stress on the child's medial foot structures (McCrea 1985; Griffin 1986). Laxity in the medial and plantar supporting ligaments would contribute to this sequela. The clinician should consider providing orthotic support for the structures of the foot as a possible way to prevent these changes and to impede any influence of foot pronation that might promote genu valgum (McCrea 1985).

In the older child and adult, while the femoral condyles are in contact, a minimum space of 3½ inches (9 cm) between the malleoli indicates abnormal genu valgum (McDade 1977; Griffin 1986). Severe genu valgum often occurs in combination with femoral retrotorsion (abnormal lateral femoral twist, or inadequate degree of medial twist for optimal function) and supination, rather than pronation, deformity in the foot.

Iliotibial band contracture—In the presence of genu valgum, evaluate for tightness of the iliotibial band by observing it on the lateral aspect of the knee joint. If, as you attempt to align the lower leg segment properly under the femur, the iliotibial band becomes taut and prominent, it is probably contracted and contributing to the valgus deformity. McCrea (1985) recommends serial casting to reduce the contracture.

Transverse Plane Motion—Lower Leg Rotation/Genicular Position

The tibia and fibula extend on the femur by a "corkscrew" motion of up to 6 degrees of lateral rotation, until congruity between the articulating surfaces at the knee is achieved (Schafer 1987). The closed-packed position of extension then blocks further tibiofibular rotation. This lateral rotation of the lower leg occurs during the final 10 degrees of knee extension. In assessing knee joint extension mobility, take this rotary motion into account (McCrea 1985; Brooks 1985).

Any degree of flexion at the knee will normally permit transverse plane (rotary) motion of the lower leg on the femur (Schafer 1987). This mobility reflects the integrity of the capsular, ligamentous, and muscular tissues surrounding the knee joint (McCrea 1985; Schafer 1987). Transverse plane mobility is significantly greater in children who are less than 3 years of age than it is in older children and adults (Valmassy 1984).

When the range of medial rotary motion of the flexed knee is excessive and lateral rotation is limited to within 10 degrees lateral to the sagittal plane, McCrea (1985) describes this phenomenon as "internal genicular position" (hereafter referred to as medial genicular position). McCrea (1985) suggests that it is maintained by limitation of length in—or by hypertonic contractions of—any or all of the five muscles that cross the knee joint to rotate the tibia medially. Only one muscle, the lateral head of the biceps femoris, can execute lateral rotation of the tibia. Ligamentous and capsular tissues within the joint adapt in similar fashion to maintain the medial rotation position of the tibia and fibula (Figure 3.13).

McDonough (1984) identifies this rotational discrepancy in young infants who are commonly very large at birth in proportion to the uterus. He describes the rotational deviation in the context of tibial torsion, however, which is a separate issue.

Neonates reveal a greater range of rotary mobility in the knee joint than do children and adults, and they typically demonstrate a propensity toward medial genicular position as a consequence of intrauterine confinement. Persistence of this deformity in later life might indicate a lack of complete resolution of this newborn biomechanical problem; it may indicate that the deformity was too severe at birth to yield fully to the corrective forces applied by normal modeling processes (McDonough 1984; McCrea 1985). Among the hypertonic neuromotor-impaired population, the lack of normal modeling forces into lateral rotation and persistence of pronation in stance contribute to persistence of this rotary deviation within the knee joint.

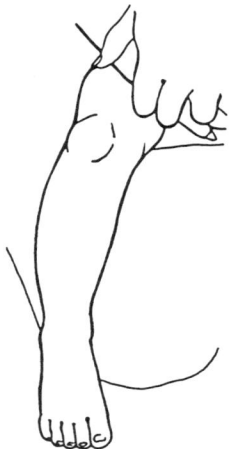

Figure 3.13
Abnormal neuromotor status, age 2 years: Medial genicular position appears with the knee flexed.

Assessing for Genicular Position

Schafer (1987) reports that approximately 10 degrees of passive tibial rotation normally occurs in both directions with the knee flexed. However, this measurement is obtained with a specially designed caliper or a comparable measuring device.

McCrea (1985) suggests that in children (of unspecified ages, but presumably less than 3 years) the knee joint normally allows 45-95 degrees of lateral rotation and 45-65 degrees of medial rotation, or slightly greater lateral than medial motion. He obtains these values by maintaining the knee in 90 degrees of flexion, with the foot held rigidly in calcaneal midposition and the ankle held rigidly at 90 degrees. He then moves the foot on the transverse plane, measuring the angles of adduction and abduction of the foot relative to the sagittal plane and comparing the findings. These values are unusually high, however. When the medial rotation range exceeds the range of lateral rotation, the presence of medial genicular position is indicated.

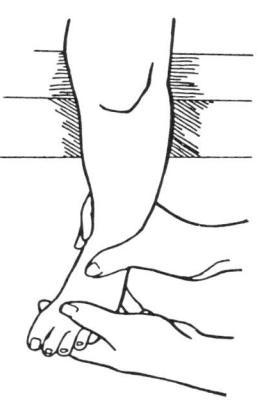

The child's flexed knee should be tested with the child positioned in both supine and sitting to determine the influence of two-joint muscle contracture as a contributing problem (McCrea 1985). When no change in ranges occurs with hip flexion and extension, the deformity is probably due more to ligamentous adaptation than to muscle tissue tightness. Medial genicular position resolves in knee extension, provided that the knee joint capsular tissues and musculature allow full extension to congruity between the tibial and femoral condyles.

McCrea (1985) recommends serial castings in 30 degrees of knee flexion to reduce soft tissue contracture. Achieving lateral rotary mobility is a way to reduce the deforming influences of this rotational abnormality at the knee, the hip, and the foot. Further, he suggests orthotic intervention to protect the distal foot structures from pronating as a compensation. Pronating the foot effectively increases the angle of gait, but it achieves this at the expense of the medial and plantar ligaments of support at the foot and ankle (McCrea 1985).

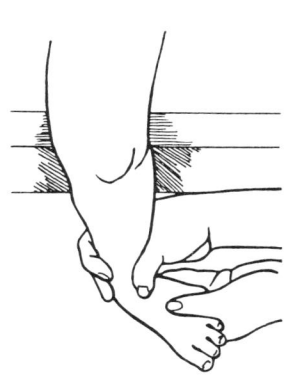

Medial genicular position can occur together with medial tibiofibular torsion. Management of the two components differs, however. Genicular deformity—because it is caused by soft-tissue adaptation—can respond to casting or night splints during early life, when chondral modeling is underway. Torsion deformity, however, does not respond to night splinting or casts because of the difficulty in securing the proximal end of the tibia and fibula against the applications of lateral torque force distally (Bleck 1982).

Stabilize both the foot and ankle in maximum congruity throughout this test while rotating the lower leg medially and laterally. Neither supinate nor pronate the foot and ankle.

Lateral genicular deformity—Although rare compared to the occurrence of excessive lateral tibial torsion (McCrea 1985), lateral genicular knee deformity might also occur in early childhood in the presence of chronic lateral torque forces of significant—and abnormal—magnitude. This may happen more often in children with neuromotor disorders who "W-sit" with both feet turned out; or who reveal "windblown" deformity of the lower legs, in which both lower legs rotate in the same direction. In these children, the patellae align on the sagittal plane in sitting, while one or both lower legs aligns in lateral rotation.

Radiologic assessment might be indicated to distinguish lateral tibiofibular torsional deformity from lateral genicular position. This assessment should take place before any intervention is undertaken to reduce the deformity. Torsional deformity requires osteotomy. Genicular deformity can be expected to respond to serial castings (Valmassy 1984; McDonough 1984; McCrea 1985). In either case, on clinical examination the range of lateral rotation of the lower leg greatly exceeds that of medial rotation when the knee is flexed 90 degrees. Both problems, genicular and torsional, place the foot in position in stance to pronate throughout the stance phase. The risk of increasing foot deformity over time is high (McCrea 1985).

The Tibia and Fibula

Tibiofibular Torsion

Medial "tibial" torsion is commonly the first concern when a child reveals in-toeing in gait. Most clinicians have found that in the presence of ankle mortice axis values less than the age-specific norms, a high incidence of in-toeing occurs (McCrea 1985; Staheli 1977, PCNA). Staheli (1977) determines tibial torsion with the knee flexed and might be observing genicular deformity as well. However, in-toeing can occur in the absence of medial tibial torsion (Bleck 1982). No clinical examination of the tibia can occur without including the fibula, which joins the tibia in housing the talus distally and directing its motion.

True lateral torsion occurs in both the tibia and fibula in normal development, as cadaver studies have revealed (Hutter and Scott 1949). The distal aspects of both bones are highly cartilaginous and pliable under torque forces early in life while rapid growth is occurring (McCrea 1985). Although muscle action generates significantly greater forces than static loading, the high incidence of medial torsion deformities in Japanese adults who are raised in Japan suggests to Hutter and Scott (1949) that static loading plays a part in bony modeling. The Japanese have few chairs in their homes and often spend hours in kneel-sitting with toes closer to the midline than the heels. Here, too, however, the determination of torsional deformity with the knee flexed might indicate a ligamentous adaptation into medial genicular position among the people of this culture.

The normal angle of gait (forward foot progression), is measured by comparing the stance-phase placement of the longitudinal bisection of the foot to the sagittal plane. This angle averages 30 degrees lateral in infants and 10 degrees in preschoolers, diminishing with increasing age to between 0 and 6 degrees in older children and adults (Scrutton 1969; Sutherland 1984). Approximately 1 to 3 percent of adults toe in significantly in gait (generating negative values for angle of gait) in relation to medial tibial torsion (measured clinically with the knee flexed). The percentage of children who toe in among school-age children is closer to 5 to 9 percent, and in 2-year-olds, 30 percent (Hutter et al. 1949; Bleck 1982).

Young children exhibit in-toeing gait more often than older children and adults, perhaps because the ankle joint axis is increasing through childhood, or because of persistence of medial genicular position. However, most infants toe out when they walk, revealing an average angle of gait approaching 30 degrees, while the pitch of the TMA is only 6 degrees lateral to the frontal plane. Thus, there is little evidence of a functional relationship between the frontal-plane pitch of the ankle joint axis and the angle of gait in young children with normal neuromotor function, except in the extremes of medial genicular position or tibiofibular torsion and of femoral antetorsion—and even these connections are not consistent.

With the knee joint extended, the normal pitch of the transmalleolar axis (TMA) to the frontal plane may be used as a clinical measure of tibiofibular torsion. Normal pitch averages 0 degrees at birth (with knee flexion imposed by contracture), approximately 6 degrees at 1 year, and 10-15 degrees at 2 years; it increases to 20 to 30 by age 5 to 7 years (McCrea 1985).

Many cases of true medial tibiofibular torsion are familial in origin and are accompanied by an apparent lateral bowing of the distal lower leg. These findings recall the Newborn's Biomechanical Problem List from Chapter 2. It is not clear what the familial tendency may be. Does the infant grow the tibia in torsion? Does the mother carry the fetus in a small womb, or does she have oversized babies? Does the child lack effective modeling mechanisms that would reduce torsional deformity?

There is good reason for pursuing the evidence regarding "true" rather than "apparent" medial tibiofibular torsion. It is important in selecting an appropriate management course for the child with neuromotor impairment if that child is not likely to resolve spontaneously the problem of immaturity in lower leg and knee joint alignment. The lateral torque forces that occur in normal gait do not occur as effectively, if at all, in the child with disabilities.

Historically, night splinting has had no significant effect on known bony torsional deformity. This is because it has not been possible to stabilize adequately the proximal epiphysis to apply torque force to the metaphysis with available splinting devices (McCrea 1985). In this case, bone surgery is needed.

However, early and consistent night splinting or progressive casting can effect change in the soft tissue structures, for better or worse (McDonough 1984). Orthotic devices can do the same if they are appropriately designed to protect the foot and ankle ligaments and if they are implemented early in life. Judicious use of these devices can, to varying degrees, improve the biomechanical interaction of the whole extremity in favor of application of more normal torque forces (McCrea 1985).

Assessing for Tibiofibular Torsion

The status of lateral torsion in the tibia and fibula is estimated clinically by identifying the transmalleolar axis (TMA)—which includes both the distal tibia and fibula—and then measuring its pitch

axis of mortice

relative to the frontal plane. The resulting measurement, usually referred to as the "axis of mortice," indicates the extent of development of lateral torsion of the tibial and fibular shafts (Root et al. 1971; McCrea 1985; Mann 1985 in Jahss; Regnauld 1986). (The axis of mortice is also the TMA, around which supination and pronation occur, featuring primary motions of plantarflexion and dorsiflexion respectively. (See Figures 3.1 and 3.4.)

Although the published average norms for the mature ankle joint range between 12 and 30 degrees (Root et al. 1971; McCrea 1985), most of the current literature claims that clinically observed (versus radiologically determined) values of between 20 and 30 degrees lateral to the frontal plane are normal (Hutter et al. 1949; Bleck 1982; McCrea 1985; Mann 1985 in Jahss; Regnauld 1986).

Most authors recommend measuring the axis of mortice with the child sitting with the knee flexed and the foot unloaded (Hutter et al. 1949; Staheli et al. 1972; Bleck 1982). Others fail to specify the evaluation procedure regarding patient position (supine, sitting, standing), STJ alignment, or foot position (Wright et al. 1964; Mann 1985 in Jahss). It is impossible to rule out the existence of medial genicular position as an alternative to—or a component of—the diagnosis of medial tibial torsion as it is determined by these authors.

When examining the lower leg for evidence of torsional deformity, consider additional factors such as femoral antetorsion, knee flexion contracture, genicular position (Figure 3.13), and talar torsion (discussed following). For example, in the presence of medial genicular position, the pitch of the TMA increases with knee extension and decreases with knee flexion. Existing knee flexion contracture would impede this finding. Also, consider evidence of apparent tibial varum, which is commonly associated with torsional deformity of hereditary origin as well as with lower leg medial rotation. Then proceed as follows:

Place the child in supine or long-sitting on the table with only the feet hanging off the end. (The same measure may be taken on a footprint taken in standing with the calcaneus in midposition and the ankle at 90 degrees.)

1. Extend the knee and align the femoral and tibial condyles on the frontal plane (Root et al. 1971; McCrea 1985) (Figure 3.14).

2. Drop your line of vision to the plantar aspect of the foot, and have an assistant dorsiflex the foot while maintaining the calcaneus in midposition, neither inverted nor everted (Valmassy 1984; McCrea 1985).

3. Palpate the distal tips of the medial and lateral malleoli and extend the palpating fingers.

4. Align both fingers in parallel formation, as if they were an arrow that was shot through the TMA (McCrea 1985; Gray 1986).

5. Measure the angle formed by your fingers and the frontal plane (represented by the edge of the table) (Figure 3.15).

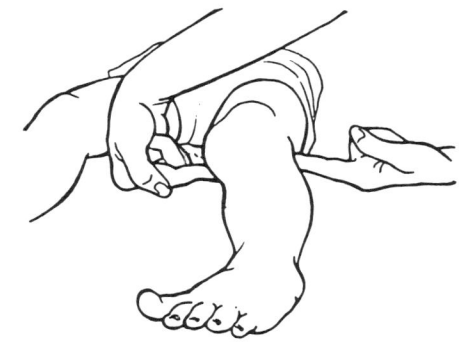

Figure 3.14 To determine clinical evidence of tibiofibular torsion, measure the transmalleolar axis (TMA). Extend the knee and align the TCA on the frontal plane and the tibial tuberosity on the sagittal plane . . .

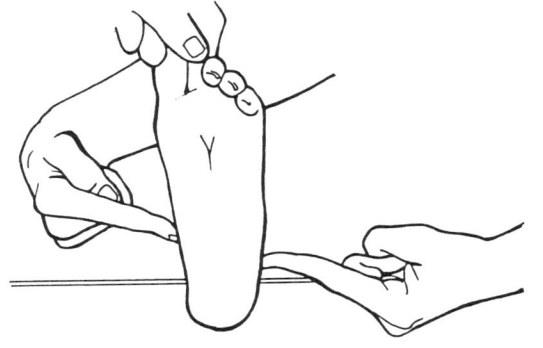

Figure 3.15 . . . then align the calcaneus in midposition and the ankle at 90 degrees. Measure the angle formed by the TMA and the frontal plane (the table surface).

If the pitch of the TMA is lower than the norms when the child's knee is extended, seek further radiologic assessment of tibial torsion to confirm a clinical finding of "medial tibiofibular torsion" or inadequate modeling into lateral tibiofibular torsion (Bleck 1982).

If the pitch of the TMA is greater than 30 degrees, lateral torsional deformity is present. Assessments of the joints and structures proximal and distal to the lower leg are likely to reveal abnormality.

Apparent Tibial Varum

The distal third of the tibia pitches medially 15-20 degrees relative to the sagittal plane at birth (Sgarlato 1971; Jordan et al. 1983). This angle reduces to approximately 6 degrees by age 1 year and is usually resolved to within 2 degrees or less by age 5 years (Jordan et al. 1983; Tax 1985). As stated previously, this deviation is neither true tibia vara nor bony curvature because the tibial shaft is normally straight at and following birth. Instead, the angle reflects evidence of persisting genu varum, residual medial leg rotation that displaces the posterior muscle bellies laterally, or incomplete lateral tibiofibular torsion, or it may be a combination of the three (McDonough 1984).

In the presence of normal foot mobility and structure, persistence of apparent distal varum past early childhood affects the subtalar joint (STJ) alignment (that is, calcaneal position) in stance. This deviation increases the position of calcaneal valgus in relation to the distal lower leg. The lateral deviation of the leg above the weight-bearing calcaneus effectively increases the STJ angle of pronation in stance.

Assessing for Apparent Tibial Varum—In Relaxed and Neutral, and in Functional Calcaneal Midposition

Begin by determining the presence of genu varum or valgum (described previously). Genu varum can contribute to a distal tibial varum measurement.

Relaxed tibial varum—Place the child in relaxed standing position—with help or positioning devices as needed—in optimum anatomical position with feet aligned at their usual angle of and base of stance or gait, and the knees in neutral flexion. Proceed as follows:

1. Measure the angle formed by the vertical bisection of the distal lower leg—between the Achilles tendon and the gastrocnemius muscle belly—and the sagittal plane.
2. Arrange the arms of a goniometer precisely on the bisection and the sagittal plane.

An inexpensive, gravity-driven roofer's level (known as an angle finder) is a good tool to use to measure this angle. The floating needle always identifies the sagittal plane. The needle floats to the top of the circular dial, which is marked in one-degree increments. The tool has two straight edges at right angles to each other, either of which can be aligned on the body segment to be assessed (in this case, the bisection of the distal lower leg). As the vertical straight edge deviates from the sagittal plane or the horizontal edge from the transverse plane, the circular dial deviates along with it. The vertically oriented needle indicates precisely the degrees of deviation. The manufacturer claims accuracy to within 1 degree. This tool has been used successfully for assessment of spinal mobility also and was recently brought to my attention by Mark Meleck, PT, in Springfield, Ohio.

Neutral tibial varum—This value reveals evidence of distal lower leg alignment when the foot structures are fully congruent. Note that by rotating the leg laterally, the posterior compartment musculature and connective tissues move around to the posterior aspect of the leg. The degree of varum typically reduces with lateral leg rotation. This value is obtained as the child remains standing (Gray 1984; Giallonardo 1988).

1. Rotate the leg while palpating the head of the talus, using Method II described later in this chapter under Assessing for Neutral (Congruent) STJ Position.
2. When the talonavicular joint is congruous, hold the leg still and measure the angle formed by the distal lower leg bisection and the sagittal plane.

Functional calcaneal midposition—This value reveals evidence of distal lower leg varum when the calcaneus is in optimum position for weight-bearing at midstance in gait. It is also obtained with the child in standing position.

1. Rotate the leg until the vertical bisection of the calcaneus is aligned within 2 degrees of the sagittal plane.
2. Hold the leg still and measure the angle formed by the distal lower leg bisection and the sagittal plane.

The Thigh-Foot Angle

Yet another dimension of the rotary structure and alignment in the lower leg and foot is the angle that the longitudinal bisection of the foot forms with the thigh. This is measured with the child in the prone position, with the hip extended and the knee flexed 90 degrees (Staheli 1977, PCNA; Bleck 1982; Engel et al. 1974; Staheli et al. 1985) (Figure 3.16). This angle is representative of a combination of features, including the tibiofibular torsional structure, the genicular position, and the position of the foot under the tibia. Therefore, this test is only a pathfinder toward the more precise determination of specific causative factors of malalignment in a child.

The normal thigh-foot angle in the newborn averages 5-10 degrees of medial deviation relative to the longitudinal bisection of the thigh. Thereafter the angle gradually increases to an average of 10 degrees lateral by the age of 5 years. This angle increases further to 12 to 18 degrees as the child enters adulthood, with a normal maximum of 30 degrees (Staheli 1977, PCNA; Staheli et al. 1985).

Assessing the Thigh-Foot Angle

Place the child in prone with knees flexed 90 degrees.

1. Align and maintain the calcaneus in midposition.
2. Dorsiflex the ankle to 90 degrees. Keep the second toe in line with the tibial crest.
3. Look down onto the sole of the foot.
4. Measure the angle formed by the longitudinal bisections of the foot and the thigh.

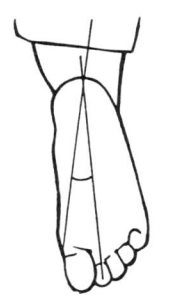

Figure 3.16
Normal values for the thigh-foot angle: Up to 10 degrees medial at birth, 10 degrees lateral after 2 years, 10 to 30 degrees in adulthood.

Talar Torsion

After ruling out the possibility of medial genicular position, medial tibial torsion, and metatarsus adductus, and after observing that the foot adducts on the transverse plane under the normally aligned tibia and fibula in stance and gait, test carefully for evidence of persistence of the adduction component of talar torsion. Use the following procedures:

Assessing for Talar Torsion

1. Check the thigh-foot angle. A negative value warrants further investigation.
2. Palpate the transmalleolar axis (TMA) to determine its pitch to the longitudinal axis of the foot. A TMA/foot angle of between 80 and 85 degrees is appropriate for a child of 1 year. As the child's age increases and the TMA migrates more laterally, the TMA/foot angle reduces to the mature value of 60-70 degrees (Staheli et al. 1985). A low (mature) TMA/foot angle, combined with a negative thigh/foot angle, suggests evidence of talar torsion.

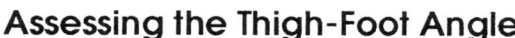

To test for evidence of persistent talar torsion:

Place the child in sitting with the knee flexed 90 degrees.

1. Grasp the entire foot in one hand and the lower leg in the other. Do not twist the leg.
2. Maintain the ankle at 90 degrees and the foot in midline inversion and eversion.
3. Have an assistant align one arm of the goniometer along the medial border of the foot and the other arm on the sagittal plane.
4. Rotate the foot laterally, abducting it on the transverse plane.
5. Measure the resulting angle.

The normal child's foot rotates into an average of 8.3 degrees of abduction under the stabilized tibia and fibula. Lack of mobility into abduction indicates a possible persistence of immature talar configuration (Bleck 1982). Radiographic assessment would confirm this clinical finding.

The torsional component of talar torsion cannot be evaluated specifically in the clinic, but it can be surmised through the assessment of forefoot supination and pronation mobility and alignment relative to the hindfoot. Researchers have suggested that the primary cause of structural forefoot varus after early childhood is incomplete resolution of the torsional deviation within the talar neck (Tiberio 1988). Chapter 2 contains more information about talar torsion.

The Ankle (Talocrural Joint)

Features of Structure and Joint Motion

The ankle is formed by the articulation between the tibia, the fibula, and the talus. The calcaneus is not included in this joint (Soderberg 1986; Hamilton 1985) (Figures 3.2, 3.3, and 3.4). As discussed previously in the context of assessment of tibiofibular torsion, the pitch of the transmalleolar axis (TMA) to the frontal and transverse planes dictates that the motions of pronation and supination occur at this joint under the following conditions: with primary dorsiflexion and plantarflexion, with secondary eversion with abduction, and secondary inversion with adduction respectively. The appearance of talocrural supination and pronation is enhanced by the same associated subtalar and midtarsal joint motions.

At birth, the transmalleolar axis aligns on both the transverse and frontal planes. As the infant develops, the lateral malleolus aligns both posteriorly and distally to the medial malleolus. After the age of 5 years, the TMA aligns at a pitch of 20 degrees of inversion to the transverse plane in the standing position, inclining upward from the lateral to the medial malleolus (Mann 1985 in Jahss; Root et al. 1977; Hicks 1953). (Figure 3.4)

The pitch of the TMA to the frontal plane averages 20-30 degrees in the mature ankle, with the knee joint extended and the calcaneus in midposition. This value approximates 6 degrees at 1 year and 10 degrees at 2 years of age. Regardless of the child's age, the TMA and the frontal plane intersect lateral to the foot (Hicks 1953; Wright et al. 1964; Frankel et al. 1980; Soderberg 1986) (Figure. 3.1). (See Assessing for Tibiofibular Torsion, above.)

The *trochlea* of the talus is its proximal articulating surface. It is shaped like a trapezoid, broader at the anterior than at the posterior aspect (Figure 3.1). Therefore as the ankle joint dorsiflexes, the degree of structural stability increases; the fit between the talus and the tibia and fibula becomes more snug (Riegger 1988; Brooks 1985; Soderberg 1986; Bahler 1986; Hamilton 1985; Frankel et al. 1980).

The medial and lateral malleoli must spread slightly to accommodate the dorsiflexing—and thus widening—talar trochlea. Because the ankle dorsiflexors (including the long toe extensors) do not attach to the fibula, it is free—within the limits of the extensibility of the tibiofibular ligaments—to separate from the tibia at its distal aspect during the motion of dorsiflexion (Soderberg 1986).

The surface of the trochlea of the talus is convex and moves under the concave surface of the tibia (Figure 3.4). The talar trochlea glides backward and medially into dorsiflexion, under the more stationary tibia, and forward and laterally into plantarflexion, in an example of the "convex on concave" rule of joint motion. This factor is an important consideration at the time that mobilization is undertaken. For example, as the ankle dorsiflexes, the distal tibiofibular ligaments must elongate to allow the fibula to separate and rotate away from the tibia. At the same time, the joint capsule and ligaments must allow room for posterior excursion of the talus (Maitland 1977; Svendsen et al. 1981; Brooks 1985; Soderberg 1986).

Because the trochlea of the talus is narrow and relatively long at the posterior aspect, the range of mobility into plantarflexion is greater than the range of mobility into dorsiflexion. In addition, the position of passive ankle plantarflexion reduces congruity between the talus and the tibia and fibula. In full passive plantarflexion, therefore, the talus can be moved on the frontal plane, which increases the apparent mobility within the subtalar joint (Root et al. 1971; Soderberg 1986).

In closed-packed positions, the talocrural joint is mobile sagittally and is more stable in the frontal than the sagittal plane. It is also more secure on the medial than the lateral aspect until the lateral malleolus grows distally. The talus is eventually held firmly by the distal tibia and fibula and by the surrounding ligaments: the anterior and posterior tibiofibular ligaments, the four components of the deltoid ligament, and the three components of the lateral collateral ligament. Together the distal tibia, the fibula, and the talus form the ankle mortice, which is a functional unit in the closed kinetic chain (Figure 3.4).

Kinesiological Considerations of the Talocrural Joint

Muscle action provides stability for the talocrural joint in plantarflexion, primarily via the posterior tibialis. Stability is aided by those plantar flexors and long toe flexors that attach to the fibula, particularly the posterior tibialis and soleus. With plantarflexion, these muscles apply a backward torque force to the fibula (into lateral rotation) and squeeze the posterior borders of the lateral and medial malleoli toward each other. This force increases the angle of the axis of mortice and closes the space between the medial and lateral malleoli, as well as the space around the narrowing talar trochlea. Evidently because of the location of the tendon of insertion of the soleus relative to the pitch of the TMA, this drawing together of the posterior malleoli increases as the TMA increases its pitch (Soderberg 1986).

Given the developmental biomechanics involved, persistent toe-standing in infancy and early childhood seems to be an effort to achieve both the mature pitch of the axis of mortice and active stability in the talocrural joint.

The triceps surae group, the peroneals, the anterior and posterior tibialis muscles, and the long toe extensors and flexors all actively contribute to stability in the ankle joint on the sagittal and frontal planes, in both stance and swing phases of gait (Sutherland et al. 1980; Hamilton 1985; Regnauld 1986; Soderberg 1986). During normal ambulatory function, the primary motions that occur in the ankle joint are dorsiflexion and plantarflexion. However, slight abduction with eversion occurs with dorsiflexion at weight assumption during the pronatory phase of stance; and adduction with inversion occurs with plantarflexion at the end of the stance phase.

After the initial 15 percent of the stance phase, the foot gradually supinates under the influence of proximal lateral torque forces. Passive ankle dorsiflexion continues, however, through midstance to terminal stance, in the presence of the increasing excursion of the lower segment into supination. Because the talocrural joint axis is pitched to allow pronation with dorsiflexion rather than supination, this combination of talocrural and foot motions in stance is evidence of overriding forces of forward momentum, weight-bearing, and lateral torque.

The ankle plantarflexors activate from 40 percent of stance through toe-off, stabilizing the tibia against falling forward over the plantigrade foot and providing force for weight shift at toe-off. Between midstance and toe-off, the foot and ankle supinate together. The usual secondary components of adduction and inversion accompany ankle plantarflexion (Wright et al. 1964; Mann 1985 in Jahss; Hamilton 1985; Gray 1986; Rodgers 1988).

Assessing Talocrural Joint Alignment

Use the same procedure for determining evidence of tibiofibular torsion as for determining the pitch of the ankle joint axis. The alignment of the TMA is identified at the distal ends of the malleoli and is measured by comparing it to the frontal and transverse planes. (See the previous discussion of Assessing for Tibiofibular Torsion.)

Features of Talocrural Joint Mobility

Infants and toddlers exhibit 20-50 degrees of dorsiflexion range, which amounts to 10-35 degrees more than the average adult (Jordan et al. 1983; McCrea 1985). By adulthood, the ankle joint usually allows between 8 and 20 degrees of dorsiflexion (McCrea 1985; Jordan et al. 1983; Frankel et al. 1980). With the foot structures aligned in neutral (congruent) position (see the discussion of The Subtalar Joint following) and the knee extended, the minimum range of ankle dorsiflexion required for normal adult walking is 5-7 degrees, although some authors report that a full 10 degrees are needed (McCrea 1985; Root et al. 1977; Perry 1974; Frankel et al. 1980). The 10-degree value is obtained with the calcaneus aligned in midposition, parallel to the distal lower leg (Root et al. 1977).

Because the range of ankle dorsiflexion decreases with increasing degrees of supination of the foot (pronation occurs with dorsiflexion around the axis of this joint), the lower minimum findings are likely to be derived from measurements taken in full congruity of the subtalar and midtarsal joints. When the foot achieves this measure of congruity in gait, the heel has usually begun to leave the ground. (See Assessing for Neutral (Congruent) STJ Position following, for more details on setting the foot structures in congruity for this test.)

This ideal dorsiflexion mobility is implemented from midstance to terminal stance in gait, as the tibia moves forward over the supinating, plantigrade foot. The result is increased stability at midstance, which is encouraged by the following factors:

- Support on a stable foot in calcaneal midposition.
- The close-packed position of the talar trochlea in the ankle mortice.
- The stabilizing influence of eccentric activation of the triceps surae group—particularly of the soleus muscle.
- The increasing rigidity of the foot structures as they achieve full congruity with continued supination through midstance to heel-off.

Plantarflexion mobility normally measures 30-45 degrees or more (Frankel et al. 1980). The minimum range of plantarflexion required for normal gait is 20 degrees (Root et al. 1971). This range of motion is seen twice in the stance phase of the gait cycle: at the moment following heel strike when the foot is lowered to the ground, and between heel-off and toe-off at the end of stance (Root et al. 1971; Root et al. 1977; Frankel et al. 1980; Sutherland et al. 1980b).

Assessing Talocrural Joint Mobility

Evaluation of ankle joint motion requires attention to the position of both the knee joint and the foot structures. The sitting or supine positions will suffice for assessment, provided that knee joint motion is not restricted.

Because talocrural joint motion occurs at the talus and is observed primarily at the calcaneus, some authors suggest that the clinician consider only the hindfoot-tibial relationship in the assessment of ankle joint mobility (Giallonardo 1988; Oatis 1988). Others suggest that by including the entire lateral pillar in the assessment, a more accurate impression of the functional range of dorsiflexion becomes evident. We dorsiflex over the entire foot in walking.

If the forefoot is fixed in plantarflexion, for example (thus constituting a forefoot equinus deformity), while the inclination of the calcaneus is steeply pitched up from the transverse plane, both the medial and lateral longitudinal arches are high. The result is a form of cavus foot in which the functional dorsiflexion range for walking is not disclosed by assessment of the hindfoot-leg angle alone. In this type of foot, excessive talocrural dorsiflexion is usually required to achieve forward progression of the tibia over the entire weight-bearing foot, the distal portion of which resists dorsiflexion (Tiberio 1988). This type of foot seems comfortable in a heeled boot that allows the hindfoot to rest on a higher level than the forefoot.

In measuring talocrural joint motion, take the following two measures:

- Include as the landmarks for placement of the arms of the goniometer the longitudinal bisection of the lateral lower leg and the lateral plantar aspect of the foot, from the posterior calcaneus to the base of the fifth toe. Align the pivot point of the goniometer at the point of convergence of the two lines.

- Measure the angle formed by the longitudinal bisection of the lower leg and the lateral aspect of the hindfoot (Oatis 1988; Giallonardo 1988). Discrepancy between the two values indicates a sagittal-plane forefoot deformity.

Accurate assessment of talocrural dorsiflexion is executed with the STJ aligned in two positions: calcaneal midposition and neutral (congruent) position. (See Assessing for Neutral (Congruent) STJ Position, following.) Pronation of the foot displaces the lower segment under the talus and allows the subtalar and midtarsal joints to express their respective dorsiflexion capability along with the dorsiflexion of the talocrural joint. The pronated foot thus appears to manifest a greater degree of talocrural dorsiflexion than is actually available.

Measurement of dorsiflexion range with the calcaneus in midposition—neither inverted not everted—will reveal the capacity for dorsiflexion through midstance in gait when, optimally, the calcaneus aligns within 2 degrees of the sagittal plane (Root et al. 1971). The normal minimum dorsiflexion for this subtalar joint position is 10 degrees past the 90-degree ankle position, or 100 degrees.

Measurement of dorsiflexion with the foot structures locked in congruity—which is usually slightly more supinated than it is in calcaneal midposition—reveals the capacity of the joint to dorsiflex through the latter stages of the stance phase. The normal minimum dorsiflexion for this test is 5-7 degrees past the 90-degree ankle position, or 95-97 degrees.

Also evaluate dorsiflexion mobility in the following two knee positions: with the knee flexed, which is intended to relax the gastrocnemius muscle, and again with the knee extended (Figures 3.17 and 3.18). If the same measurement is obtained in both knee positions and that measurement is less than the minimums described above, limitation is evident in both the gastrocnemius and soleus muscles.

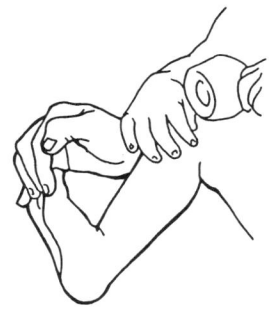 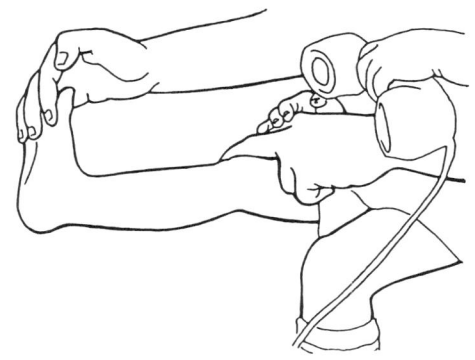

Figure 3.17
Align the subtalar joint (STJ) in neutral (congruent) position, then assess ankle dorsiflexion with the knee flexed . . .

Figure 3.18 . . . and with the knee extended, to detect any possible influence of the gastrocnemius muscle on limitation of motion.
(Normal range of dorsiflexion = 8-15 degrees; minimum = 5-7 degrees.)

Consider, too, the presence of hypertonus, a bony block, or capsular limitation at the ankle joint (Jordan et al. 1983; McCrea 1985; Brooks 1985).

Take two measures in each knee and foot position: initial endpoint (connective tissue and resting muscle length) and final endpoint (passive tissue extensibility). The initial finding is more significant to function than the final measure.

The Subtalar Joint

Features of Subtalar Joint (STJ) Structure and Alignment

The subtalar joint (STJ) includes only the talus and the calcaneus and their articulating surfaces. The STJ is designed to afford the foot a high degree of adaptability to rotary forces from the body above and from the ground below. The STJ communicates those rotary forces via supination and pronation from the leg to the forefoot and vice versa through its biomechanical interconnections with the lower leg (rearfoot complex) and the midtarsal joint (MTJ). In the normal foot, the motions of supination and pronation—as they occur at both the STJ and MTJ—help maintain a balance of the arches of the foot. The muscles that execute each motion counterbalance each other in the effort to maintain stability in the foot in gait, especially on difficult terrain (Salek 1977; Hamilton 1985; Regnauld 1986).

The STJ axis is triplanar, aligning within all three planes. The axis lies at an average of 42 degrees relative to the transverse plane, with a normal range of 21-69 degrees (Figure 3.19). It lies at an average of 16 degrees relative to the sagittal plane, with a normal range of 4-47 degrees (Figure 3.20) (Root et al. 1971; Wright et al. 1964; Mann

Figure 3.19 STJ Axis (frontal plane view). Average pitch = 42 degrees to the transverse plane. Lower pitch to the transverse plane produces increased mobility of the frontal plane component of supination and pronation: inversion and eversion. Higher pitch reduces frontal plane mobility and increases the transverse plane component: abduction and adduction.

Figure 3.20 STJ Axis (overhead view). Average pitch = 16 degrees medial to the sagittal plane. Lower pitch to the sagittal and transverse planes produces increased frontal plane (inversion and eversion) mobility. Higher pitch to the sagittal plane (closer to the frontal plane) increases sagittal plane mobility (dorsiflexion/plantarflexion).

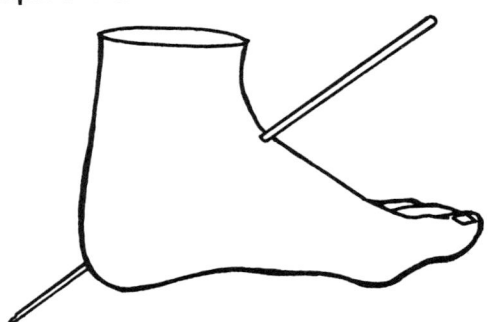

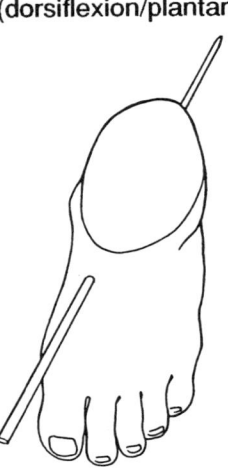

Figure 3.21 STJ Axis. Note inversion and eversion capability around the axis.

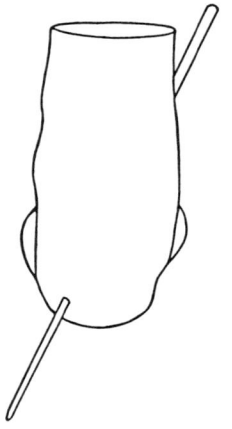

Figure 3.22 STJ Axis. Note the abduction and adduction capability around the axis (with minimal dorsiflexion/ plantarflexion).

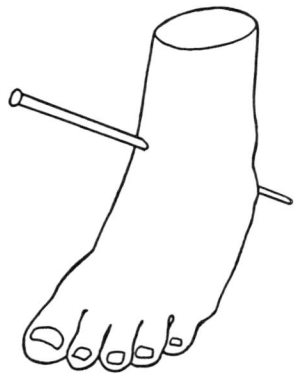

1985 in Jahss; Hicks 1953; Frankel et al. 1980). The location and pitch of this triplanar axis allows the calcaneus to move, thus combining primary calcaneal inversion and eversion, secondary transverse plane abduction and adduction, and minimal dorsiflexion and plantarflexion. These conditions are evident in Figures 3.21 and 3.22. If the pitch to the transverse plane were increased, mobility into inversion and eversion would decrease and abduction and adduction (or transverse plane mobility) would increase. Axial pitch is a function of the structure of the calcaneus and the talus and their articulations (Root et al. 1977).

Posterior talocalcaneal articulation—The frontal plane stability of the hindfoot depends upon sagittal plane alignment of the posterior talus on the calcaneus, within a small degree of deviation (Frankel et al. 1980; McCrea 1985; Regnauld 1986). The posterior facets of both the talus and the calcaneus are contoured so that the center of the calcaneal surface is convex, and the talar surface is concave (Figure 3.4). This configuration requires that the motions of inversion and eversion follow a modified rule of convex and concave. In the open-chain, as the calcaneus everts and inverts, the proximal posterior calcaneus glides on the more stationary talar body. In the closed-chain, the talus and calcaneus glide against each other in opposite directions. A small measure of rotary motion on the transverse plane (abduction and adduction) also occurs at this articulation (Riegger 1988).

Anterior/medial talocalcaneal articulation—The anterior talar facet is convex and can be divided into medial and lateral subsections. The adjoining facets on the calcaneus are curved together into a concavity, cupping the talar facets while allowing the talus to slide forward and backward in a diagonal trough that angles the medial to the sagittal plane. The medial anterior talar facet articulates with the superior supporting surface of the shelf-like sustentaculum tali of the calcaneus. The lateral anterior talar facet is located on the plantar-lateral aspect of the neck of the talus, where it articulates with an inclined ridge on the distal dorsal-superior surface of the calcaneus (Hamilton 1985).

Radiologic Assessment

Weight-bearing roentgenograms of the foot structures can be enlightening to the clinician who is gathering objective data about the effectiveness of various interventions to reduce foot deformity. A growing body of normative data is accumulating in the literature and will contribute significantly to the clinical significance of radiographic findings, of which there are many, including the following:

Calcaneal inclination—When the sagittally aligned foot is viewed on the frontal plane, the plantar border of the calcaneus forms an angle of inclination with the transverse plane (Figure 3.23). This angle increases from an average of 12 degrees in the newborn to approximately 22 degrees in the adult (Regnauld 1986; Vanderwilde et al. 1988). Tachdjian (1985) suggests, however, that the normal calcaneal inclination angle in children is 20-25 degrees, and approaches abnormality at 30 degrees. McCrea (1985) reports that the normal calcaneal inclination falls within a range of 15-30 degrees.

Talar declination—On a frontal plane view, the talus seats on the calcaneus in a position of plantarflexion. The angle formed by the longitudinal bisection of the talus and the transverse plane increases with pronation and reduces with supination in the closed-chain.

Radiologic assessment reveals that in calcaneal midposition, the average pitch is 26.5 degrees (S.D. 5.3 degrees) to the transverse plane by the age of 8 years (Bleck et al. 1977; Tachdjian 1985). This pitch diminishes linearly from a starting angle of approximately 35 degrees in infancy to an average adult value of 21.5 degrees (DiGiovanni et al. 1976; Regnauld 1986; Vanderwilde et al. 1988) (Figure 3.23).

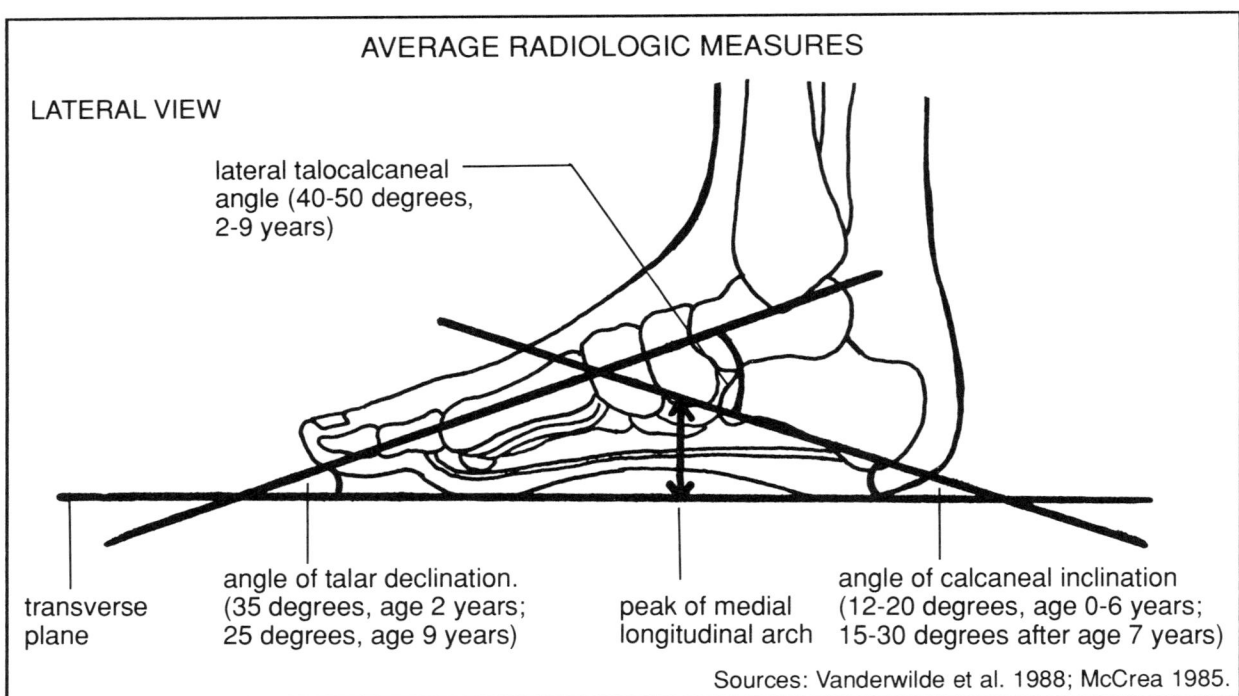

AVERAGE RADIOLOGIC MEASURES

LATERAL VIEW

lateral talocalcaneal angle (40-50 degrees, 2-9 years)

transverse plane

angle of talar declination. (35 degrees, age 2 years; 25 degrees, age 9 years)

peak of medial longitudinal arch

angle of calcaneal inclination (12-20 degrees, age 0-6 years; 15-30 degrees after age 7 years)

Sources: Vanderwilde et al. 1988; McCrea 1985.

Figure 3.23

Lateral talocalcaneal angle—On a frontal plane view of the foot, the lines formed by the longitudinal bisection of the talus with the calcaneal inclination intersect to form the lateral talocalcaneal angle. The angle remains close to a mean of approximately 40 degrees (with a range as wide as 15-60 degrees) throughout infancy and childhood. DiGiovanni et al. (1976) determined that this angle averages 45 degrees in adults. It reduces with supination and equinus deviations, and it increases with subtalar joint pronation (McCrea 1985; Vanderwilde et al. 1988).

Dorsoplantar talocalcaneal angle—From an overhead (dorsoplantar) view, the talocalcaneal angle is determined by the intersection of the longitudinal axes of the calcaneus and the talus. DiGiovanni et al. (1976) and Bleck et al. (1977) measure this angle by intersecting a line bisecting the head and neck of the talus with a line drawn parallel with the lateral surface of the calcaneus.

Vanderwilde et al. (1988) report a linear decline in the mean for this angle. On a graph of findings, this mean value approximates 42 degrees at birth and lowers to approximately 22 degrees at age 9 years. McCrea (1985) reports a normal angle of 15-20 degrees. Both DiGiovanni et al. (1976) and Bleck et al. (1977) report norms of 18 degrees.

Features of Subtalar Joint Motion

The STJ allows supination and pronation around its triplanar axis. The pitch of the axis to the various planes determines the relative proportions of the components of these motions: inversion and eversion; adduction and abduction; and plantarflexion and dorsiflexion.

Open-chain STJ motion—Off weight-bearing, STJ motions of supination and pronation result primarily in movement of the lower segment (calcaneus and forefoot) on the more stationary talus. The tibia and fibula do not alter alignment in response to these open-chain foot motions. The distal segment is free.

Closed-chain STJ motion—With the calcaneus loaded (as in standing and during the stance phase of gait), the closed kinetic chain operates to maneuver the talus within all three planes simultaneously, and, thus, within no pure plane at any time. With pronation, the talus rotates into adduction while plantarflexing as it slides forward and medially on a diagonal. With supination, the talus abducts (rotates laterally) while dorsiflexing as it slides posterolaterally on a diagonal.

During the motion of pronation, the calcaneus simultaneously everts and adducts (rotates medially) under the sliding talus while it plantarflexes to varying degrees. With supination, the calcaneus inverts and abducts under the talus while it dorsiflexes. Therefore, although the calcaneus is weight-loaded in the closed-chain, it is only distally "fixed" against moving its location on the ground (Root et al. 1977).

When bone structure is normal, the following factors are essential to the efficient function of the STJ:

- Integrity of the supporting ligaments.
- Balanced muscle power.
- Well-organized weight shifts (Jones 1975; Salek 1977; Root et al. 1977; Frankel et al. 1980; Jordan et al. 1983; Jordan 1984; McCrea 1985; Gray 1986; Regnauld 1986; Franco 1987).

Assessing the Foot—Special Considerations

The foot is a complicated and intricate instrument of support and movement. Standardization of observations regarding its alignment and motions is necessary to the decision-making processes that apply to intervention, as well as to effective communication of findings among members of the management team. To date, such standardization does not exist. Researchers have found that the reliability quotients of goniometric measurements of the structural and mobility status of the ankle and foot joints is poor among different examiners, falling to as low as .17 (Oatis 1988). This poverty of interrater reliability suggests that the segments are being manipulated, viewed, and measured in variable ways.

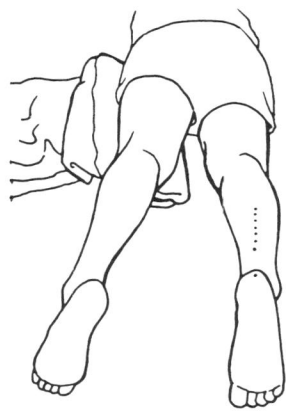

Figure 3.24
Positioning in prone for open-chain STJ assessment with the knee extended. Align the foot on the sagittal plane by elevating the opposite side of the pelvis.

Observe the motions of the hindfoot and forefoot from a sagittal plane perspective. To minimize factors that would reduce goniometric reliability, position the patient in prone with the feet hanging off the end of a table. Then, if needed, flex and abduct the opposite leg (or insert a folded towel under the opposite hip) in order to align the posterior tuberosities of the calcaneus on the frontal plane (Figure 3.24). For goniometric assessment, this is the preferred testing position (Oatis 1988).

Maintain a true sagittal plane view of the leg and foot while assessing foot joint motions. It is imperative that the child's body segments, as well as the examiner's eyes, not move from their alignment on the sagittal plane of the segment. Oblique perspectives are useless in determining STJ and MTJ structural integrity and alignment.

Full plantarflexion of the ankle moves the narrow end of the talus into the tibiofibular mortice, and frontal plane motion of the talus is possible. Such talar motion distorts or exaggerates any findings and must be avoided. Maintain the ankle joint in a comfortable angle of dorsiflexion during STJ assessment to seat the talar trochlea in the ankle mortice.

If you have observed limitation of ankle dorsiflexion only with the child's knee extended, then position the child in prone with the knee flexed 90 degrees. This will eliminate any hindering of calcaneal motion by a shortened gastrocnemius muscle. Align the viewing angle accordingly (to the posterior aspect of the leg and foot), and be careful to maintain the raised lower leg on the sagittal and frontal planes.

When undertaking open-chain assessments in this position, I use an angle finder as a measurement tool (described previously—see Assessing for Apparent Tibial Varum). I repeatedly check to ensure that the distal lower leg is aligned on the sagittal plane before I measure the calcaneal and forefoot positions. (For more details of STJ assessment procedures with the angle finder, see Chapter 7.)

Assessing STJ Mobility

Assess subtalar motion by moving the calcaneus on the frontal plane into inversion and eversion, with the distal lower leg stabilized and the ankle dorsiflexed gently (Figures 3.25 and 3.26). Apply only gentle pressure to move the calcaneus. Do not force it. While maintaining the calcaneus at the endpoint of inversion:

- Align one arm of the goniometer on the distal lower leg bisection.
- Align the other arm of the goniometer on the vertical calcaneal bisection.
- Let the joint of the goniometer fall accordingly, after placing the arms on the bisections.
- Repeat the procedure with the calcaneus aligned in maximum eversion.

The resulting angles measured between the vertical bisection of the calcaneus and the vertical bisection of the distal lower leg indicate the total range of frontal-plane mobility. This total range averages close to 45 degrees in newborns, and 25-30 degrees in the mature foot. The normal range varies widely, however, from 20-60 degrees (Oatis 1988). The average range allows 15-25 degrees of inversion and 4-6 degrees of eversion, relative to calcaneal midposition. The minimum total range needed for normal walking is somewhere between 8 and 12 degrees, including at least 4 degrees of eversion past calcaneal midposition. This eversion mobility is needed for adequate absorption of shock at initial foot contact and weight assumption (Root et al. 1971).

Figure 3.25 Assessing STJ mobility in a 4-year-old child. Set the calcaneal bisection parallel with the lower leg bisection. Stabilize the ankle in dorsiflexion (unforced). Invert the calcaneus; measure the angle formed by the posterior, vertical calcaneal and lower leg bisections. (In the illustration, the calcaneus inverts 20 degrees.)

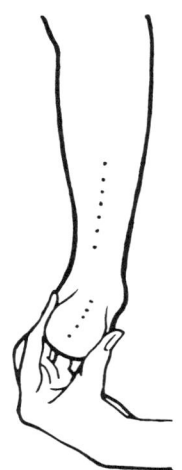

Figure 3.26 . . . Then evert the calcaneus and measure. (The figure reveals 9 degrees of eversion.) Note the 2:1 relationship between the measurements as a ratio of inversion to eversion, relative to calcaneal midposition. Given full extensibility of the surrounding tissues, these ranges indicate that STJ neutral (STN) is 0, as the heel everts 1/3 of the total range past STN.

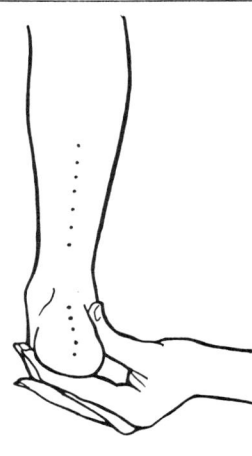

Two methods exist to determine the existing amount of inversion and eversion within the total range:

1. Use calcaneal midposition as the starting position. From this starting point, the range of inversion normally exceeds the range of eversion by a minimum ratio of 2:1. Reported norms show ratios as high as 10:1 (Root et al. 1971; Frankel et al. 1980; Jordan et al. 1983; Mann 1985 in Jahss; Oatis 1988). Oatis (1988) states that Root et al. (1971) "reported that pronation normally contributes two-thirds of the total STJ motion" (p. 1818). Presumably, Oatis intended to use the word "supination" instead of "pronation," which is inaccurate in this context. Root et al. (1971) define STJ neutral position as one of calcaneal midposition and use calcaneal midposition as the starting position.

2. Gray (1984) uses the STJ neutral (congruent) position as the starting position for evaluating frontal plane mobility. Gray (1984) and Giallonardo (1988) perform this assessment by first "locking" the foot structures into neutral (congruent) position. (See Determining Neutral Foot Position, page 156.) Most other authors do not lock the foot structures during this test. This maneuver might alter the starting position and thus the results by a few degrees.

Assessing for Neutral (Congruent) STJ Position

Root et al. (1971 and 1977) define "neutral subtalar position" in the context of external alignment features, in such a way that the foot is neither supinated nor pronated. By their definition, the calcaneus is perpendicular to the ground and parallel to the distal third of the leg (within 2 degrees), as it is optimally during midstance in gait. They state that STJ neutral position is the only one in which the forefoot will "lock" on the hindfoot. They omit the concept of talar head palpation and talonavicular congruity from their definition of neutrality, although they do suggest that some feet exhibit an abnormal neutral position.

Since 1977, most authors of podiatric and physical therapy literature regarding the biomechanics of the foot include a palpations test for talonavicular congruity as a criterion for determining STJ neutral (or maximally congruent) position (Jordan et al. 1983; Gray 1984; Oatis 1988; Giallonardo 1988; Milgrom et al. 1985; Tiberio 1988). However, many of these authors seem to use Root's concept of *ideal* STJ neutral interchangeable with the patient's *actual* STJ neutral position. It is now known that when the STJ is aligned in congruity, the calcaneus is typically aligned in varus position relative to the bisection of the distal lower leg. This alignment averages 10 degrees in infants and 2 to 3 degrees in the mature foot (Sgarlato 1971; Jordan et al. 1983; Valmassy 1984; Milgrom et al. 1985; Tiberio 1988). Persistence of this varus configuration might be related to unresolved calcaneal torsion, or it may be related to our evolutionary past, in which we climbed trees using our hands and feet and walked on soft ground. Since then, we have gained maximum weight-bearing stability by lowering both calcaneal tubercles onto the floor. This lowering occurs with the calcaneus aligned perpendicular to the ground.

Because the calcaneal varus values commonly seen in neutral foot position in the open chain do not normally occur in the closed chain, I propose to reduce the definition of STJ neutrality to mean maximum congruity of subtalar and talonavicular joint structures. This congruity might be determined clinically by palpation.

I use the term *calcaneal midposition* to set the alignment of the vertical calcaneal bisection within 2 degrees of the sagittal plane. In open-chain assessment of STJ mobility, calcaneal midposition is the point of reference in which the vertical calcaneal bisection is aligned parallel both to the sagittal plane and to the bisection of the distal third of the lower leg.

In the closed chain, the calcaneus is optimally aligned within 2 degrees of the sagittal plane in relaxed stance and at midstance in gait. It is the stable foot position of Root et al. (1977) The calcaneal plantar tubercles are plantigrade. It is the ideal midpoint of the subtle rotary excursions of the foot and leg that occur in the stance cycle. The angle of *functional calcaneal midposition* is formed by the bisections of the calcaneus in midposition and the distal third of the lower leg in stance. The value recorded for functional calcaneal midposition is frequently used in molding splints and casts for orthoses for children with neuromotor impairment. (The calcaneus might be set in 2 degrees varus within this context.)

I urge that a cross-disciplinary congress of informed clinicians gather at an outstanding medical library to spend time together to sort out the conflicting meanings within the terms that are currently in use and to agree upon a new list of working definitions. Until then (as was done previously with anteversion and antetorsion in this text), the terms listed above, which describe the various STJ or calcaneal positions of congruity and function, will be used in this text.

The determination of STJ congruity (that is, neutrality) is made more easily in the mature foot (after the age of 7 years) than in the foot of a very young child. The child's changing long bone structure and joint alignment—including talar torsion and tibial plafond eversion as well as the presence of fatty tissue under the foot—might interfere with palpations of the talar head and might render precise clinical measurement of STJ neutrality unattainable, or the findings somewhat debatable (Bahler 1986). The lack of ossification in the young child's foot and ankle bones also reduces the visibility of the bone structures on radiologic examination. With these limitations in mind, three methods of clinical assessment are presented here (Jordan et al. 1983; Gray 1984; Oatis 1988; Giallonardo 1988).

Method I—Open-chain palpation of the head of the talus

When the STJ and the MTJ are neutrally aligned, 80-90 percent of the talar head is covered by the proximal navicular and the supporting ligamentous bands (McCrea 1985). Therefore, the talar head cannot be palpated easily in its neutral (that is, maximally congruent) position.

Because the lower segment dorsiflexes, everts, and abducts with pronation, and it plantarflexes, inverts, and adducts with supination, these motions of the lower segment uncover the head of the talus. It becomes prominent on the medial side of the foot with pronation and on the dorsum of the foot with supination. (Refer to Figures 3.27 and 3.28 for assistance in identifying bony landmarks and articulations.)

First, find the navicular on the midpoint of the medial aspect of the foot. It is usually located between 2 and 3 cm (1 to 1½ inches) diagonally below and distal (anterior) to the apex of the medial malleolus. It forms the keystone of the longitudinal arch. Its tuberosity is usually easy to see as well as to palpate. In the infant and small child, the navicular is undersized and cartilaginous and is often covered with fatty tissue (McCrea 1985; Tachdjian 1985).

Find the talar head just proximal to the navicular, with which it articulates. Pronation of the lower segment is usually required to expose the talar head enough to be palpable. With pronation, the medial talar head protrudes from behind the navicular articulation as the latter moves away from the talar head (Jordan et al. 1983; Gray 1986). At the same time, a sulcus appears on the dorsum of the foot, left by the displaced head of the talus (Jordan et al. 1983).

The lateral aspect of the talar head is uncovered with supination of the lower segment. The talar head appears and is easily palpated on the proximal dorsum of the foot, just lateral to the midline and under the tendon of the long toe extensors after it crosses the ankle joint. The medial side of the head of the talus disappears, leaving a sulcus behind the tuberosity of the navicular when the foot is supinated (Jordan et al. 1983).

At the midpoint where the medial and lateral sides of the head of the talus cannot be palpated, congruency—or STJ and MTJ neutrality—is achieved (Jordan et al. 1983; Gray 1984; Giallonardo 1988). If the talar head is large, a slight protrusion might remain evident on both sides. The talar head is the only bone in the foot that protrudes and recedes with motion.

IDENTIFYING AND PALPATING THE BONES AND JOINTS OF THE FOOT AND ANKLE

MEDIAL ASPECT

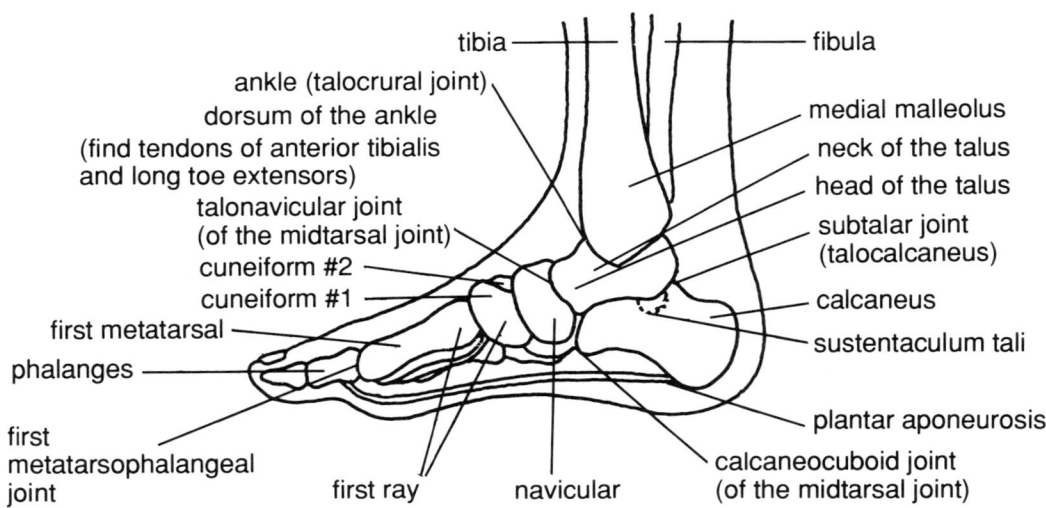

- Locate the medial malleolus.

- Palpate the sustentaculum tali 2 cm directly below the medial malleolus. (It is usually sensitive, and pressure on it is painful.)

- Divide the medial aspect of the foot in half, excluding toes. Find the navicular tuberosity at the center. It is often prominent and visibly detectable.

- The head of the talus lies directly proximal to the navicular, because the two bones form the talonavicular joint within the midtarsal joint. The talar head is difficult to palpate with the foot in neutral position. This is because the talar head fits into the navicular facet that covers up to 90 percent of the talar head surface. To palpate the talar head, *pronate* the foot. A small rounded convexity appears proximal to the navicular tuberosity with pronation.

- Palpate the narrow seam formed at the talonavicular joint, and follow the seam to the dorsum of the foot. Note the proximity of the MTJ to the ankle.

- The first ray includes the first cuneiform and first metatarsal. Palpate the navicular and move your finger distally toward the great toe. The first cuneiform articulates proximally with the navicular, where the motions of dorsiflexion/inversion and plantarflexion/eversion occur.

- Hyperextend the hallux (great toe). Note concurrent first ray plantarflexion and the windlass effect by which increased tension on the medial plantar aponeurosis raises the height of the arch (by first ray plantarflexion) and draws the calcaneus into inversion with dorsiflexion.

Figure 3.27

IDENTIFYING AND PALPATING
THE BONES AND JOINT OF THE FOOT

LATERAL ASPECT

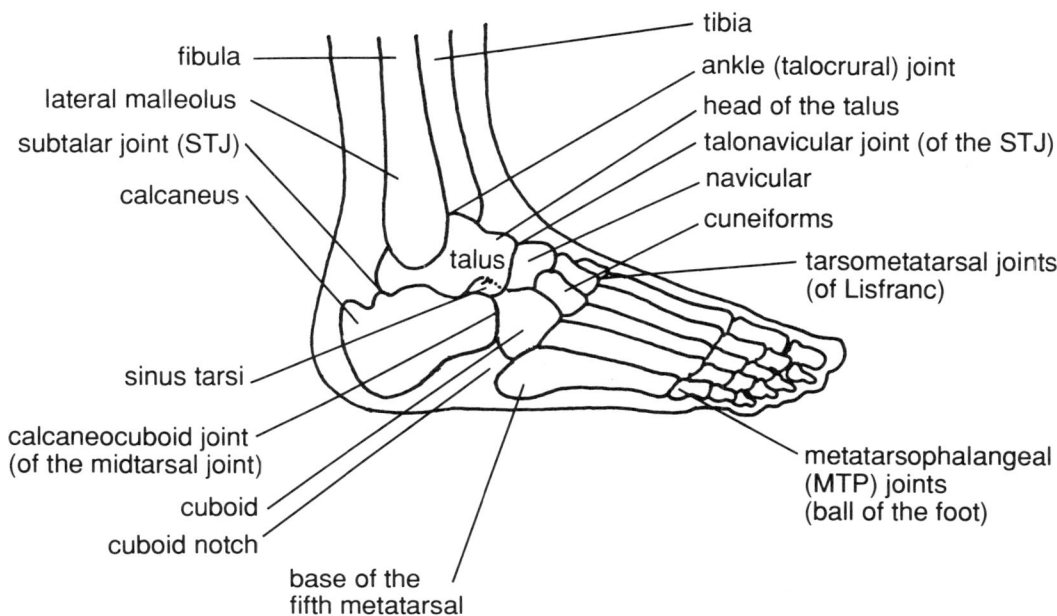

Adapted from M. Tachdjian, *The Child's Foot.* 1985. Philadelphia, PA: W. B. Saunders Co.

- Locate the lateral malleolus and find its distal anterior edge.

- Move diagonally down and forward approximately 2 cm (3/4-inch) to find a small hole — the sinus tarsi — not evident in infants and preschoolers. This opening between the talus and the calcaneus closes while the lower segment pronates.

- Find the base of the fifth metatarsal, in the center of the lateral plantar surface of the foot. It protrudes.

- Move your finger posterior to it to locate the cuboid, at the peak of the cuboid notch. Palpate the cuboid bone. It is broad and flat.

- Try to feel the groove of the calcaneal cuboid joint within the cuboid notch.

Figure 3.28

With the STJ thus aligned in neutral position, the following angles should be measured and noted:

- The angle formed by the vertical bisection of the calcaneus and the distal lower leg.
- The angle formed by the plantar plane of the metatarsal heads and the vertical calcaneal bisection.

These measures will be replicated at the time of molding when progressive casts are made to reduce equinovalgus deformity. The measurements will also be used in mathematical reference and adjusted as needed to achieve functional calcaneal midposition when molding the foot and ankle for devices needed for functional stance and gait. These measurements are useful when preparing splints and certain types of orthoses.

Method II—Closed-chain talar head palpation

Position the child in standing.

- Palpate the talar head as described above.
- Rotate the leg (or the trunk) medially and laterally until you achieve talonavicular joint congruity.
- Measure the angle formed by the vertical bisections of the calcaneus and the distal third of the lower leg. This measurement should agree with what you obtained in open-chain assessment. (To use an angle finder to take this measure, see Chapter 7.)

Method III—Open- or closed-chain palpation of the ankle joint dorsal depressions

At times, the talar head is difficult to palpate with certainty. A useful secondary method of determining neutral position of the STJ and the foot structures is to palpate gently the depth of the two depressions (sulci) that appear in the skin at the dorsum of the ankle joint (Price 1982). These depressions are found beside—not between—the tendons of the anterior tibialis and the long toe extensor muscles. Unlike talar head palpations, the dorsal ankle depressions are not a feature of the subtalar joint. They are simply representative of the distribution of soft tissue on the dorsum of the ankle in varying foot positions (Figure 3.29).

- Keep the child's ankle joint comfortably dorsiflexed.
- Place the broad palmar surface of the tips of your thumb and forefinger on the dorsal depressions. Do not create the depressions—merely observe them.
- Move the child's foot through the arc of supination and pronation (Figure 3.30).
- Note the relative depth of the depressions as the foot position changes. With supination, the medial depression deepens and the lateral one fills. The opposite occurs with pronation.
- When you perceive the depth of both depressions to be equal, presume that the STJ is congruent. Measure the calcaneal-lower leg bisection angle. This is STJ neutral position.

Figure 3.29
Determining STJ neutrality, Method III—Dorsal Depressions. Dorsiflex the ankle to a comfortable end point and locate the dorsal depressions, which are the large indentations beside (not between) the tendons of the anterior tibialis and long toe extensors . . .

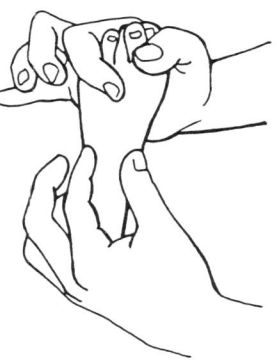

Figure 3.30
. . . Rock the lower segment slowly into supination and pronation, palpating the depressions until the depth is comparatively symmetrical. At the same time, watch the plantar surface of the foot move throught the arc of supination and pronation, and stop at the peak of the arc.

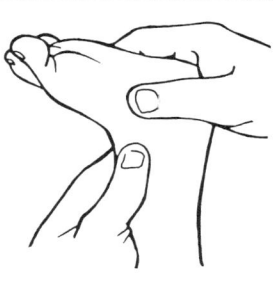

Figure 3.31 "Lock" the forefoot on the hindfoot by gently dorsiflexing the fourth and fifth metatarsal heads on the neutrally aligned STJ and talonavicular joint. Do not abduct nor adduct the forefoot. Keep the second toe in line with the tibial crest.

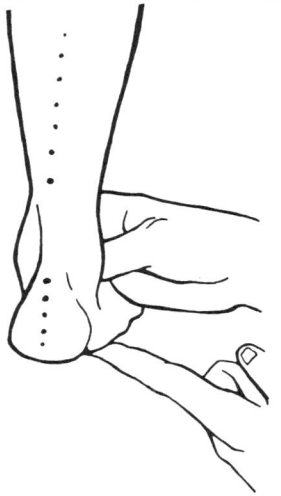

- Repeat the same procedure in the closed chain, using Method II, palpating the dorsal ankle depressions to achieve equal depth.

- Maintain the hindfoot in neutral position, and gently dorsiflex the fourth and fifth metatarsal heads on the sagittal plane. Do not abduct nor adduct the forefoot. Keep the second toe in line with the tibial crest (Figure 3.31).

- You will feel the MTJ and the STJ "lock" in congruity on each other with this maneuver. This locked position is the neutral position of the foot. As discussed previously, it is also used to determine talocrural joint mobility, as a second dorsiflexion mobility test position, in addition to the test for calcaneal mid-position.

Various degrees of calcaneal varus in neutral position are expected in infants and young children (Valmassy 1984; D'Amico 1984). The average newborn foot is congruous with the calcaneus aligned in 10 degrees of varus. This is because of persistent calcaneal torsion. Varus deviation in STN can be exaggerated when using the talo-navicular joint palpation test if talar torsion does not resolve. The lower segment must be inverted to gain congruity between the (undersized) navicular and the talar head. This varus deviation diminishes with age until it approaches 4 degrees by age 5 years, and 2 to 3 degrees at and after the age of 7 years (Jordan et al. 1983; Tiberio 1988).

Rearfoot Complex—The Foot/Leg Connection in the Closed Chain

A significant feature of the STJ is the mortice formed by the talus, the tibia, and the fibula (Figure 3.4). Any closed-chain motion that affects the position of the talus is reflected in a concurrent motion at the lower leg. The triplanar axes of the talocrural and subtalar joints—which together form the rearfoot complex—combine to provide motion in all three body planes, allowing the unrestricted motions of the hip joint to communicate with those of the rearfoot and ankle in the kinematic chain.

During pronation initiated at the foot, calcaneal eversion occurs with medial rotary talar migration, which induces medial deviation and medial rotation at the lower leg via the ankle mortice. The knee joint mechanically flexes (Root et al. 1977; Brooks 1985; Soderberg 1986; Gray 1986; Bahler 1986; Schafer 1987; Rodgers 1988). The proximal consequences include femoral medial rotation, hip adduction with flexion, and anterior pelvic tilt (Jordan et al. 1983) (Figures 3.32 and 3.33). By palpating the greater trochanter of the femur, its anterior and posterior migration is perceptible with minimal degrees of pronation and supination, respectively (Schafer 1987).

During supination of the foot, the dorsal/posterior migration of the talus induces tibial lateral rotation and knee extension (Figure 3.34). More proximally, hip lateral rotation and extension occur as well. The pelvis tilts posteriorly with bilateral foot supination.

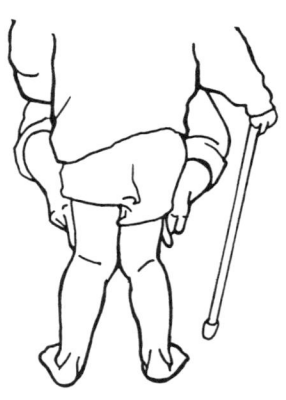

Figure 3.32
Closed-chain pronation (exaggerated)—rear view. Note calcaneal eversion, medial deviation and rotation of the lower legs, hip and knee flexion, hip adduction and medial rotation. (Normal neuromotor status, age 3 years.)

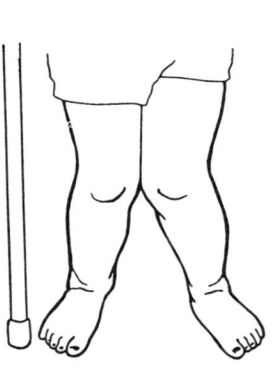

Figure 3.33
Closed-chain pronation (exaggerated)—anterior view. Note forefoot abduction, passive dorsiflexion of the first ray, and toe grasp.

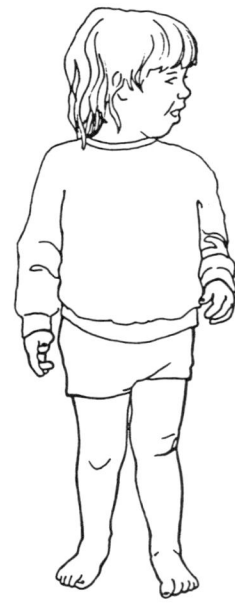

Figure 3.34 Closed-chain supination (evident in the left leg). Note forefoot adduction, lateral/posterior deviation with rotation of the lower leg, knee hyperextension, hip lateral rotation, and pelvic retraction (elevation with lateral rotation).

Subtalar Joint Complex—The STJ/MTJ Connection in the Closed Chain

(Refer to Figures 3.35-3.43.)

The orientation of the axes of the STJ and the midtarsal joint (MTJ) combine to provide the foot structures with ample motion on all three body planes. The closed-chain motions of supination and pronation of the STJ (as described previously) cannot occur without the participation of the midtarsal joint as it affects the forefoot. (For more detail regarding the structure and function of the MTJ, see Midtarsal Joint, following.) The following discussion examines the changes occurring in the alignment of both joints as the foot pronates and supinates.

Pronation—When the balanced foot pronates, as it does during the initial 15 percent of the stance phase of gait, the entire foot is involved. At the STJ, calcaneal eversion up to 6 degrees and talar plantarflexion with adduction predominate. The dome of the medial arch lowers as a result, and topples medially. The distal medial pillar dorsiflexes and abducts around the MTJ and the first ray articulations (Figures 3.35, 3.38, and 3.41). The congruity of the STJ is disrupted. The calcaneus and talus cannot offer the forefoot a secure structural base. The foot becomes a loose adapter for shock absorption and efficient adjustment to uneven terrain (Root et al. 1977; Frankel et al. 1980; Jordan et al. 1983; Mann 1985 in Jahss; Gray 1986).

Supination—The motion of supination also involves the whole foot. At the STJ, talar abduction with dorsiflexion occurs with calcaneal inversion. The proximal medial pillar elevates while the distal segments plantarflex and adduct. The dome of the medial longitudinal arch rises. The distal lateral pillar (cuboid and fourth and fifth metatarsals) dorsiflexes under weight-bearing compression (Figures 3.37, 3.40, and 3.43). Tension is applied to the short plantar calcaneocuboid ligament, to the lateral bands of the long plantar ligament (located between the calcaneus and the bases of the lateral four metatarsals), and to the plantar tarsometatarsal ligaments. The foot structures stabilize at the endpoint of the extensibility of the tendons of support.

Supination moves the foot structures into congruity. The neutrally aligned STJ provides a stable base for the forefoot to achieve congruous articulation. The forefoot "locks" on the neutrally aligned hindfoot. Weight-bearing in neutral position uses the foot as a rigid lever for efficient carriage of the body over the foot between terminal stance and toe-off. The magic of the rapid conversion from pronated loose adapter in early stance to supinated rigid lever at late stance is the weight shift of the center of gravity over the stance foot, combined with the descending lateral rotary forces that are initiated at the hip joint (Root et al. 1977; Jordan et al. 1983; Sutherland 1984; Gray 1986).

Figure 3.35 Pronation (right foot, medial view). Compare to Figure 3.36. Note tibiofibular medial rotation and talar plantarflexion as components of the rearfoot complex. Note forefoot dorsiflexion at the talonavicular joint, and first ray dorsiflexion at the naviculocuneiform joint.

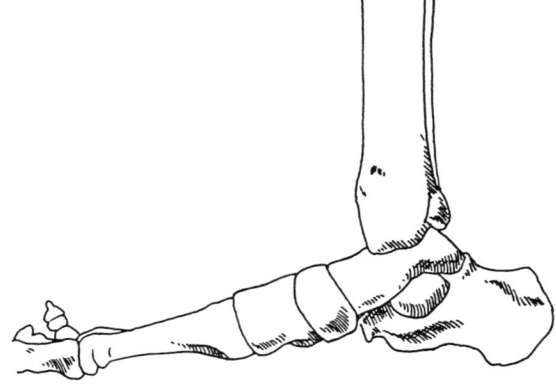

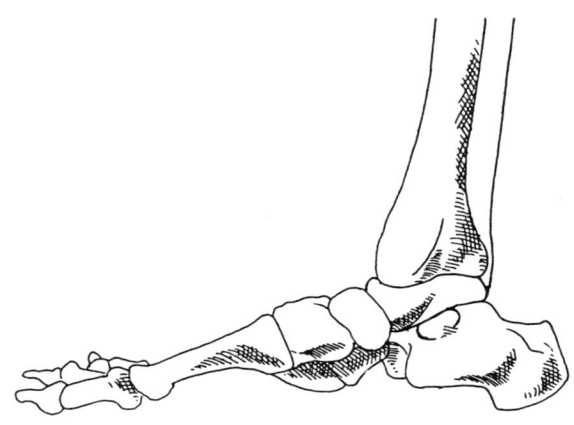

Figure 3.36 Calcaneal midposition (right foot, medial view).

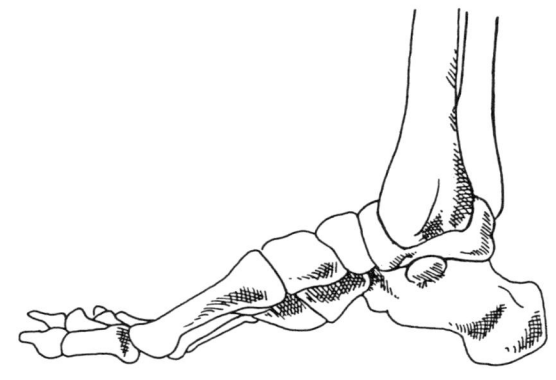

Figure 3.37 Supination (right foot, medial view). Note tibiofibular lateral rotation and posterior deviation, and talar dorsiflexion. The medial longitudinal arch is increased in height. The first ray plantarflexes to maintain contact with the ground.

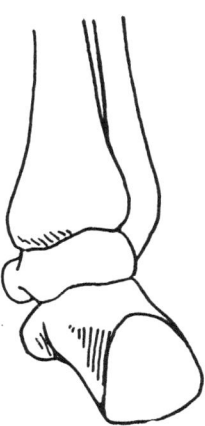
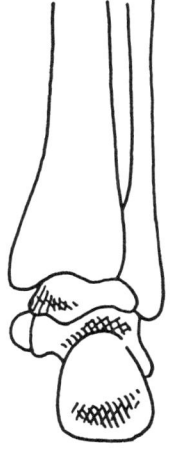
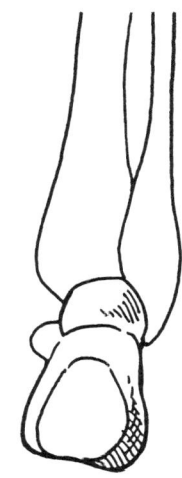

Fig 3.38
Pronation (right foot, posterior view—extreme). Note talar adduction and calcaneal eversion.

Figure 3.39
Calcaneal midposition (right foot, posterior view). Note the sustentaculum tali on medial calcaneus. Note the contour of the posterior talocalcaneal articulation.

Figure 3.40
Supination (right foot, posterior view). Note lateral tibiofibular rotation and lateral deviation, and calcaneal inversion.

Figure 3.41   Pronation (right foot, overhead view). Note forefoot (MTJ) and first ray dorsiflexion, MTJ dorsiflexion with abduction, and talar adduction.

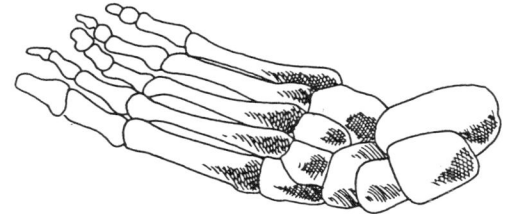

Figure 3.42   Neutral foot position (right foot, overhead view). Note congruity between talar head and navicular.

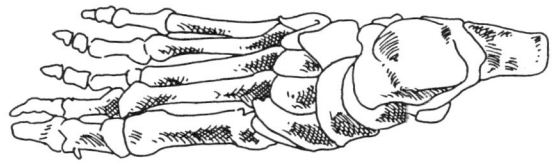

Figure 3.43   Supination (right foot, overhead view). Note MTJ adduction and plantarflexion, dorsiflexion of the lateral rays, and talar abduction.

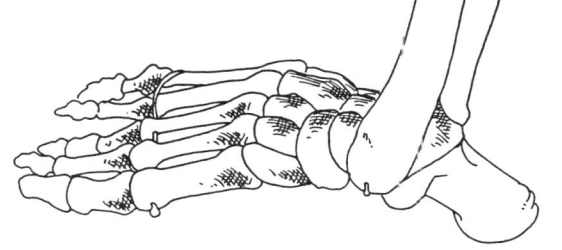

The Midtarsal Joint (Transverse Tarsal)

Features of Structure and Joint Function

The MTJ divides the forefoot and midfoot from the hindfoot (Jordan et al. 1983). (Figure 3.1) It minimizes rotary forces from the ground to the leg. It also communicates and accommodates—via its interaction with the STJ—rotary forces that descend from the proximal joints to the metatarsal heads (Root et al. 1977; Jordan et al. 1983; Regnauld 1986).

Four bones, rather than two, comprise the midtarsal joint (MTJ). These four bones—the talus, the navicular, the calcaneus, and the cuboid—articulate with each other to form two sets of axes: anatomical (between the articulating bones joining the hindfoot and the forefoot) and functional (incorporating the hindfoot and forefoot segments of the entire MTJ).

The anatomical joints are:

- The talonavicular joint, a multiaxial ball-and-socket joint formed by the articulation between the talus and navicular and the surrounding bands of the plantar and deltoid ligaments.

- The calcaneocuboid joint, a saddle-shaped joint between the calcaneus and the cuboid bones (Figures 3.1, 3.2, and 3.3).

Each of these joints within the MTJ has an axis that aligns in the frontal plane, as their articulating surfaces fall on the frontal plane and perpendicular to the subtalar joint (Hicks 1953) (Figures 3.2 and 3.3). The available mobility within the MTJ is dependent upon STJ alignment. As discussed previously, when the STJ is pronated, MTJ mobility increases in all directions, while the supinated STJ imposes restriction on MTJ mobility (Root et al. 1971; Frankel et al. 1980; Jordan et al. 1983; Mann 1985 in Jahss). These changes occur because the change of position of the calcaneus and talus in pronation alters the pitch of the talonavicular and calcaneocuboid axes, which become parallel to each other. In this way, the combined axes increase their potential for mobility. In supination, the same axes lose this parallel relationship, approximating each other at the medial ends, and motion is prohibited around either of them (Frankel et al. 1980; Mann 1985 in Atlas).

The Functional Axes

The navicular and cuboid tend to operate in a state of relative congruity with each other. Because of this, they are considered as a single structural component of the entire MTJ and its two functional axes, both of which are oblique to all three pure body planes. Supination and pronation occur around each of these axes, in proportions relative to their respective planar pitches.

Planar pitch of the axes can vary between individual feet also, with variations in bone structure (Root et al. 1977). The closer an axis lies in proximity to a pure plane, the greater the capacity for motion in the plane that is perpendicular to the axis.

The oblique axis—The position of the oblique axis resembles the TMA and lies anterior to it, though closer than the TMA in proximity to the sagittal plane (Figure 3.44). The oblique axis forms an average pitch of 52 degrees to the transverse plane (Figure 3.45), and 57 degrees medial to the sagittal plane (or 33 degrees lateral to the frontal plane). The close proximity of the oblique axis to the frontal plane results in primary motion on the sagittal plane. This produces primary dorsiflexion and plantarflexion of both the navicular and the cuboid, with concurrent secondary abduction and adduction, and negligible inversion or eversion (Root et al. 1977). The mobility around this axis can be expected to approach a combined total of 22 degrees of dorsiflexion and plantarflexion with abduction and adduction (Hicks 1953).

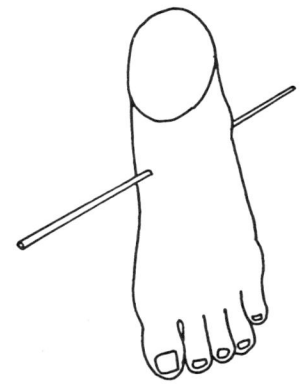

Figure 3.44 Midtarsal joint (MTJ)—oblique axis (overhead view). Average pitch = 33 degrees lateral to the frontal plane. (Note similarity to ankle axis.) Allows primary dorsiflexion/plantarflexion with secondary abduction and adduction and minimal eversion/inversion. A decrease in pitch to the frontal plane increases primary sagittal plane mobility.

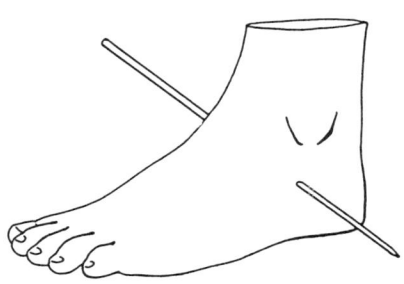

Figure 3.45 MTJ—oblique axis (lateral view). Average pitch = 52 degrees to the transverse plane. Note transverse plane motion (abduction and adduction) capability. A decrease in the pitch reduces transverse plane mobility and increases it on the frontal plane.

The longitudinal axis—This axis lies at an average pitch of 15 degrees to the transverse plane (Figure 3.46), and 9 degrees medial to the sagittal plane (Figure 3.47). The primary motion of frontal plane rotation—inversion and eversion of the navicular and cuboid on the hindfoot—occurs around this axis because of its close proximity to the transverse plane. The rotary mobility in the forefoot can be expected to total 8 degrees (Hicks 1953). The minimum range of forefoot inversion mobility required for normal function of the foot is 4 to 6 degrees, to allow adequate compensation for the 4 to 6 degrees of calcaneal eversion that occurs optimally during the pronatory phase of stance in gait (Root et al. 1977). This finding of 8 degrees of

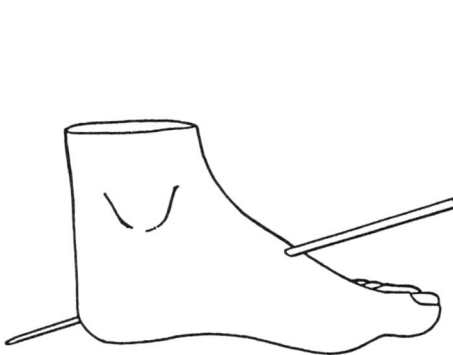

Figure 3.46 MTJ—longitudinal axis (medial view). Average pitch = 15 degrees to transverse plane. Note primary frontal plane motion (inversion and eversion) potential, which increases by reducing the pitch. The secondary motions of supination and pronation are minimal around this axis.

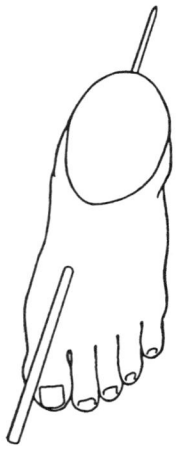

Figure 3.47 MTJ—longitudinal axis (overhead view). Average pitch = 9 degrees medial to the sagittal plane. Note the potential for frontal plane motion.

normal MTJ mobility, however, can be expanded considerably by adding both of the following:

- The normal 10-22 degrees of movement of the first ray into plantarflexion with open-chain pronation and into dorsiflexion with open-chain supination.

- The normal 10 degrees of flexion with supination and of extension with pronation observed in the fifth ray in the open chain (Root et al. 1977; Hicks 1953).

The two functional MTJ axes thus combine to provide movement within the foot on all three planes.

STJ/MTJ Stability—Maintaining the Arches

By aligning the feet adjacent to each other with the medial surfaces contacting, the longitudinal and transverse arches together form a wide-mouthed, short cone. The body weight is distributed around the perimeter of this cone, on the lateral pillars and the metatarsal heads (Schafer 1987). The arches that form the cone are compliant by design; they yield to the myriad of forces imposed upon them. This flexibility serves to minimize the influence of those forces on the body's equilibrium.

The longitudinal and transverse arches are intrinsically stable because of the shape of the bones and their intimate congruity in the close-packed position. The bones are designed to deviate in predictable patterns of supination and pronation in response to externally applied rotary forces (Mann 1985 in Jahss). The longitudinal arch can be divided longitudinally into medial and lateral pillars that function differently in the normal foot.

The medial longitudinal arch includes the medial pillar of the foot and the medial calcaneus. It is the dynamic aspect of the foot, altering its alignment and configuration to accommodate the compressive forces incurred in gait (Mann 1985 in Jahss). Supination of the foot increases the height of the medial arch, while pronation reduces it.

The lateral longitudinal arch lies within the lateral pillar and consists of the lateral calcaneus, the cuboid, and the lateral two rays. It is significantly lower in height than the medial arch. The lateral arch typically flattens in the closed chain because of the distribution of weight about the cone's border (Mann 1985 in Jahss). The lateral pillar functions as the point of stability for medial foot motions because body weight is taken on the lateral pillar during most of the stance phase of gait (Mann 1985 in Jahss; Gray 1986). Supination of the foot lowers this arch by forcing the lateral rays—including the cuboid and the fourth and fifth metatarsals—into dorsiflexion.

Integrity of the supporting ligaments is essential to the proper alignment and function of the subtalar joint complex, which incorporates the longitudinal arches (Salek 1977; Bleck et al. 1977; Jordan et al. 1983; Mann 1985 in Jahss; Regnauld 1986; Franco 1987; Riegger 1988). An abundance of ligaments serve to stabilize the talar body on the calcaneus and to maintain the arc of the medial longitudinal arches. Most of these ligaments cross the medial and plantar aspects of the ankle, STJ, and MTJ. In crossing, they restrict pronation strains beyond the normal 4-6 degrees that occur in the earliest phase of the stance cycle (Root et al. 1977; Hamilton 1985; Regnauld 1986; Soderberg 1986; Riegger 1988).

Functional efficiency of the foot depends upon the integrity of these ligaments, which include the following (Hamilton 1985; Regnauld 1986; Soderberg 1986; Franco 1987; Riegger 1988):

- The four large bands of the deltoid ligament medially (Figure 3.48).
- The short plantar calcaneonavicular (spring) ligament (Figure 3.48).
- The long plantar calcaneocuboid ligament (not shown).
- The anterior talofibular ligament laterally (Figure 3.49).
- The ligaments that envelop the talar head and neck: the medial, lateral, posterior, and interosseus talocalcaneal ligaments, and the dorsal talonavicular ligaments.

The medial aspect of the plantar aponeurosis—which connects the medial-plantar aspect of the calcaneal tuberosity with the proximal phalanx of the great toe—aids these ligaments in their supporting function (Figure 3.48). The aponeurosis and the plantar ligaments together bear most of the tension strain imposed on the foot in standing. They maintain a limited distance between the calcaneus and the metatarsal heads and prevent the dome of the longitudinal arch from lowering abnormally. As the great toe hyperextends—as it does during the push-off phase of stance in gait—the plantar

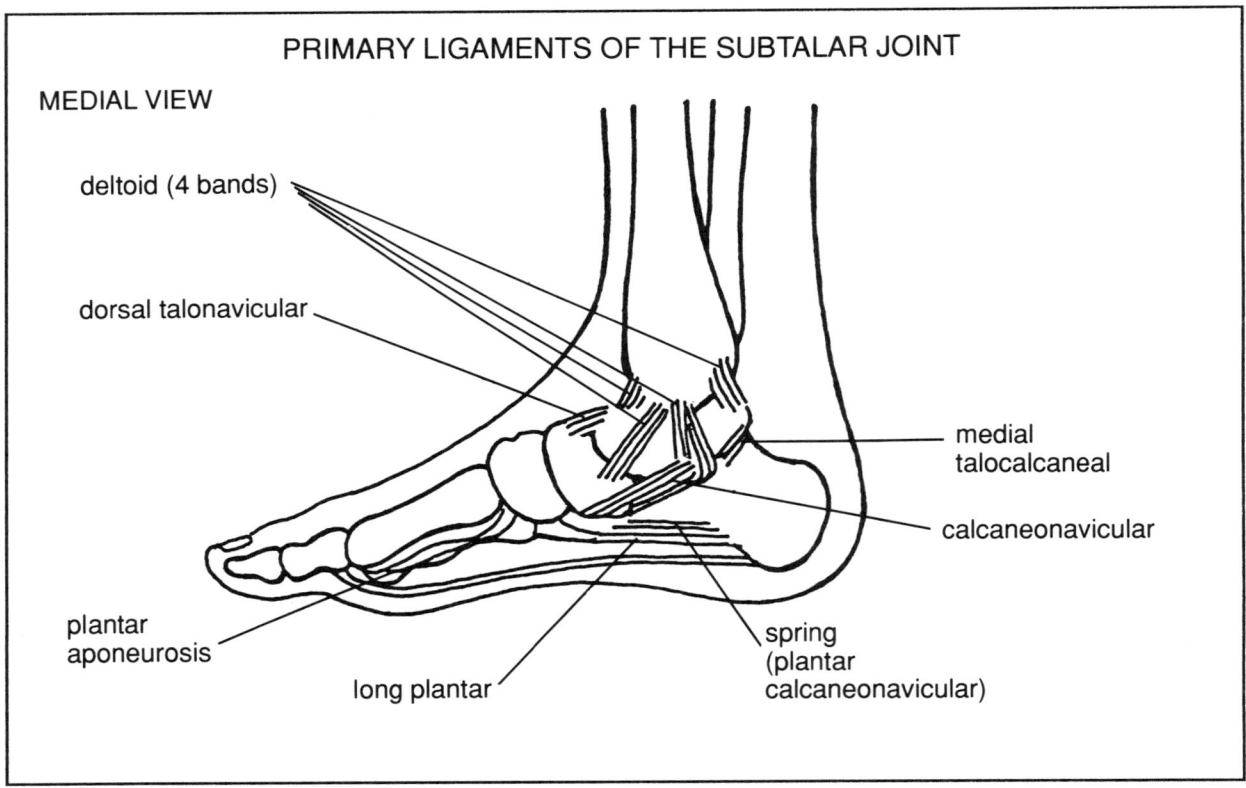

Figure 3.48

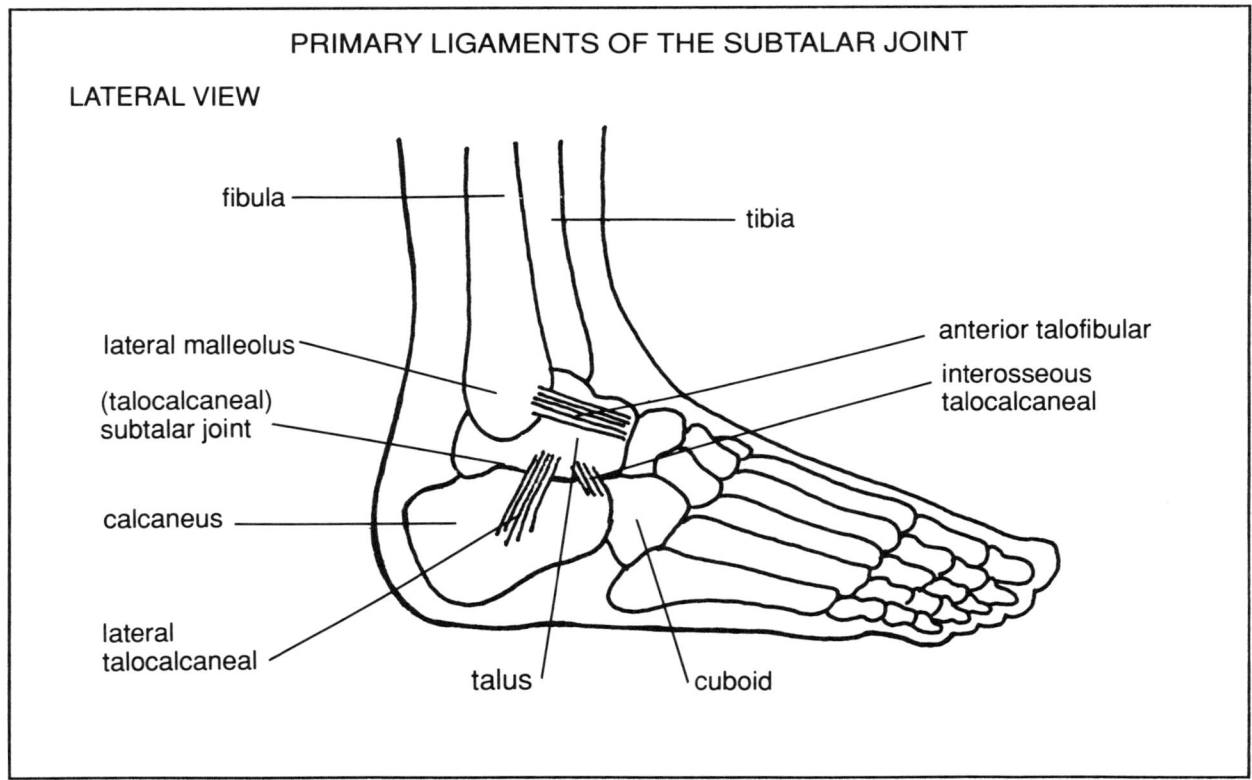

Figure 3.49

aponeurosis exhibits a "windlass effect" in which hyperextension of the first phalanx (together with plantarflexion of the first ray) applies tension to the aponeurosis. At that point the aponeurosis pulls the calcaneus into dorsiflexion and inversion. The windlass effect thereby increases the height of the medial longitudinal arch between the heel-off and toe-off stages of the stance phase of gait. During those stages, the foot is supinating (Salek 1977; Jordan et al. 1983; Soderberg 1986; Gray 1986; Franco 1987; Riegger 1988).

The STJ is inherently more stable medially than laterally, as its medial and plantar aspects are more abundantly endowed with ligamentous support than the lateral aspect (Riegger 1988) (Figure 3.49). Furthermore, the normal range of motion into supination greatly exceeds the normal range into pronation (Hamilton 1985; Oatis 1988). With supination of the foot, lateral rotation of the tibia and fibula occurs with calcaneal inversion and talar abduction. The foot becomes rigid. The increased pitch of the TMA to the frontal plane converts its sagittal-plane primary motion into an inversion motion. Collapse into extreme supination on weight-bearing is a likely event, together with anterior talofibular ligament sprains.

Kinesiological Considerations in Maintaining the Arches

From 12-20 percent of the strain of weight-bearing on the foot is borne by the posterior tibialis and peroneal muscles. Because of their cross-diagonal tendons of insertion on the plantar aspect of the foot, these muscles function like an active stirrup, balancing the medial and lateral muscle forces for inversion and eversion that are needed to maintain equilibrium (Schafer 1987). The peroneus longus muscle tendon of insertion courses around the lateral calcaneus to attach on the plantar surface of the first cuneiform and the base of the first metatarsal. Therefore it stabilizes the first ray in plantarflexion and prohibits it from dorsiflexing abnormally on the navicular. The plantarflexion function of the peroneus longus maintains the pitch of the first ray. Thus it contributes to maintenance of the height of the medial longitudinal arch (Regnauld 1986; Soderberg 1986).

The posterior tibialis courses behind and under the medial malleolus to attach to the plantar aspects of the first cuneiform and the navicular tuberosity, with slips to the bases of the second and fourth metatarsals and the second cuneiform. This muscle provides supinatory forces in stance. The long toe flexors aid these forces by compressing the distal long bones into the tarsals, in accordance with the line of pull of their tendons of insertion. The intrinsics participate in stabilization in stance as well, giving the foot its fluid equilibrium capability (Regnauld 1986; Schafer 1987; Schenkman 1988).

Assessing the Longitudinal Arch

Generate an outline of the weight-bearing foot, either by drawing it with a marker on paper or by forming a footprint out of chalk or ink. The footprint reveals changes that occur with maturation, as pronation diminishes and the plantar fat pad (if present) dissolves. The mean proportional width of the area of the arches relative to that of the heel reduces by small increments approximating:

- 100 percent at age 1 year
- 95 percent at 2 years
- 90 percent at 3 years
- 80 percent at 4 years
- 75 percent at 5 years
- 70 percent at 6-7 years

There is a continuing decline in width percentage until mid-adolescence, at which time the decline ceases and the mean width of the arch approaches 60 percent of the mean width of the heel (Staheli et al. 1987).

By the age of 5 (or earlier in some children) the normal foot in stance is straight on the entire lateral aspect, and the toes are parallel to each other and to their adjacent metatarsals (Root et al. 1971; Jordan et al. 1983). The medial longitudinal arch is visible in weight-bearing; its peak at the navicular bone is approximately 15 mm above the floor (Aharonson et al. 1980).

Determining evidence of pronation—Using chalk or ink, obtain the child's footprints in standing and walking. Notice the configuration of each footprint. On a broad foot, the space between the navicular and a line drawn adjacent to the medial calcaneus and the medial first metatarsal head measures 1 cm or less (Rose et al. 1985). Broad configurations are common among infants and very young children (Rose et al. 1985; Staheli et al. 1987). A concave lateral border together with a convex (bulging) medial border indicate pronatory abnormality in children older than 5 years (Root et al. 1971; Rose et al. 1985).

Heel oval bisection—Outline the heel oval on the footprints for both stance and gait. Bisect the heel oval from anterior to posterior ends, and extend the bisection line to the toes. (See Assessing TMT Alignment on the Transverse Plane, following.) A heel oval that points medially to the great toe is an indication of abnormality in school-age children and adults, but it is not uncommon in preschoolers (Rose et al. 1985).

Valgus index—The valgus index is a mathematical calculation of "percentage shift" of the malleoli to determine their relative versus frontal-plane distance from the heel oval midpoint. Measures are taken on the static footprint. This procedure requires that a set square be used to mark the location of the malleoli on the footprint. Rose derived the valgus index in 1962 as a measure of severity of pronation deformity. He regards it as a significant indicator of abnormality, although he states that the most significant test is the great toe hyperextension test (described following). The higher valgus index values of between 15 and 19 commonly occur together with broad foot types in the school-age child and adult, but the average valgus index for this population is between 9 and 11 percent. The study by Rose et al. (1985) contains details about calculating the ankle joint valgus index from the stance footprint.

Leg rotations—Rotate the weight-bearing lower extremity and observe the influence on the foot. If lateral rotation of the hip joint while maintaining the knee extended elicits supination in the foot and a significant increase in the height of the arch, the STJ is a component of the flattened arch deformity. If no response is evident in the arch, the deviation is more likely a fixed osseous deformity.

Great toe hyperextension—Hyperextend the great toe in the *open chain,* and look for evidence of the windlass effect of the plantar aponeurosis. With toe hyperextension, the medial arch increases dramatically in height, and the calcaneus inverts. If the plantar aponeurosis is permanently overstretched, hyperextension of the great toe does not elicit the windlass effect.

Repeat great toe hyperextension in the *closed chain* and watch again for the normal response of elevation of the medial longitudinal arch combined with lateral rotation of the lower leg. Some children show only one component of the response—a mild elevation of the arch (Rose et al. 1985). Where no response occurs, Rose et al. (1985) state that the existing pronation of the first ray in closed-chain foot pronation shifts the pitch of the first ray axis closer to the sagittal plane, where it prohibits the first ray plantarflexion that is a feature of the windlass effect of the plantar aponeurosis.

Feiss line test—Flexible pes planus is easily distinguished from structural flat foot by this test. If the navicular aligns with the medial malleolus and the first metatarsal head when the foot is off weight-bearing, and it lowers in standing, the deformity is flexible (Giallonardo 1988).

Determining evidence of cavus deformity—There are several varieties of cavus foot—all of which include an abnormal fixed component of supination or varus deformity. The high-arched foot in which the range of STJ eversion past midline is limited is abnormally rigid in stance. Clinical evidence of the lateral longitudinal arch in the closed chain indicates a high calcaneal inclination relative to the transverse plane. This evidence also indicates plantarflexion of the forefoot around the oblique axis of the MTJ and of the first ray as the forefoot seeks contact with the ground.

Footprint evaluation—A static footprint of a cavus-type foot reveals little or no evidence of connection between the hindfoot and the metatarsal heads, because of elevation of the medial and lateral longitudinal arches.

MTJ Function

In considering the forefoot, the primary concern is the midtarsal joint function. In static stance, weight is distributed over the heel, the calcaneocuboid junction, and all the metatarsal heads (Salek 1977; Regnauld 1986; Cavanagh et al. 1987). In a study involving adults, Cavanagh et al. (1987) substantiated the findings of Aharonson et al. (1980) regarding pressure distribution under the foot in relaxed standing. Both researchers found that the heel bears 61 percent of body weight; the forefoot, 28-35 percent; and the midfoot, 4-8 percent. Aharonson's study group included only children at age 4 years.

In gait, the weight is distributed more evenly between the heel and the entire forefoot. In both gait and stance, the forefoot offers the widest—and therefore the most positionally stable—support base. The rule that demands consistent attention, therefore, with regard to the forefoot is this: *The metatarsal heads always seek full contact with the ground.* Regardless of hindfoot function, hindfoot alignment, or the influence on alignment of the proximal segments, the metatarsal heads will attempt to lower to the ground during weight-bearing and walking activities (Root et al. 1977; Jordan et al. 1983; Gray 1984; Gray 1986).

If the forefoot is malaligned relative to the hindfoot, a compensatory malalignment will be imposed at the hindfoot in standing (STJ mobility permitting) to accommodate the rule of forefoot contact (Root et al. 1977; Jordan et al. 1983; McCrea 1985; Bahler 1986; Franco 1987). For example, a varus forefoot may impede the normal and timely conversion of the foot from loose adapter to rigid lever. The lack of mobility into forefoot eversion would cause the hindfoot to remain in pronation throughout the stance phase of gait (Root et al. 1977; Jordan et al. 1983; Gray 1986; Tiberio 1988).

Assessing the MTJ—Longitudinal Axis

I often make this assessment with the child positioned in prone with the knee flexed. I use a gravity-operated angle finder, described previously and illustrated in Figure 3.50, to gather data pertaining to lower leg and foot structures in the following sequence:

1. The lower leg alignment, setting the distal third on the sagittal plane.
2. The calcaneal bisection angle—with the lower leg positioned precisely on the sagittal plane.
3. The forefoot position relative to the transverse plane (Figure 3.50). (For more details about using the angle finder, see Chapter 7.)

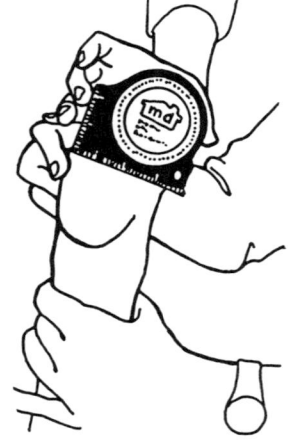

Figure 3.50 Using a gravity-driven angle finder to determine neutral foot position in prone, maintain the knee flexed and the distal lower leg on the sagittal plane. Use the vertical straight edge to measure calcaneal (STN) angle (not shown). Use the horizontal straight edge to determine total transverse plane deviation of the metatarsal heads. Subtract the calcaneal value from the metatarsal heads value to determine forefoot-to-hindfoot alignment.

To undertake goniometric evaluation, as described previously under Assessing for Neutral (Congruent) STJ Position, begin this assessment with the child lying prone, with the foot extending off the support surface and the calcaneal tubercles aligned on the frontal plane. (Roll the leg and pelvis as needed.) (Refer to Figure 3.24.) Maintain a strict sagittal/transverse plane perspective of the plantar surface of the foot throughout this procedure (Root et al. 1971; Jordan et al. 1983; Gray 1984) (Figure 3.51). Proceed as follows:

1. Secure a neutral (congruent) STJ position by palpating the talonavicular joint and/or relative dorsal depression depth.

2. With your thumb on the plantar surface of the fourth and fifth metatarsal heads, gently dorsiflex them on the sagittal plane until you feel resistance where the MTJ locks on the congruent STJ. Be sure you neither abduct nor adduct the forefoot. Maintain the second toe in line with the tibial crest. (For those who cannot resist dorsiflexing the talocrural joint or deviating from the sagittal plane with this procedure, some clinicians suggest that the fourth and fifth toes be distracted on their respective metatarsals by pulling them in a line parallel with the connecting metatarsals.)

3. While holding the lateral rays in dorsiflexion (loaded), look at the plantar surface of the foot. Maintain a strict sagittal and transverse plane orientation.

4. Compare the plane of the forefoot to the calcaneal bisection with the first measure.
   a. Have an assistant place the stationary arm of the goniometer parallel with the vertical calcaneal bisection.
   b. Place the moving arm parallel with the plane of the plantar surface of all five metatarsal heads.
      In the balanced foot, this calcaneal-forefoot measurement is within 90-92 degrees (Root et al. 1971; Jordan et al. 1983).

5. Compare the plantar plane of the forefoot to the transverse plane with the second measurement. This value reveals the degree of excursion required for all five metatarsal heads to move from congruity to full contact with the ground in the closed chain. There are no published norms for this measurement, although it broadens the clinician's perspective on the existing function of the foot structures in stance.
   a. Maintain the foot in congruity.
   b. Have an assistant align the stationary arm of the goniometer parallel with either the seam in the tiles on the floor below, or with the edge of the table, both of which should be perpendicular to the lower leg bisection. The stationary arm corresponds with the transverse plane.
   c. The moving arm is then aligned on the plantar surface of all five metatarsal heads.

If, in either of these assessments, the first or fifth metatarsal heads are not on the same plane as the central metatarsal heads, repeat the measurements using the central three metatarsal heads (Gray 1984).

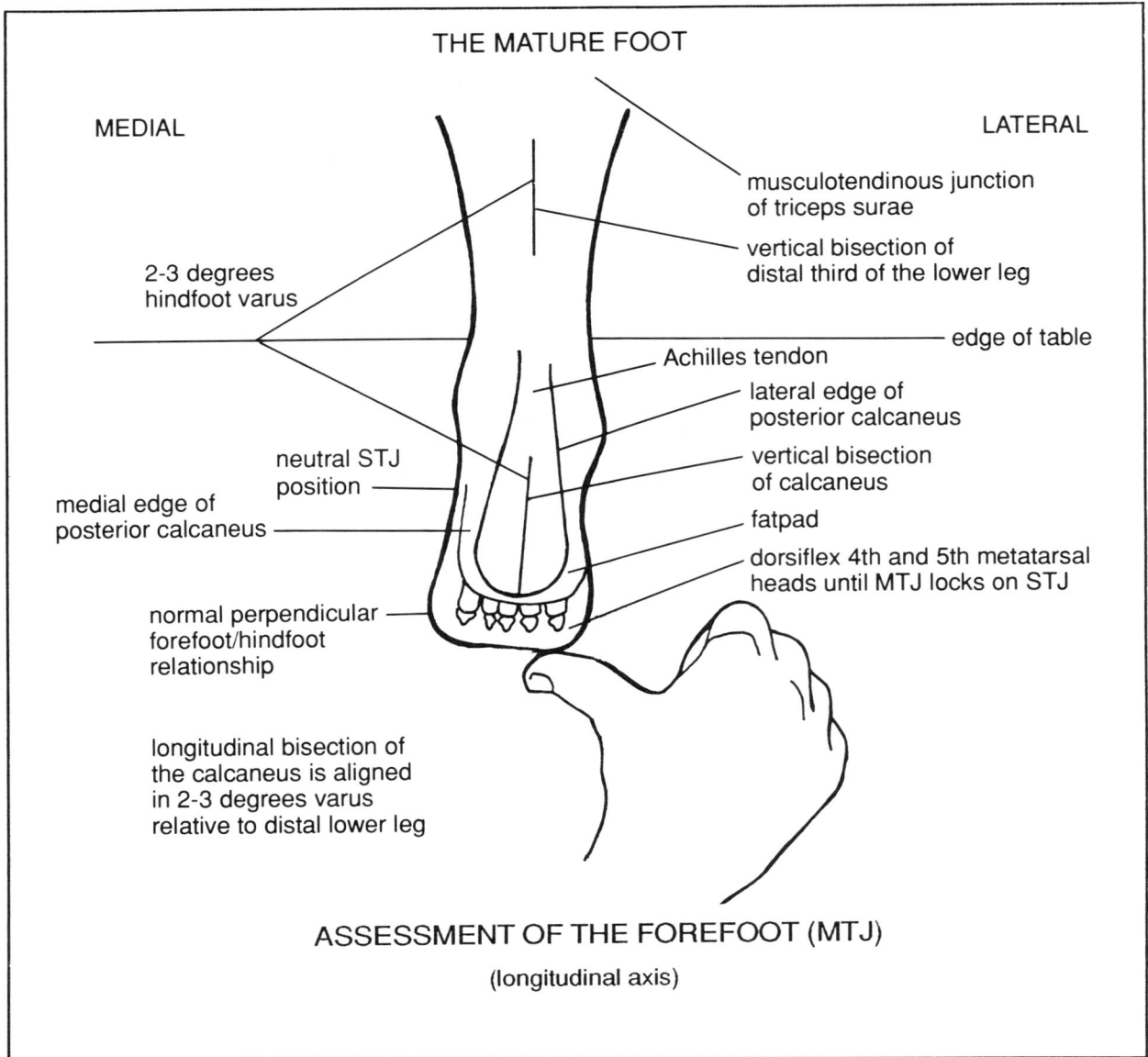

THE MATURE FOOT

MEDIAL

LATERAL

musculotendinous junction
of triceps surae

vertical bisection of
distal third of the lower leg

2-3 degrees
hindfoot varus

edge of table

Achilles tendon

lateral edge of
posterior calcaneus

neutral STJ
position

vertical bisection
of calcaneus

medial edge of
posterior calcaneus

fatpad

dorsiflex 4th and 5th metatarsal
heads until MTJ locks on STJ

normal perpendicular
forefoot/hindfoot
relationship

longitudinal bisection of
the calcaneus is aligned
in 2-3 degrees varus
relative to distal lower leg

ASSESSMENT OF THE FOREFOOT (MTJ)

(longitudinal axis)

Figure 3.51

Determining Neutral Foot Position

The same procedure for determining MTJ status around the longitudinal axis reveals the neutral foot position. The foot structures are locked in full congruity (See Assessing the MTJ—Longitudinal Axis, Figures 3.50 and 3.51, discussed previously.) Varus deviations are often observed at both the calcaneus and the forefoot in children when the subtalar joint is congruous. This fully congruent foot resists any ground reaction forces on the forefoot in the direction of further MTJ dorsiflexion, abduction, or eversion.

Abnormal Findings of MTJ Assessment

Forefoot varus—If the endpoint of dorsiflexion of the fourth and fifth rays is reached early—before obtaining an angle of 90-92 degrees between the plantar plane of the metatarsal heads and the calcaneal bisection—the problem of forefoot varus is identified. The condition indicates that the plane of the forefoot is structurally inverted on the hindfoot. This malalignment is rarely evident in standing because the forefoot typically lowers to contact the ground fully (Root et al. 1971; McCrea 1985). In quiet stance, however, many people with forefoot varus roll one or both feet into supination, evidently to relieve pronatory stresses.

Persistent structural forefoot varus deviation into maturity influences the hindfoot—and thus the entire closed kinetic chain—by disrupting the timing of conversion of the foot from loose adapter to rigid lever during the stance phase of gait. The inverted forefoot must pronate to achieve ground contact. The pronation forces are communicated to the STJ, which, mobility permitting, also pronates to accommodate the floor reaction forces imposed from the forefoot. The pronated foot thus remains hypermobile during stance rather than converting to the rigid lever needed for efficient transfer of weight at toe-off. The prolonged pronatory phase interrupts the normal operation of the closed chain and promotes persistence of medial rotation in the lower leg and femur and flexion at the knee and hip joints (Tiberio 1988).

Forefoot varus deformity is a common finding in children of all ages with neuromotor impairment. This deformity may be a significant factor in the prevalence of pronation deformities among children in that group.

Forefoot valgus—If the end point of passive dorsiflexion of the fourth and fifth rays occurs after they pass into eversion—so the first and fifth metatarsal heads form an angle greater than 92 degrees relative to the calcaneal bisection—forefoot valgus deformity has been identified (Root et al. 1971; Jordan et al. 1983). This deformity generally occurs as a long-term consequence of unyielding varus deviation at the hindfoot. Forefoot valgus also fosters persistence of hindfoot varus by causing the foot to roll laterally on weight-bearing.

A plantarflexed first ray must be identified and ruled out or it may falsely suggest that the forefoot is in valgus deformity (Tiberio 1988). In this case, the central metatarsal heads should be measured as a group, separate from the first metatarsal head. First ray abnormalities are discussed later in this chapter.

The Metatarsal System

The cuneiforms, the cuboid, the metatarsals, and the toes comprise the metatarsal system. It includes the rays that are formed by the metatarsals and their proximal adjacent tarsal bones, with the exception of the fifth ray, which includes only the fifth metatarsal (Oatis 1988). It is in the metatarsal system that balance of the forces imposed on the foot—both from the ground and from the body—is finally executed (Regnauld 1986). This system is directly influenced by the MTJ, the rays, and the tarsometatarsal joints (TMTJ), which derive their biomechanical function from the rearfoot and subtalar joint complexes (Regnauld 1986). Around their combined axes, the MTJ, the rays, and the TMTJ permit the motions of *plantarflexion* during supination, *dorsiflexion* during pronation, and *rotation* during both (Jones 1975; Root et al. 1977; McCrea 1985; Regnauld 1986).

The first and fifth rays each have a unique axis of motion. Together they are capable of approximating each other in the same way as the metatarsals of the thumb and fifth finger on the hand.

The First Ray

The first ray, as described above, consists of the first cuneiform and the first metatarsal. Its mobility is similar to the thumb on the hand. The axis of motion of the first ray takes a course of progression through the foot that is the opposite of the other, more proximal axes discussed previously in this chapter. The first ray axis is more proximal on the posterior aspect, progressing medial to lateral through the foot from the navicular tuberosity through the base of the third metatarsal, and forming a pitch approximating 10 degrees to the transverse plane. (The other axes in the foot and ankle lie in the opposite direction to this axis.) The close proximity of the first ray axis to the transverse plane indicates that it has a high degree of frontal plane mobility (Hicks 1953).

The first ray axis also aligns at nearly 50 degrees lateral (rather than medial) to the sagittal plane. This pitch, which is closer to the frontal plane than the sagittal plane, favors sagittal plane motion of the first ray. Thus, the first ray dorsiflexes and plantarflexes equal distances above and below the second ray through an arc of 10 degrees, with concurrent secondary adduction and inversion, and abduction and eversion, respectively (Root et al. 1977).

The average pitch of the first ray to the transverse plane falls between 12 and 21 degrees in children, increasing in adults to between 18 and 30 degrees (McCrea 1985; Regnauld 1986; Vanderwilde et al. 1988). Tachdjian (1985) suggests that the first ray normally aligns parallel with the longitudinal bisection of the talus, at the same pitch to the transverse plane when viewed from a frontal plane perspective. Vanderwilde et al. (1988) use graphs to indicate that the pitch of the talus with the transverse plane approaches a mean of 34 degrees at birth and decreases steadily throughout childhood to an average of 26 degrees at age 9 years.

Vanderwilde et al. (1988) also describe evidence of varying angles formed by the talus and the first metatarsal as the child grows older. Their views thus differ from Tachdjian's view.

The talo-first-metatarsal angle apparently ranges between a mean of approximately 18 degrees at birth to approximately 9 degrees at age 9, essentially leveling off after 5 years of age. These values reveal evidence of decreasing dorsiflexion of the first ray relative to the talus.

In the closed chain the first ray pitch to the transverse plane changes together with the pitch of the calcaneal inclination, though to a greater degree. With supination, the first ray plantarflexes along with the second and third rays, and the MTJ around its oblique axis. The first ray pitch increases, as does the pitch of the calcaneal inclination. The medial longitudinal arch thus increases in height. The lateral rays dorsiflex concurrently, under the strain of weight-bearing. Prolonged supination eventually results in a valgus forefoot deformity (Hicks 1953). Meanwhile, the talar declination angle decreases with supination. Talar dorsiflexion occurs in supination.

All of these changes in pitch reverse in pronation. In pronation the medial longitudinal arch lowers in height (Hicks 1953). The medial rays dorsiflex, the lateral rays plantarflex, and the talar declination angle increases. A varus forefoot deformity either results from or is worsened by prolonged pronation.

Assessing First Ray Status and Motion

This is a simple assessment but is highly significant in determining appropriate intervention with splints or orthoses (Root et al. 1971; McCrea 1985; Gray 1986).

Place the child in sitting or supine on a table with the ankle dorsiflexed to neutral.

1. Align the subtalar joint in neutral position, and view the foot from its anterior aspect.

   > In reviewing the writings of all of the authors, particularly those of Root et al. (1971), I have determined that the "neutral STJ" position to which they refer for this test is actually the calcaneal midposition. This is a test of flexibility of the first ray around the stable, plantigrade foot that optimally appears in midstance in gait. Calcaneal midposition is not necessarily a position of neutrality.

2. Stabilize the forefoot by dorsiflexing the lateral four rays. Be careful not to abduct the forefoot, because this will induce pronation.
3. Observe and palpate the location of the central three metatarsal heads relative to the hindfoot. Be sure to look for varus or valgus inclination in these metatarsals. They ideally align to within 2-3 degrees of the transverse plane when the calcaneus aligns on the sagittal plane.

4. Grasp the entire first metatarsal head between your thumb and forefinger.

5. Dorsiflex and plantarflex the first ray.

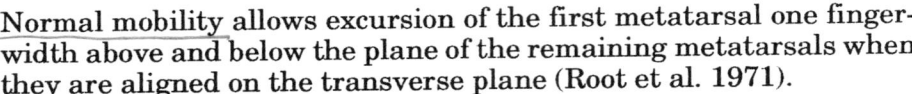
Normal mobility allows excursion of the first metatarsal one finger-width above and below the plane of the remaining metatarsals when they are aligned on the transverse plane (Root et al. 1971).

Abnormal Findings of First Ray Assessment

Hypermobile first ray—While maintaining the calcaneus in midposition and stabilizing the lateral four metatarsal heads, the first metatarsal may sometimes be dorsiflexed more than one finger-width above the second. When that happens, the first ray is hypermobile into dorsiflexion and is a source of pronatory instability and fatigue in gait.

Plantarflexed first ray (rigid or semi-rigid)—Forefoot eversion or valgus deformity might be caused by a plantarflexed first ray, which resists passive dorsiflexion past the second metatarsal head, while the remaining metatarsal heads maintain a neutral or varus-deviated orientation relative to the hindfoot. This deformity typically occurs with varus hindfoot deformity in which the range of motion into calcaneal eversion is abnormally limited. The first ray might be plantarflexed by genetic disposition to a cavus-shaped foot or to a high calcaneal inclination. The result is that the foot cannot adequately pronate (Jordan et al. 1983; Root et al. 1977; Gray 1986; Tiberio 1988).

This compensation is common in children with spastic hemiplegia and quadriplegia who reveal equinovarus deformity at the ankle and hindfoot. The medial plantar fascial and ligament structures eventually shorten with growth and continued supinatory deviation.

Plantarflexed first ray (flexible)—In the presence of a varus hindfoot and forefoot (including the lateral four metatarsal heads), compensatory plantarflexion of the first ray is a common active stabilizing mechanism (Gray 1986). By remaining flexible, the deformity resolves with stress-induced dorsiflexion into alignment with the other metatarsal heads. When the metatarsal heads 2 through 4 align in varus and the first ray can be dorsiflexed to align with them, the forefoot deformity is actually one of varus—rather than valgus—deviation.

The Transverse Arch

The transverse arch is evident in the metatarsal heads in the open chain. The metatarsals form a similar arc across the dome of the foot, rising toward the medial aspect of the foot. The transverse arch at the metatarsal heads flattens in stance and contributes to the springiness in the forefoot for weight-bearing and transfers (Mann 1985 in Jahss; Cavanagh et al. 1987; Riegger 1988). The transverse arch is sustained primarily by the interosseus and plantar ligaments and the short muscles of the first toe, particularly the transverse head of the adductor halluces, the short muscles of the fifth toe, and the peroneus longus (Schafer 1987).

The Metatarsals

The metatarsals are designed to distribute body weight efficiently over the foot in stance and gait. Their relative length contributes to the smooth carriage of the center of gravity in the stance phase of gait, from the heel to the lateral border to the forefoot. Weight is carried across the metatarsal heads, from the shorter lateral to the longer medial forefoot, at the toe-off stage of the stance phase. The stance phase terminates on either the first metatarsal head or on the first and second metatarsal heads together. The first metatarsal is only slightly shorter than the second, which favors a smooth diagonal weight transfer to the opposite foot. The efficient and refined reciprocal stabilizing action of the antagonistic muscle groups that cross these joints require precise and balanced alignment of the metatarsals and distal tarsal bones (Jones 1975; Root et al. 1977; Salek 1977; Regnauld 1986; Gray 1986; Franco 1987; Schafer 1987; Riegger 1988).

Morton's foot, which features an abnormally short first ray, causes an excessive distribution of loading forces to the second metatarsal head. The first ray is too short to arrive on the ground in proper time. The common results are first ray pronation with abduction away from the second ray; plantarflexion; and compensatory hallux valgus with bunion formation (Gray 1986; Rodgers 1988).

The Tarsometatarsal Joint (TMTJ)

The TMTJ is a collective joint comprised of the articulations between the three cuneiforms and the cuboid that make up the proximal bar, as well as the bases of the metatarsals on the distal bar (Figure 3.1). Its axis is situated obliquely along the same orientation as the oblique axis of the TMA, STJ, and MTJ, and it lies close to the frontal plane. Thus the TMTJ allows small deflectionary movements into dorsiflexion and plantarflexion to occur. This gives the forefoot elasticity under pressure and better adaptability to uneven surfaces (Bahler 1986). It is at this articulation that transverse plane deviations in structural alignment—such as metatarsus adductus—occur.

The TMTJ axis aligns closer to the frontal plane in the infant than in the adult. This affords the infant foot a greater capacity for sagittal plane motion at that joint. In both infants and adults, a dorsoplantar view reveals that the lateral four metatarsals align parallel to each other, while the first ray (the first cuneiform and metatarsal) deviates medially from the second ray between 8 and 15 degrees in the newborn, and between 5 and 10 degrees in the mature foot. The navicular and talus align with the first ray, which deviates medially as a result of the adduction component of residual talar torsion.

Pronation produces abduction of the forefoot; supination results in adduction (Figures 3.41, 3.42, and 3.43). These motions displace not only the navicular, cuboid, and cuneiforms, but the metatarsals as well. Thus the motions involve the TMTJ.

Assessing TMT Alignment on the Transverse Plane

Adduction and abduction occur on the transverse plane in the foot. Footprint assessment (a drawing of the perimeter of the weight-bearing foot) reveals that when the foot is aligned in calcaneal midstance position, the metatarsals align parallel with the sagittal-plane bisection of the heel. A line drawn through the center of the heel oval to the toes falls either through the second toe, or between the second and third toes (Root et al. 1971; Root et al. 1977; Aharonson et al. 1980; McCrea 1985; Rose et al. 1985; Gray 1986) (Figure 3.52). The foot is straight on the lateral surface.

Relaxed standing footprints of many children younger than 5 years show a bisection line that falls medial to the second or even first toe. This is because their closed-chain foot position is pronation. When the bisection line falls medial to the great toe in the child age 5 or over, it is considered a sign of abnormality (Rose et al. 1985).

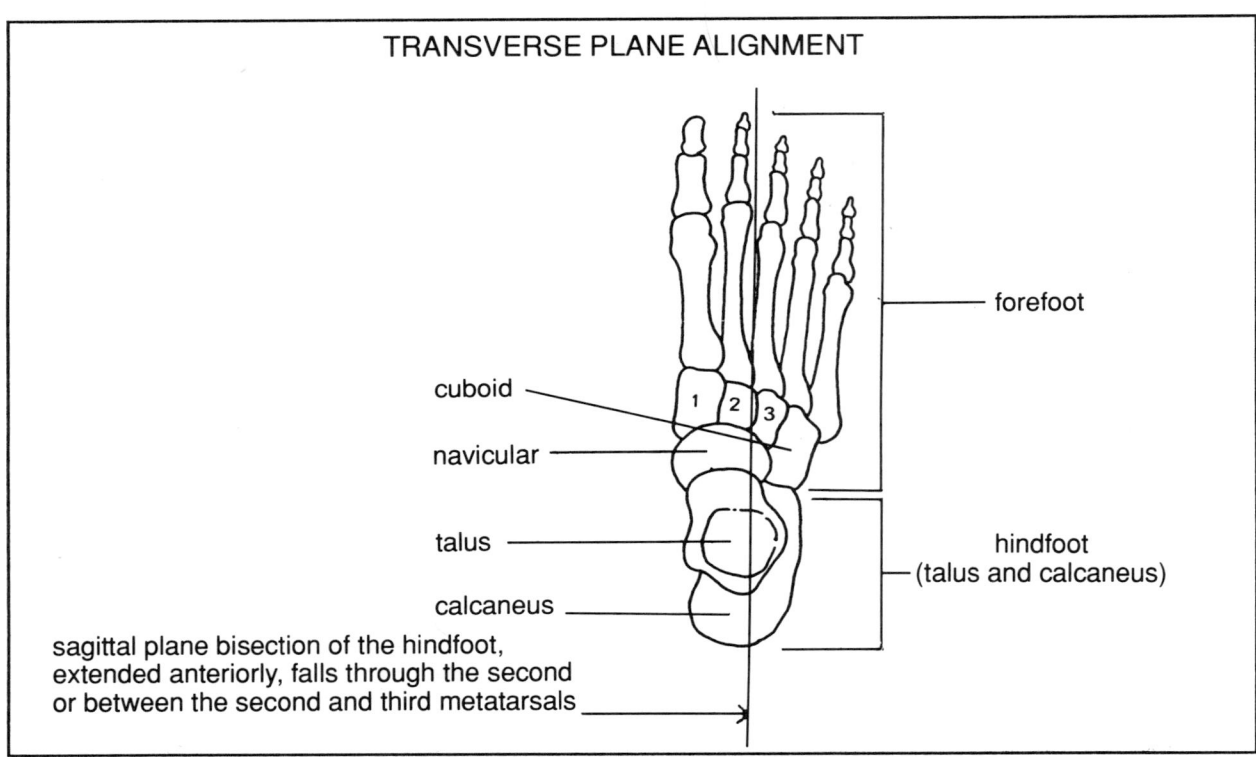

Figure 3.52

Abnormal Findings in TMT Assessment

Metatarsus adductus—Metatarsus adductus is a structural medial deviation of the metatarsals at the tarsometatarsal articulation, relative to the sagittal plane. As discussed previously, metatarsus adductus is not normal (Agnew 1988). There is speculation about the subject, but it is not yet known whether some metatarsus adductus deformities resolve spontaneously or whether they become "skewfoot" deformities by adulthood. Such a deformity would develop as a child compensates for the in-toeing caused by the adductus by turning the entire foot laterally in stance. In forward progression, this position imposes extraordinary pronatory force on the loaded subtalar joint (Agnew 1988).

Metatarsus adductus is evident when clinical examination of the foot reveals a convexity on the lateral aspect with the apex at the base of the fifth metatarsal, and a concavity and high arch on the medial aspect. When the entire foot is viewed from the plantar aspect, it takes the shape of a comma or the letter "C." The deformity is rigid in some cases and flexible (correctable by manipulation) in others. It is likely to be a result of intrauterine positioning (Hensinger et al. 1982; McCrea 1985).

Forefoot adductus—The term "forefoot adductus" is accurate only when the medial deviation of the metatarsals includes the navicular and cuboid and occurs at the midtarsal joint. This is because the forefoot includes the tarsal bones by some definitions, and forefoot motions are understood to occur around the MTJ (McCrea 1985). Pure adductus cannot occur at the MTJ without osseous abnormality. Forefoot adductus is often accompanied by supination.

The Metatarsophalangeal (MTP) Joints

The metatarsophalangeal (MTP) joints are formed by the articulation between the heads of the metatarsals and the bases of the proximal phalanges. They comprise the "ball of the foot," as it is commonly known, and the "break" across which the foot progresses at the end of the stance phase. The MTP joints are limited spheroid joints, which renders them capable of limited motion on the transverse plane (abduction and adduction) in addition to their primary function as hinges for motions of extension and flexion on the sagittal plane (Schafer 1987; Oatis 1988).

The MTP joints are supple and strong and function as the final transmitter of the forces of weight-bearing. They allow dorsiflexion of 65-90 degrees, and plantarflexion of up to 50 degrees (Figure 3.53) (Root et al. 1977; Regnauld 1986; Oatis 1988). The minimum range of hyperextension required for normal locomotion at the first MTP joint is 65-75 degrees. Slightly less than 65 degrees is needed at the latter MTP joints because they lift off the ground sooner than the great toe at the end of the stance phase of gait (Root et al. 1977; Mann et al. 1979). These hyperextension values are achieved by concurrent plantarflexion of the rays against the rising phalanges. If the distal metatarsals are dorsiflexed manually, passive toe hyperextension mobility reduces to 30-40 degrees, and the true length of the flexor muscles and of the plantar aponeurosis as a stabilizing ligament becomes evident.

Figure 3.53 Great toe hyperextension: Note the windlass action of the plantar aponeurosis, evident in the heightened longitudinal arch. Repeat this assessment in relaxed stance (not shown).

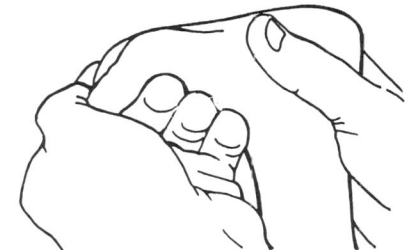

Two small sesamoid bones are embedded in the tendon of insertion of the flexor halluces brevis as it crosses the plantar aspect of the distal first metatarsal. They increase the magnitude of tension force for the flexor halluces longus in the same way that the patella enhances the tensile power of the quadriceps. In toe-standing, the sesamoids act as a footstool for the first metatarsal, giving it increased height (Grant 1962). During the stance phase of gait, prior to heel-off, the phalanges remain in 20 degrees of passive dorsiflexion on the metatarsals (Mann et al. 1979).

Kinesiological Considerations Regarding the MTP Joints in Gait

The two extrinsic toe extensors are active throughout swing. They assist the ankle dorsiflexors in aligning the foot on the sagittal plane and in controlling the lowering of the foot following initial contact. Their activity during the stance phase is minimal (Mann et al. 1979). The long toe extensors apply compressive stabilization forces to the phalanges and metatarsals because of the line of pull of the distal tendons. Between foot contact and heel-off, the extrinsic toe flexor muscles activate eccentrically as stabilizers, translating (compressing) the phalanges and metatarsals into the tarsus (Root et al. 1977; Schenkman 1988).

The intrinsic toe flexors and abductors arise within the foot itself and activate together during the stance phase, between the assumption of weight and toe-off. The intrinsic muscles contribute both to maintenance of toe contact with the ground and to stabilization of the arches during stance (Mann et al. 1979; Riegger 1988). The intrinsics are active at 35 percent of the gait cycle, which includes the onset of heel rise, the beginning of foot supination, and the concentration of body weight on the metatarsal heads (Rodgers 1988).

Between the heel-off and toe-off stages of stance, the pendulous weight of the swing leg contributes to the forward momentum of the body over the stance foot. The toes passively dorsiflex further, while at the same time downward compressive forces plantarflex the first ray against the hyperextending first phalanx (Root et al. 1977). The resulting hyperextension of the toes, particularly of the great toe, draws on the plantar aponeurosis. The plantar aponeurosis, by its windlass action, elevates and stabilizes the longitudinal arch in preparation for weight transfer to the opposite foot (Mann et al. 1979).

The significance of the availability of passive toe extension beyond neutral is readily apparent to anyone who attempts to walk normally while maintaining the toes in flexion throughout the stance phase of gait. The limitation on hip extension and stride length is obvious and should be considered seriously at the time a splint or cast is modified for walking. However, ambulation has been shown to be quite possible without the toes at all (Mann et al. 1979). Prolonged and increased activity into flexion, however, can affect the quality of gait by restricting push-off (Schafer 1987).

Assessing the MTP Joints

Begin an assessment of the toes by observing their alignment on the transverse plane, relative to each other and to their adjacent metatarsals.

- Look for hallux valgus and evidence of bunion formation.
- Flex and extend the toes. Note the differences in toe extension range with and without stabilization of the distal metatarsals.

Leg Length

After examining all the structural features of the lower extremity that might affect its functional or actual length in weight-bearing, a close look at the leg length relationship is essential, both before and after intervention with splints or orthoses.

Multiple factors can alter leg length in stance and gait, including:

- Scoliosis
- Pelvic obliquity
- Hip flexion contracture (as a limiting force on full hyperextension to terminal stance)
- Genu valgum or varum
- Knee flexion contracture
- Subtalar joint pronation
- Ankle equinus
- Plantar/dorsiflexion of the first ray

In addition, proximal subluxation of the femur from the acetabulum induces a functional leg length discrepancy.

Assessing Leg Length in Supine

After determining radiologically that hip subluxation is not a contributing factor, clinical assessment of relative leg lengths requires extreme precision and attention to details of pelvic alignment, joint position, and landmarks. Even a bone scan can be inaccurate if these details are overlooked during the procedure.

Use the following first five procedures to detect structural limb length inequality in infants and children. The remaining procedures are intended for children older than 3 years of age.

Place the child in supine position (Vogel 1984).

1. Level the pelvis perpendicular to the midline of the trunk.
2. Flex both hips and knees and place the plantar aspects of the feet on the surface (bridging position).
3. Align the knees in 90 degrees of flexion.
4. Compare the height of the knee joints. If one knee is higher, the tibia is longer in that limb (Allis sign).

5. Compare the longitudinal alignment of the knees. If you measure one knee to be further forward than the other, the femur is possibly longer in that limb (Galeazzi's sign).

6. Measure *anatomic length* of the lower extremity by extending fully the hips and knees. Use as landmarks the proximal edge of the greater trochanter and the distal end of the lateral malleolus (Vogel 1984).

7. Measure lower segment length with the child in prone position, with hips extended and knees flexed 90 degrees.

   a. Align the lower legs on the sagittal and frontal planes.

   b. Measure the distance from the medial intercondylar articulation at the knee joint to the distal border of the medial malleolus.

   c. Measure the distance from the proximal border of the fibula to the distal border of the lateral malleolus.

   d. Measure the distance from the medial intercondylar articulation to the plantar plane of the heel.

   e. Repeat the measures for the opposite leg.

8. Use the following procedures to detect *clinical limb length,* which acknowledges the position of the femoral head relative to the acetabulum:

   a. Palpate the anterior superior iliac spine. Find a replicable landmark on it, such as the inferior border, and place one end of your tape measure on that landmark.

   b. If necessary, have an assistant maintain extended and neutral alignment of the hip and knee joints.

   c. Pull the tape measure to the distal edge of the lateral malleolus.

   d. Repeat the procedure on the other leg.

   e. Compare these findings to those for anatomic length.

Consider variables such as frontal plane deviations at the knee joint; differences in leg circumference; pelvic defects; joint contractures and foot deformities; and problems of palpation of landmarks. All of these variables can diminish a direct clinical measurement of leg length (Vogel 1984).

Assessing Leg Length in Standing

Continue leg length assessment with the patient in a standing position, if possible. It is in the standing position that the effects of limb length difference are apparent. Place the patient in anatomical position, with weight evenly distributed between the feet. (Use a standing table, tilt table, or prone board, if needed, and carefully align the extremities.) Note the following postural features:

- True limb shortening produces a lowering of the pelvis on the short side, which becomes entirely evident with both knees fully extended (though not hyperextended). Palpate the upper border of the iliac crests as accurately as possible, with your line of vision lowered to the same level as the crests.

- The shoulder on the same side as the shortened leg might also be lower, if compensatory scoliosis has not occurred.
- The longer limb might show genu valgum of greater degree than the shorter limb.
- Compensatory pronation deformity is evident commonly in the foot of the longer leg, which results from an effort to reduce the length inequality and its resulting obliquity at the pelvis (McCrea 1985; Schafer 1987).

Features of Optimum Mature Leg and Foot Position in Standing

The observations and principles reviewed in this chapter are summarized in the following list of features of structure and alignment in the lower extremities of a child of age 5 years or more. These features are noted with the child positioned in relaxed standing at the normal angle and base of gait.

- The sagittal plane curvatures of the spine and pelvis are within normal, age-appropriate limits, neither exaggerated nor reduced (Regnauld 1986).
- The pelvis is level—parallel with the transverse plane.
- The hips are adequately extended, with neutral rotation, allowing the femoral transcondylar axis (TCA) to lie within 10 degrees of the frontal plane (McCrea 1985).
- The articulating surfaces of the femoral and tibial condyles lie on the transverse plane (Root et al. 1971).
- The tibiofemoral angle is within an age-appropriate value of valgum relative to the sagittal plane (McCrea 1985; McDade 1977).
- The knees are extended to 0 degrees relative to the frontal plane.
- The longitudinal bisection of the distal third of the lower leg aligns on the sagittal plane (Root et al. 1971; Jordan et al. 1983; Tax 1985).
- The transmalleolar axis (TMA) aligns 20-30 degrees lateral to the frontal plane (McCrea 1985).
- The vertical calcaneal bisection aligns in midposition—within 2 degrees of the sagittal plane (Root et al. 1971; Frankel et al. 1980; Aharonson et al. 1980; Valmassy 1984; McCrea 1985).
- The plantar surface of the metatarsal heads fully contacts the ground (Root et al. 1971; Aharonson et al. 1980).
- The longitudinal arch is apparent (Aharonson et al. 1980; Tax 1985; Regnauld 1986; Staheli et al. 1987).
- The lateral surface of the foot is straight in the area of the calcaneocuboid joint (Root et al. 1971; McCrea 1985).

- Concavities of equal depth are apparent on the skin surfaces above and beneath the lateral malleolus (Root et al. 1971).
- The metatarsals are parallel to each other and to the longitudinal bisection of the hindfoot (Aharonson et al. 1980).
- The toes are straight and parallel to the metatarsals.

A Pediatric Biomechanical Assessment Form has been included as Appendix 5 as a means of assisting the clinician in conducting a thorough biomechanical assessment as a necessary prerequisite to intervening for the management of functional and structural problems in children with neuromotor deficit, using splints, casts, or orthoses.

Summary

A systematic, carefully conducted assessment of the mobility and alignment features of the pelvis and lower extremities can reveal many significant findings to the pediatric clinician. Such factors as persistent hip flexion contracture, femoral torsional deformity, hamstrings contracture, forefoot varus deformity, forefoot equinus deformity, or a plantarflexed first ray can significantly diminish the mechanical advantages of a custom-molded splint or orthosis. When these findings are uncovered, the management team can make more knowledgeable judgments concerning the potential outcome of an intervention effort that uses casts, splints, or orthoses. The team can also identify specific needs for muscle strength and for such specialized procedures as joint mobilization or surgery.

The next chapter examines some of the problems of alignment and function that commonly occur in children with neuromotor disorders, particularly those involving hypertonus and hypotonia.

References

Agnew, P., DPM. December 8, 1988. Personal communication, Richmond, VA.

Aharonson, Z., A. Voloshin, T. V. Steinbach, M. A. Brull, and I. Farine. 1980. Normal foot-ground pressure pattern in children. *Clinical Orthopaedics and Related Research* 150:220-223.

Asher, C. 1975. *Postural variations in childhood*. Boston, MA: Butterworths.

Bahler, A. 1986. The biomechanics of the foot. *Clinical Prosthetics and Orthotics* 10(1):8-14.

Beals, R. K. 1969. Developmental changes in the femur and acetabulum in spastic paraplegia and diplegia. *Developmental Medicine and Child Neurology* 11:303-313.

Bernhardt, D. B. 1988. Prenatal and postnatal growth and development of the foot and ankle. *Physical Therapy* 68(12):1831-1839.

Bleck, E. E. 1982. Developmental orthopaedics. III: Toddlers. *Developmental Medicine and Child Neurology* 24:533-555.

Bleck, E. E. 1987. Orthopaedic management in cerebral palsy. *Clinics in Developmental Medicine, no. 99/100.* Philadelphia, PA: J. B. Lippincott.

Bleck, E. E., and U. J. Berzins. 1977. Conservative management of pes valgus with plantar flexed talus, flexible. *Clinical Orthopaedics and Related Research* 122:85-92.

Brooks, S. 1985. *Joint mobilization applied to the neurologically involved child.* Lecture notes and instructional materials from training course, Dallas, TX.

Cavanagh, P. R., M. M. Rodgers, and A. Iiboshi. 1987. Pressure distribution under symptom-free feet during barefoot standing. *Foot & Ankle* 7(5):262-276.

D'Amico, J. C. 1984. Developmental flatfoot. In *Symposium on podopediatrics—Clinics in podiatry,* edited by J. V. Ganley, 535-546. Philadelphia, PA: W. B. Saunders.

DiGiovanni, J. E., and S. D. Smith. 1976. Normal biomechanics of the adult rearfoot: A radiographic analysis. *Journal of the American Podiatry Association* 66(11):(unnumbered reprint).

Engel, G. M., and L. T. Staheli. 1974. The natural history of torsion and other factors influencing gait in childhood. *Clinical Orthopaedics and Related Research* 99:12-17.

Fabry, G., G. D. McEwen, and A. R. Shands. 1973. Torsion of the femur: A follow-up study in normal and abnormal conditions. *Journal of Bone and Joint Surgery* 55-A(8):1726-1738.

Franco, A. H. 1987. Pes cavus and pes planus: Analyses and treatment. *Physical Therapy* 67(5):688-694.

Frankel, V. H., and M. Nordin. 1980. Biomechanics of the foot. In *Basic biomechanics of the skeletal system,* edited by V. H. Frankel and M. Nordin, 192-219. Philadelphia, PA: Lea & Febiger.

Giallonardo, L. M. 1988. Clinical evaluation of foot and ankle dysfunction. *Physical Therapy* 68(12):1850-1866.

Grant, J. C. B. 1962. *An atlas of anatomy, 5th ed.* Baltimore, MD: Williams and Wilkins.

Gray, G. W. 1984. *Functional locomotor biomechanical examination.* Toledo, OH: American Physical Rehabilitation Network.

Gray, G. W. 1986. *Enhancing clinical skills through biomechanics.* Lecture notes and instructional materials. South Carolina American Physical Therapy Association annual meeting, Charleston, SC, May 17.

Griffin, P. P. 1986. The lower limb. In *Pediatric orthopaedics, 2d ed.,* edited by W. W. Lovell and R. B. Winter, 865-893. Philadelphia, PA: J. B. Lippincott.

Gross, R. H. 1987. *Orthopedic problems in children.* Lecture and personal communication. Medical University of South Carolina, Charleston, SC.

Hamilton, W. G. 1985. Surgical anatomy of the foot and ankle. *Clinical symposia* monograph (CIBA):37(3).

Hensinger, R. N., and E. T. Jones. 1982. Developmental orthopaedics I: The lower limb. *Developmental Medicine and Child Neurology* 24:95-116.

Hicks, J. H. 1953. The mechanics of the foot, I: The joints. *Journal of Anatomy* 87:345-357.

Hutter, C. G., and M. D. Scott. 1949. Tibial torsion. *Journal of Bone and Joint Surgery* 31-A(3):511-518.

Jones, B. S. 1975. Flat foot: A preliminary report of an operation for severe cases. *Journal of Bone and Joint Surgery* 57-B(3):279-282.

Jordan, R. P. 1984. Therapeutic considerations of the feet and lower extremities in the cerebral palsied child. *Symposium on podopediatrics—Clinics in podiatry,* edited by J. V. Ganley, 547-561. Philadelphia, PA: W. B. Saunders.

Jordan, R. P., J. Cusack, and B. Rosseque. 1983. *Foot function and its relationship to posture in the pediatric patient with cerebral palsy and other neuromuscular disorders.* Lecture notes and instructional materials. Sponsored by the Neurodevelopmental Treatment Association, New York, May 20-22.

Maitland, G. D. 1977. *Peripheral manipulation, 2d ed.* Boston, MA: Butterworths.

Mann, R. A. 1985. Biomechanics of the foot. In *Atlas of orthotics, 2d ed.,* edited by W. H. Bunch and other members of the American Academy of Orthopedic Surgeons, 112-125. St. Louis, MO: C. V. Mosby.

Mann, R. A. 1985. Biomechanics. In *Disorders of the foot, vol. 1,* edited by M. H. Jahss, 37-67. Philadelphia, PA: W. B. Saunders.

Mann, R. A., and J. L. Gahy. 1979. The function of the toes in walking, jogging, and running. *Clinical Orthopaedics and Related Research* 142:24-29.

McCrea, J. 1985. *Pediatric orthopedics of the lower extremity: An instructional handbook.* Mount Kisco, NY: Futura.

McDade, W. 1977. Bow legs and knock knees. *Pediatric Clinics of North America* 24(4):825-839.

McDonough, M. W. 1984. Angular and axial deformities of the legs of children. In *Symposium on podopediatrics—Clinics in podiatry,* edited by J. V. Ganley, 601-620. Philadelphia, PA: W. B. Saunders.

Milgrom, C., M. Giladi, A. Simkin, M. Stein, H. Kashtan, J. Margulies, R. Steinberg, and Z. Aharonson. 1985. The normal range of subtalar inversion and eversion in young males as measured by three different techniques. *Foot & Ankle* 6(3):143-145.

Murphy, S. B., S. R. Simon, P. K. Kijewski, R. H. Wilkinson, and N. T. Griscom. 1987. Femoral anteversion. *Journal of Bone and Joint Surgery* 69-A(8):1169-1176.

Oatis, C. A. 1988. Biomechanics of the foot and ankle under static conditions. *Physical Therapy* 68(12):1815-1821.

Perry, J. 1974. Kinesiology of lower extremity bracing. *Clinical Orthopaedics and Related Research* 102:19-31.

Perry, J., M. M. Hoffer, D. Antonelli, J. Plut, G. Lewis, and R. Greenberg. 1976. Electromyography before and after surgery for hip deformity in children with cerebral palsy. *Journal of Bone and Joint Surgery* 58-A(2):201-206.

Phelps, E., L. J. Smith, and A. Hallum. 1985. Normal ranges of hip motion of infants between nine and 24 months of age. *Developmental Medicine and Child Neurology* 27:785-792.

Pitkow, R. B. 1975. External rotation contracture of the extended hip. *Clinical Orthopaedics and Related Research* 110:139-145.

Price, Lawrence, DPM. 1982. Personal consultation. March 28.

Rang, M., R. Silver, and J. de la Garza. 1986. Cerabral palsy. In *Pediatric orthopaedics, 2d ed.,* edited by W. W. Lovell and R. B. Winter. Philadelphia, PA:J. B. Lippincott Co.

Ray, R. L., and M. G. Erlich. 1979. Lateral hamstring transfer and gait improvement in the cerebral palsy patient. *Journal of Bone and Joint Surgery* 61-A(5):719-723.

Regnauld, B. 1986. *The foot: Pathology, aetiology, semiology, clinical investigation and therapy.* New York, NY: Springer-Verlag.

Riegger, C. L. 1988. Anatomy of the ankle and foot. *Physical Therapy* 68(12):1802-1814.

Rodgers, M. M. 1988. Dynamic biomechanics of the normal foot and ankle during walking and running. *Physical Therapy* 68(12):1822-1830.

Root, M. L., W. P. Orien, and J. H. Weed. 1977. *Normal and abnormal function of the foot: Clinical biomechanics, vol. 2.* Los Angeles, CA: Clinical Biomechanics Corporation.

Root, M. L., W. P. Orien, J. H. Weed, and R. J. Hughes. 1971. *Biomechanical examination of the foot, vol. 1.* Los Angeles, CA: Clinical Biomechanics Corp.

Rose, G. K., E. A. Welton, and T. Marshall. 1985. The diagnosis of flat foot in the child. *Journal of Bone and Joint Surgery* 67-B(1):71-78.

Ryder, C. T., and L. Crane. 1953. Measuring femoral anteversion: The problem and a method. *Journal of Bone and Joint Surgery* 35-A:321-328.

Salek, B. 1977. *The significance of structural and functional development in the normal foot and therapeutic implications thereof in the child with neuromotor disorder.* Unpublished monograph. Commack, NY: Suffolk Rehabilitation Center.

Schafer, R. C. 1987. *Clinical biomechanics: Musculoskeletal actions and reactions, 2d ed.* Baltimore, MD: Williams and Wilkins.

Schenkman, M. 1988. *Taking it a step further.* Lecture notes and instructional materials. American Physical Rehabilitation Network, Indianapolis, IN: November 11-13.

Scrutton, D. 1969. Footprint sequences of normal children under five years old. *Developmental Medicine and Child Neurology* 11:44-53.

Sgarlato, T. E. 1971. *A compendium of biomechanics.* San Fransico, CA: California College of Podiatric Medicine.

Soderberg, G. L. 1986. *Kinesiology: Application to pathological motion.* Baltimore, MD: Williams and Wilkins.

Staheli, L. T. 1977. The prone hip extension test. *Clinical Orthopaedics and Related Research* 123:12-15.

Staheli, L. T. 1977. Torsional deformity. *Pediatric Clinics of North America* 24(4):799-811.

Staheli, L. T., and G. M. Engel. 1972. Tibial torsion: A method of assessment and a survey of normal children. *Clinical Orthopaedics and Related Research* 86:183-186.

Staheli, L. T., D. E. Chew, and M. Corbett. 1987. The longitudinal arch: A survey of eight-hundred and eighty-two feet in normal children and adults. *Journal of Bone and Joint Surgery* 69-A(3):426-428.

Staheli, L. T., M. Corbett, W. Craig, and H. King. 1985. Lower-extremity rotational problems in children. *Journal of Bone and Joint Surgery* 67-A:39-44.

Staheli, L. T., W. R. Duncan, and E. Schaefer. 1968. Growth alterations in the hemiplegic child. *Clinical Orthopaedics and Related Research* 40:205-212.

Sutherland, D. H. 1984. *Gait disorders in childhood and adolescence.* Baltimore, MD: Williams and Wilkins.

Sutherland, D. H., L. Cooper, and D. Daniel. 1980b. The role of the ankle plantar flexors in normal walking. *Journal of Bone and Joint Surgery* 62-A(3):354-363.

Sutherland, D. H., R. Olshen, L. Cooper, and S. L-Y. Woo. 1980a. The development of mature gait. *Journal of Bone and Joint Surgery* 62-A(3):336-353.

Svendsen, B., T. M. Kjell, and R. Merritt. 1981. *Joint mobilization laboratory manual: Extremity joint testing and selected treatment techniques.* Bryn Mawr, PA: Noreq.

Tachdjian, M. 1985. *The child's foot.* Philadelphia, PA: W. B. Saunders.

Tardieu, G., and C. Tardieu. 1987. Cerebral palsy: Mechanical evaluation and conservative correction of limb joint contractures. *Clinical Orthopaedics and Related Research* 219:63-70.

Tardieu, G., C. Tardieu, P. Cobeau-Justin, and A. Lespargot. 1982. Muscle hypoextensibility in children with cerebral palsy: II. Therapeutic implications. *Archives of Physical Medicine and Rehabilition* 63:103-107.

Tax, H. R. 1985. *Podopediatrics, 2d ed.* Baltimore, MD: Williams and Wilkins.

Tiberio, D. 1988. Pathomechanics of structural foot deformities. *Physical Therapy* 68(12):1840-1849.

Valmassy, R. L. 1984. Biomechanical evaluation of the child. *Symposium on podopediatrics—Clinics in podiatry,* edited by J. V. Ganley, 563-579. Philadelphia, PA: W. B. Saunders.

Vanderwilde, R., L. T. Staheli, D. E. Chew, and V. Malagon. 1988. Measurements on radiographs of the foot in normal infants and children. *Journal of Bone and Joint Surgery* 70-A:407-415.

Vogel, F. 1984. Short leg syndrome. In *Symposium on podopediatrics—Clinics in podiatry,* edited by J. V. Ganley, 581-599. Philadelphia, PA: W. B. Saunders.

Waters, R. L., and B. R. Lunsford. 1985. Energy expenditure of normal and pathologic gait: Application to orthotic prescription. In *Atlas of orthotics, 2d ed.,* edited by W. H. Bunch and others of the American Academy of Orthopedic Surgeons. St. Louis, MO: C. V. Mosby.

Wright, D. G., S. M. Desai, and W. H. Henderson. 1964. Action of the subtalar and ankle-joint complex during the stance phase of walking. *Journal of Bone and Joint Surgery* 46-A:361-464.

CHAPTER 4

Common Features of Alignment in Children with Neuromotor Disorders

---

Objectives for the Reader

- To differentiate between two causative factors in promoting anterior pelvic tilt: hyperextension through the lumbar spine and lumbosacral hyper-extension as a function of hip flexion contracture.

- To describe the functional and kinesiological relationship between anterior pelvic tilt, hip flexion contracture, femoral antetorsion, and activation of the gluteus maximus as a torque force.

- To explain the closed-chain relationship between femoral antetorsion and pronation of the foot.

- To specify the distinguishing alignment features of the following deformities: equinus, equinovalgus, equinovarus, flexible pes planus, and crouch.

- To suggest the primary functional limitations imposed by the problems associated with equinus, equinovalgus, equinovarus, flexible pes planus, and crouch.

This chapter will explore the structural and functional consequences of the chronic application of deforming forces frequently observed in children with abnormal neuromotor function. The chapter will discuss problems in cephalocaudal sequence, beginning with those related to persistent hypertonus, followed by those that commonly occur with crouch deformity, and closing with generalized hypotonia.

Children with a neuromotor deficit struggle to distribute body weight as efficiently as possible over a small base of support and around their center of gravity. Their task is made more difficult, however, because they must compensate for biomechanical problems. These problems are imposed by abnormal muscle and weight-bearing forces that have resulted in shortening and overstretching of various soft tissues, distortions in the outcome of the skeletal modeling process, and imbalances of muscle power.

Hypertonus

Estimated Ambulatory Potential

It has been estimated that 85 percent of children with spastic diplegia will walk by the age of 4 years. Of that percentage, 20 percent will use assistive devices. Virtually all children with hemiplegia will walk by the age of 3 years. Of those with spastic quadriplegia, 66 percent will probably become ambulatory with or without some sort of assistive devices; most of those will do so after the age of 4 years (Molnar 1985; Molnar 1986; Wilson 1987). The achievement of independent sitting by 2 years of age seems to be a positive indicator that walking will develop, while postponement of independent sitting until after the age of 4 years correlates with low expectations for ambulation (Molnar 1985; Molnar 1986; Wilson 1987).

In a study of 50 children with spastic diplegia, which spanned a follow-up duration of 4-16 years, Badell-Ribera (1985) noted the age of acquisition of three styles of sitting, of symmetrical crawling (bunny-hopping) and reciprocal crawling as the main means of locomotion, and of sitting from supine. She also noted the age of acquisition of four levels of ambulation:

    I. Exercise ambulation.

    II. Household ambulation—low endurance.

    III. Household ambulation—high endurance.

    IV. Community ambulation.

All of the children received physical therapy almost daily from the time of early diagnosis until they achieved their levels of ambulatory function. In all of these cases, the available motor control at 1½ to 2½ years of age was predictive of locomotor prognosis. Specifically, those children (18) who achieved reciprocal crawling and who never used the bunny-hopping pattern achieved Level IV, community ambulation, without aids by 3½ to 6 years of age. The eight high-endurance household ambulators (Level III) were able to assume sitting from prone (rather than from supine) and used symmetrical hopping between ages 1½ and 2½ years. These children attained reciprocal crawling after age 3 years. Five children who achieved Level II, low-endurance household ambulation, never crawled reciprocally. These children used symmetrical hopping by age 2½ years and attained crutch ambulation by age 5½ years.

Common Features of Alignment in the Presence of Hypertonus

The following discussion pertains primarily to the child with spastic diplegia. As was done in Chapter 3, this chapter will review the alignment features that commonly occur in this population in a proximal-to-distal progression, except where clarity in describing certain biomechanical relationships requires diverting from this track. Problems related to hip subluxation will not be considered in this discussion.

The Pelvis and Lumbar Spine

Deviations in pelvic alignment in the standing position are a common problem in children with neuromotor disorder. A major goal of movement training for the pediatric therapist is the achievement of reciprocal control of the pelvis by the trunk musculature. The goal is to obtain an easy interplay between the abdominal obliques, the rectus abdominous, the quadratus lumborum, and the lumbar extensor muscles. Optimum antigravity function of the posterolateral hip musculature depends upon the controlled pelvis as a stable point of stability.

However lordotic, young children normally achieve this interplay. This is evident in their increasingly competent antics on riding toys, jungle gyms, slides, roller skates, and other types of playground equipment. Young children normally gain their anterior pelvic tilt from hyperextension through the entire lumbar spine (Asher 1975).

Many children with spastic diplegia fail to resolve the neonatal lumbar kyphosis. They retain a posterior pelvic tilt by maintaining the lumbar spine in flexion. Others might fail to resolve the neonatal hip flexion contracture. They might tilt the pelvis anteriorly at the lumbosacral joint, with or without persistent lumbar flexion (Bleck 1987; Brooks 1985). Children with spastic quadriparesis typically reveal asymmetric distribution of hypertonus through the trunk and extremities. They also develop pelvic obliquity with subsequent apparent leg length discrepancy (Bleck 1987). Children with spastic hemiplegia commonly elevate and rotate the pelvis toward the more affected side, creating a pelvic obliquity which results in apparent (often combined with true) leg length discrepancy (Bobath et al. 1976; Staheli et al. 1968).

Pelvis/Hip Joint Connection

Each of these deviations in pelvic alignment diminishes the efficiency of hip muscle function by altering the line of pull of the hip musculature. For example, the normal sacrofemoral angle, which is derived radiographically by intersecting lines drawn parallel to the femur and to the proximal edge of the sacrum, falls within 45-65 degrees. Tilting the pelvis forward at the lumbosacral joint effectively reduces this angle; this occurs in contracture of the iliopsoas muscle (Staheli 1977, CORR). Bleck (1987) uses a sacrofemoral angle of less than 50 degrees, combined with clinical evaluation results, as indication for surgery. Proximal to the sacrum, the lumbar spine might be in any of the following positions: flexed, normally aligned, or hyperextended. Lumbar hyperextension indicates participation by the psoas and the lumbar extensor muscles in the reduction of neonatal primary kyphosis. These muscles may also abnormally compensate for weakness in the trunk flexors and hip extensors (Bly 1983).

The gluteus maximus functions optimally as a lateral rotator of the hip with the hip in extension (Soderberg 1986). The position of hip flexion imposed by anterior pelvic tilt actually converts the upper fibers of the same muscle into medial rotators of the hip. The iliopsoas is also a medial hip rotator in stance position; this is because of the location of the vertical axis of hip rotation at the head of the femur (Soderberg 1986). Active or passive shortening of the iliopsoas muscle produces an anterior pelvic tilt and facilitates femoral medial rotation while impeding the activity of the gluteus maximus as a lateral rotator. Thus the magnitude of lateral torque forces on the growing femur is significantly compromised. Bleck (1987) reports that his studies of the relationship between hip extension and lateral rotation and derotation of the proximal end of the femur indicate "that the earlier hip extension is obtained, the more likely correction of torsion will occur" (p. 332).

Furthermore, the action of the gluteus medius is compromised by the change in pelvic alignment. Thus the greater trochanter, whose creation through cartilage modeling relies upon tensile forces applied by the gluteus medius, fails to form appropriately, and neonatal coxa valga commonly persists (Staheli et al. 1968; Bleck 1987). Ryder's test for femoral torsional deformity becomes difficult to conduct because the greater trochanter is not clearly palpable. The acetabulum remains shallow.

Finally, the tendon of insertion of the psoas muscle cups the distal femoral head en route to the lesser trochanter. When the psoas muscle is shortened, the tendon of insertion restricts the head of the femur from gliding distally with hip abduction. In this way, iliopsoas contracture contributes to hip subluxation and poverty of abduction strength.

Distal Consequences of Pelvic Malalignment

Problems associated with anterior pelvic tilt

The closed chain dictates that persistent hip flexion contracture (such as the type present with anterior pelvic tilt) combines with femoral antetorsion to promote medial hip rotation (or a lack of lateral rotation). After the neonatal lateral rotation contracture is resolved

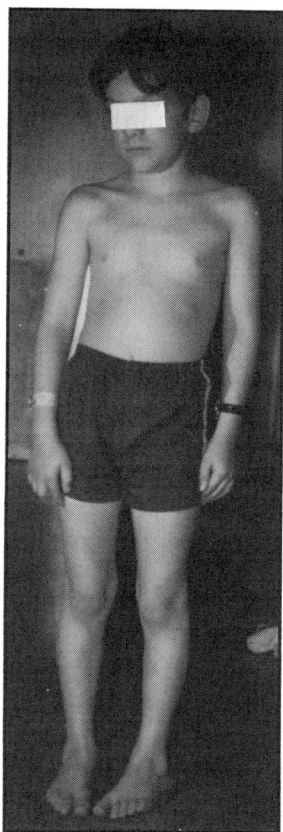

Figure 4.1 Evidence of femoral antetorsion: patella aligns medial to sagittal plane of the leg. Note that feet are adducted (in-toed), which protects them from pronating. Age 9 years.

(or, in the case of the premature infant who might not have developed the full extent of contracture, when adequate medial hip rotation mobility is available), the head and neck of the femur attempt to align in maximum congruity with the acetabulum. Consequently, the transcondylar axis aligns in medial rotation relative to the frontal plane. The patella also aligns medial to the sagittal plane bisection of the knee joint (Figure 4.1).

Problems associated with medial femoral torsion

The lower leg initially aligns in congruity with the medially deviated femoral condyles. This alignment reduces the angle of the transmalleolar axis (TMA or the axis of mortice) relative to the frontal plane (Figures 4.2 and 4.3).

Relative to these medial rotational deviations, the angle of gait and the width of the base of support vary in accordance with the child's compensatory mechanisms. The distal segments either follow suit and rotate medially along with the femoral condyles, or they compensate by rotating laterally.

Figure 4.2 Pronation in conjunction with femoral antetorsion (in-toeing corrected): tibial medial rotation and reduced axis of mortice; peroneals and long toe extensors activated as forefoot abductors/evertors (Same child as seen in Figure 4.1).

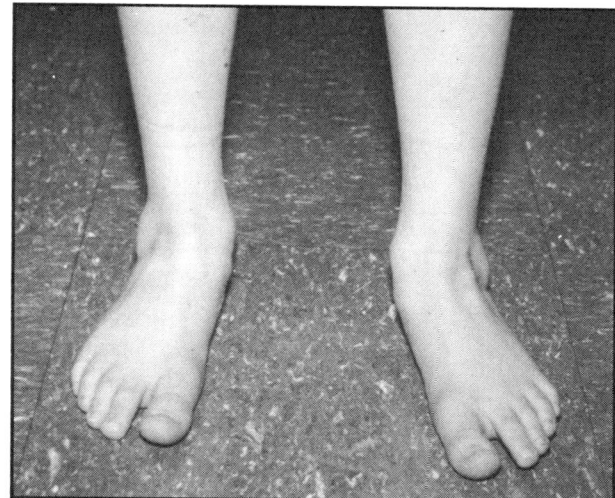

Figure 4.3 Pronation: calcaneal valgus deviation, concave lateral foot surface; reduced axis of mortice. Normal calcaneal valgus = 0-2 degrees after 5 years of age.

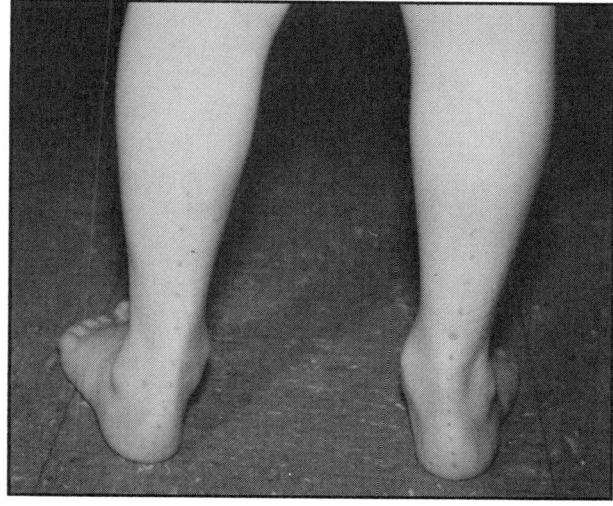

Reduced angle of gait—Some children adduct the foot, or "toe-in," while maintaining a measure of sagittal plane alignment between the foot and the lower leg (Staheli 1977, CORR; King et al. 1984). These children typically develop minimal pronation deformity because they distribute much of their body weight over the lateral borders of the feet in stance and gait (Tachdjian 1985) (Figure 4.1). They do, however, load the foot abnormally and achieve push-off over the lateral aspect of the forefoot rather than over the medial. The medial deviation is aggravated by supination deformity secondary to a spastic posterior tibialis (King et al. 1984).

Increased angle of gait with pronation—Other children eventually succeed in counteracting the proximal medial femoral torsion by increasing the lateral torsional declination in the lower leg bones. This action produces an increased angle of gait at the foot, or "toe-out," while the patellae align medially (Staheli et al. 1985; King et al. 1984). The result is an excessive distribution of weight onto the medial aspect of the foot. These children typically develop significant pronation deformity (McCrea 1985; Root et al. 1977) (Figure 4.3).

If the child seeks stability by maintaining the feet in abduction in standing, the medially rotated lower leg imposes pronatory forces on the foot as the ankle mortice carries the talus into adduction on the calcaneus. The existing subtalar joint (STJ) configuration dictates that the adducting talus also plantarflexes, adducts, and slides anteriorly on the calcaneus. This action disrupts STJ stability. The lower leg accompanies the talus in these excursions, and the knee flexes as it rotates medially over the foot (Jordan et al. 1983; Regnauld 1986).

Compensatory equinus—Anterior displacement of the center of gravity commonly occurs with anterior pelvic tilt. This happens because the antigravity trunk flexors are typically underdeveloped. The truncal balance of power favors the more efficient and primitive extensors. The normal distal equilibrium response to anterior weight shift is toe-standing, which, if persistent, can result in compensatory equinus deformity (Bly et al. 1980).

Problems associated with posterior pelvic tilt
Persistent lumbar flexion, uncompensated by hyperextension at the lumbosacral joint, might be accompanied either by a reduction of anterior pelvic tilt or by actual posterior pelvic tilt. As the child with this problem tries to stand erect, the capsular structures tighten about the extending hips as they approach the close-packed position for weight-bearing. As the closed chain operates from proximal to distal segments, lumber flexion causes a posterior tilt of the pelvis to occur together biomechanically with hip extension and knee flexion. The hips and pelvis become a unit in extension, and the backward tip of the proximal pelvis moves the acetabulae and adjacent femoral heads down and forward. The distal femoral shafts deviate anteriorly.

The child with incomplete lumbar extension, a posterior pelvic tilt, and hypertonus is inclined to stand with knees flexed. Persistence of this posture generally leads to flexion contracture at the knees and patella alta. Patella alta (elongation and narrowing of the patella) results from the profoundly increased force required of the quadriceps to maintain standing in knee flexion (Bleck 1987; Waters et al. 1985; Perry et al. 1975). The compensations at the feet are variable; they depend upon the degree of equinus deformity and the arrangement of the feet relative to the sagittal plane.

Problems associated with pelvic obliquity
Pelvic obliquity requires the expression of a rotary component in the spine because the vertebrae normally accomplish lateral flexion only with rotation. Elevation of one side of the pelvis produces an ipsilateral functional leg-length reduction and reduces the weight distribution onto the same "shorter" leg. Functional leg length and consequent step length are further reduced by maintaining the pelvis in lateral rotation, which limits anterior excursion of the leg during the swing phase of gait.

The ambulatory child with obliquity and lateral rotation of the pelvis toward the more affected side commonly attempts to achieve adequate leg length for stance and terminal swing by extending the ankle joint. The result is compensatory equinus, or toe-standing (Cerny 1984). When accompanied by hip lateral rotation (typical in young children), pronation develops at the foot; this produces equinovalgus deformity. When accompanied by the medial rotation of the hip joint that develops in older children, the foot supinates with equinus; this produces equinovarus deformity. In either case, the equinus compensation perpetuates the pelvic malalignment. In the presence of inadequate weight-bearing on the affected limb, actual leg-length discrepancy frequently results (Staheli et al. 1968).

The presence of spasticity in the lower extremity usually favors ankle plantarflexion. This happens because of the disproportionate strength and lever arms for muscle force in the calf musculature rather than in the ankle and toe dorsiflexors (Silver et al. 1985). Unilateral or asymmetric spastic ankle plantarflexion on a rigid, supinated foot can drive the pelvis into elevation and lateral rotation on the more affected side; it is modified to varying degrees by the weight-bearing angle of knee flexion or hyperextension (Winters et al. 1987).

Laxity of the supporting ligaments in the knee, ankle, and foot must be considered in addressing problems of alignment. Laxity can occur with either hypertonus or weakness. Ligamentous laxity can be the primary cause of failure of the supporting structures, or it can be induced by chronic application of deforming forces (Regnauld 1986; Schafer 1987; McCrea 1985; Bleck 1987; Root et al. 1977; Rodgers et al. 1984; LeVeau et al. 1984).

The Knee

Problems associated with knee flexion contracture
Neonatal knee flexion contracture is usually resolved before the age of 12 months, which allows the infant to sit with a vertical pelvis and both knees extended. Failure to resolve this contracture through antigravity flexion skills results in persistence of the flexion contracture (Bly et al. 1980).

In children with hypertonus, antigravity trunk flexion strength and control typically is underdeveloped, which results in a lack of equilibrium responses to backward weight shift. Consistent anterior displacement of the center of gravity over the feet promotes activity in the hamstrings and gastrocnemius/soleus as a component of equilibrium. This displacement also promotes knee flexion contracture and the inefficient use of the quadriceps in the flexed knee position. Patella alta is a common modeling consequence of such overwork by the quadriceps (Bleck 1987; Lotman 1976).

Problems of knee flexion contracture associated with medial genicular deformity

Because knee flexion permits transverse plane motion of the lower leg on the femur, neonatal medial genicular knee position also commonly persists in spastic diplegia and quadriplegia, along with an increased rotary mobility of the lower leg in the femur (McCrea 1985; Valmassy 1984). Persistent medial genicular position prohibits the achievement of normal knee extension. This is because the contracture hinders the normal corkscrew motion of the lower leg into lateral rotation with the terminal 10 degrees of knee extension.

The Lower Leg

Problems associated with tibiofibular torsion

Lateral tibiofibular torsion, perhaps accompanied by soft tissue changes in the knee joint, can evidently result from postures (such as W-sitting) in which the lower leg twists outward. It can also result from persistence of femoral antetorsion, as a compensation (McDonough 1984) (Figure 4.4). When medial torsion and/or genicular knee in one leg occurs together with lateral torsion and/or genicular position in the other leg, the legs appear "windblown" (Figure 4.5).

The Talocrural Joint

Problems associated with equinus deformity

Although commonly considered in the context of obligatory toe-standing (Figure 4.6), equinus is defined as the lack of 5-10 degrees of talocrural dorsiflexion beyond a 90-degree angle, while maintaining the STJ in neutral position (Root et al. 1971; McCrea 1985; Root et al. 1977). Both the soleus and gastrocnemius muscles are usually involved. Equinus is the most common problem of foot and ankle alignment and function in children with hypertonus; it imposes significant biomechanical problems of adjustment on the foot and the knee both in standing and in gait (Baker et al. 1964; Jordan et al. 1983; Bleck 1987; Root et al. 1977; Cerny 1984; Perry 1975; Goldner 1982; Rosenthal 1984; Rosenthal et al. 1975; Redford 1986).

Equinus-Related Deformities and Compensatory Patterns

Knee flexion contracture—Equinus deformity in spastic diplegia is frequently accompanied and enhanced by tightness in flexion at the knee joint (Rang et al. 1986; Hicks et al. 1988). It is caused by prolonged activity in, or lack of elongation of, either (or both) the gastrocnemius or the hamstring muscles (McCrea 1985; Bleck 1987; Csongradi et al. 1979; Perry 1975; Westin et al. 1983) (Figure 4.7). The swing phase is consequently clipped in length and limited in the force of forward momentum.

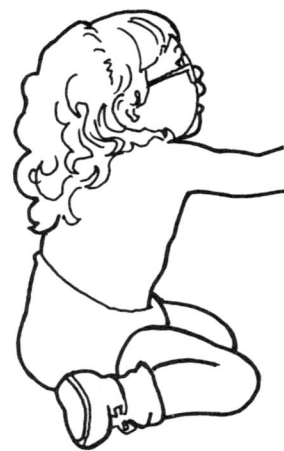

Figure 4.4
W-sitting: promotes femoral antetorsion and lateral rotary and torsional deviation in the lower legs.

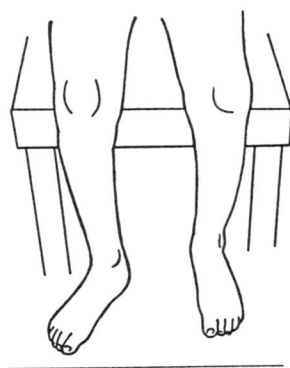

Figure 4.5
"Windblown" posture—evidence of medial (the child's left) and lateral (the child's right) genicular position.

If knee extension mobility is limited, intervention to reduce equinus deformity must include efforts to regain this mobility (Rang et al. 1986) (Figure 4.8). The following methods are commonly used, singularly or in combination, to regain extension mobility at the knee:

- Mobilization
- Night-splinting
- Long-leg serial casting
- Positioning
- Surgical lengthening, often in combination with distal rectus femoris transfer (McCrea 1985; Cary et al. 1975; Soderberg 1986; Perry 1975; Westin et al. 1983)

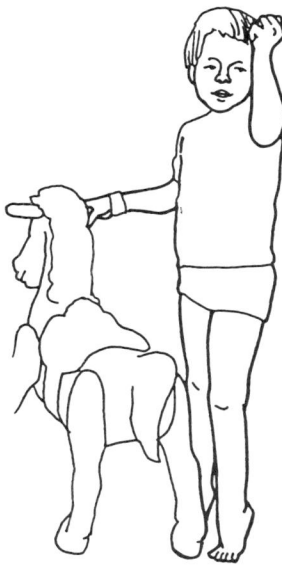

Figure 4.6
Equinus deformity (extreme).

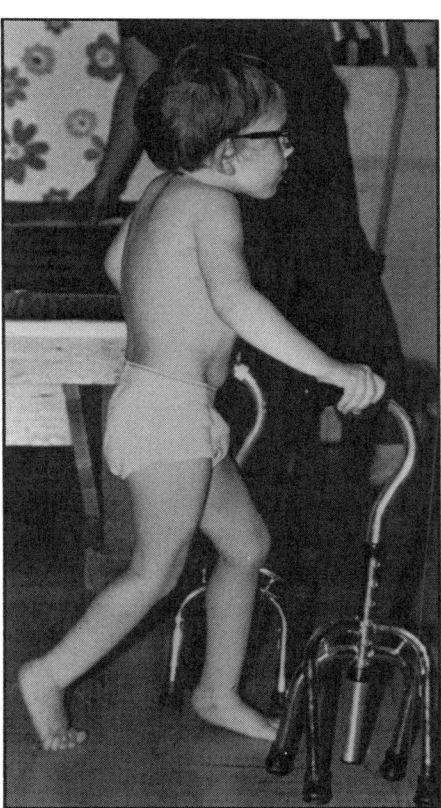

Figure 4.7
Equinus gait with knee flexion contracture. Note limited stride length and lack of plantigrade foot contact. Also note thoracic kyphosis with lumbar flexion (the lack of antigravity extension).

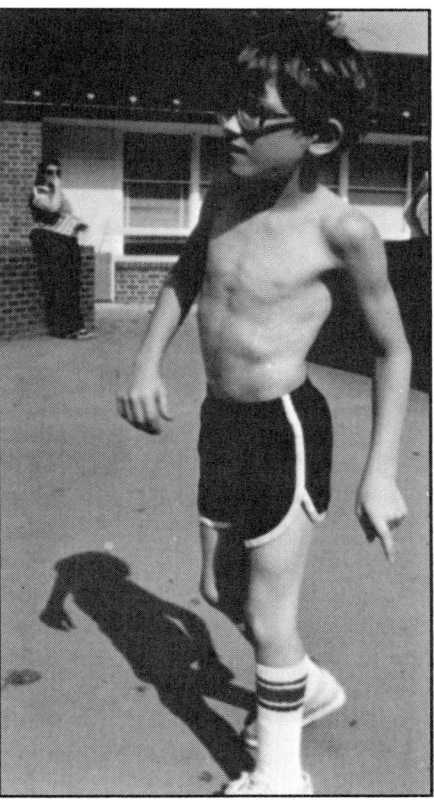

Figure 4.8
(Same child as in Figure 4.7.) Long-term (six-year) result of reduction of unilateral proximal hamstrings contracture and equinus deformity, with casting, orthoses, and a consistent program of positioning and therapeutic exercise at home and school.

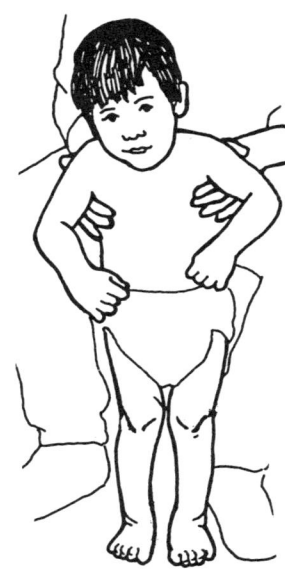

Figure 4.9
Knee hyperextension,
associated with
equinus deformity.

Knee hyperextension (Figure 4.9)—Stressing the knee joint beyond its normal range of extension is a common adjustment to the lack of dorsiflexion mobility at the ankle joint. This occurs as the child attempts to lower the heel of the affected foot to the ground while standing on it (McCrea 1985; Perry 1974; Root et al. 1977; Rosenthal 1984; Rosenthal et al. 1975; Cerny 1984; Westin et al. 1983; Cary et al. 1975; Valmassy 1984). The proximal tibial plateau is retroverted in childhood, which also contributes to this inclination to hyperextend the knee (Bernhardt 1988). Rang et al. (1986) suggest that a little knee flexion is better than recurvatum.

Equinovalgus Deformity

One study observed equinovalgus deformity, combining equinus with pronation, in 64 percent of children with bilateral hypertonus and equinus (Bennet et al. 1982). (The term valgus refers to the frontal-plane calcaneal component, which aligns in eversion beyond the normal range.) Equinovalgus deformity persists throughout the stance phase of the gait cycle in those who ambulate. Most of the body weight is taken on the medial forefoot, as the bones of the foot and leg deviate in any of the following ways (Baker and Hill 1964; Perry 1975; Jordan et al. 1983; Bleck 1987; Root et al. 1977; Cerny 1984) (Figures 4.10 and 4.11).

- The calcaneus plantarflexes and everts under the talus.
- The talus plantarflexes, adducts, and migrates medially and forward.
- Depending upon the pitch of the MTJ oblique axis and the status of the forefoot structures the forefoot dorsiflexes, abducts, and everts, uncovering most of the medial surface of the head of the talus. If the MTJ oblique axis is pitched close to the frontal plane, the forefoot dorsiflexes significantly on the hindfoot. This action creates a "rocker bottom" foot in which the navicular replaces the calcaneus as the posterior point of loading (Figure 4.12).
- In other cases, particularly those in which the angle of gait is abnormally increased, structural forefoot varus deformity is evident off weight-bearing, and in the closed chain, this inverted forefoot merely lowers to the ground. Eversion is minimal.
- The talus protrudes proximal to the navicular tuberosity.
- The tibia and fibula rotate medially on the calcaneus, riding along with the motion of the body of the talus.
- The knee either flexes with an elevated calcaneus or hyperextends as the calcaneus is lowered to the ground. The quality of knee hyperextension is abnormal because of the lack of lateral rotation of the tibia on the femur, which is needed for proper knee extension.
- The toes claw and deviate laterally.

The equilibrium responses to backward and rotary weight shifts are usually absent or underdeveloped. The lack of reciprocal action in the distal musculature results in sluggish and ineffective responses to shifts of weight over the feet (Gunsolus et al. 1975; Salek 1977; Scherzer et al. 1982). The hypertonic foot is fixed both by the pronatory collapse and by the hyperactivity in the plantarflexors, long toe flexors, and peroneals as the child seems to grasp at the ground for stability. The pronated position of the foot increases its flexibility and thus its structural instability. This position further increases the demand for stabilization. If one thinks about the proprioceptive and biomechanical circumstances involved, the child with equinovalgus deformity might have a sense of standing and walking on bags filled with jelly.

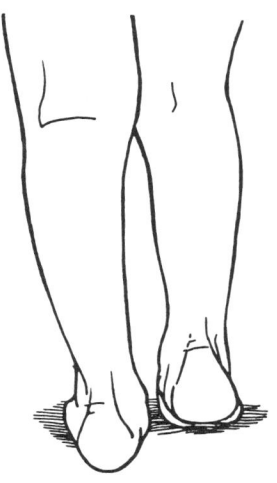

Figure 4.10
Equinovalgus deformity (posterior view). Combines pronation with equinus.

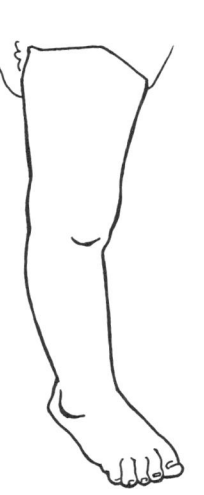

Figure 4.11
Equinovalgus deformity. Note creases at lateral ankle and lateral toe grasping.

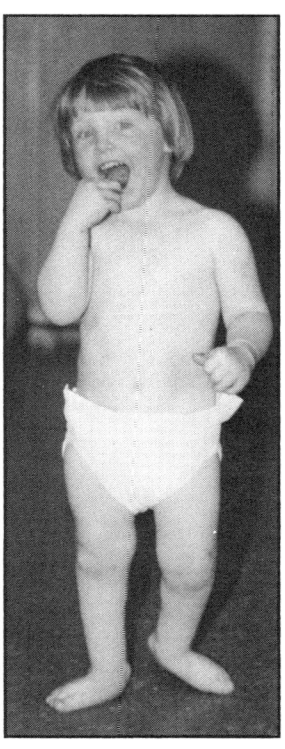

Figure 4.12
"Rocker bottom" foot deformity: primary dorsiflexion occurs at the oblique axis of the MTJ rather than at the talocrural joint.

Forefoot varus deformity—This malalignment is not evident in standing because the metatarsal heads lower to contact the ground. Usually, available joint mobility permitting, this occurs with a compensatory, equivalent pronation of the hindfoot (McCrea 1985; Root et al. 1977; Tiberio 1988). Closed-chain hindfoot valgus deformity, with or without accompanying equinus, typically occurs together with persistent immature forefoot varus deformity, or enhances it.

Hypermobile first ray—Exaggerated first ray dorsiflexion mobility reduces the efficiency of weight transfer over the foot at the latter part of the stance cycle. The result is a pronation inclination within the foot at the end of the stance phase, when maximum supination is desired. The second and third metatarsals endure extraordinary shear forces as the final stable point of contact at toe-off.

Hallux valgus and toe claw deformity—Anterior and medial displacement of body weight over the feet imposes significant loading stresses on the first ray and on the toes. Because the axis of the first ray aligns in the opposite direction to the other primary joint axes in the foot, the first ray can plantarflex and evert or dorsiflex and invert around the axis. In closed-chain equinovalgus deformity, the first ray inverts as it dorsiflexes on the navicular. However, the plantar/medial border of the metatarsal head bears most of the body weight. Shear forces occur at the first metatarsophalangeal joint (MTP), while the great toe is forced laterally by loading. The long-term result is bunion formation, in response to shear and forces applied to the skin that rubs on the shoe, and hallux valgus (Rodgers 1988; Gray 1986; Rose et al. 1985).

As stated in Chapter 3, hallux valgus also occurs as a long-term consequence of Morton's foot, in which the first ray is abnormally short. The first ray plantarflexes and everts, abducting away from the second ray in the closed chain. The long toe muscles and tendons of insertion become laterally displaced relative to the MTP joint.

After chronically flexing excessively as a compensatory balance-seeking mechanism, made more powerful by the advantageous pronatory alteration in axial direction and line of pull of the long toe flexors, the remaining toes develop claw deformity, or flexion contracture of all of the toe joints (Schenkman 1988).

Causes of Equinovalgus Deformity

The kinesiological view

It used to be generally presumed that equinovalgus occurs in response to chronic hyperactivity in the triceps surae muscle group, eventually resulting in contracture. The triceps surae are considered to be secondary supinators of the foot. When the foot is properly aligned, the tendon attaches medial to both the transmalleolar and the subtalar joint axes. However, it was thought that this tendon shortening produces a bowstring effect at the hindfoot, which causes the calcaneus to evert into valgus position. A substitute dorsiflexion with abduction was recognized as it occurred to varying degrees in the midtarsal joint around its oblique axis (Bleck 1987; Jordan et al. 1983).

Other viewpoints have appeared in current literature. Some hold that spastic peroneal muscles sometimes impose the significant deforming force. These peroneals continuously abduct the forefoot, subluxing the navicular off of the talus and drawing it laterally, and stretching the medial plantar ligaments that support the talar head (Bleck 1987). According to this view, the resulting talar plantarflexion compromises further the integrity of the subtalar joint. Bennet et al. (1982) used EMG analysis to determine that a relationship, which the authors suggest is causal, exists between the frontal plane deviations of varus and valgus components of equinus deformity and the nature of activity in the posterior tibialis muscle. Varus occurred with evidence of posterior tibialis activity. Valgus occurred with evidence of inactivity. Skinner et al. (1985) used dynamic EMG to determine other possible contributing forces to the valgus hindfoot in spastic cerebral palsy and found three patterns of abnormal muscle activity:

1. Hyperactive peroneals with strong posterior tibialis.
2. Hyperactive peroneals with weak posterior tibialis.
3. Hyperactive long toe extensors.

The triceps surae musculature was included in the study but was not mentioned as an etiological factor. This study raises the possibility that the long toe extensors are a causative force.

The biomechanical view
The biomechanical perspective sheds another dimension of light on the etiology of equinovalgus. By considering the influences of structural and postural alignment, aberrant loading forces, alterations in pitch of the axes of motion within the foot and ankle, changes in direction and strength of contractile forces in the muscles that cross those modified axes, ligamentous laxity—either original or acquired—and adaptive shortening of connective and muscle tissues, the compensatory element in dysphasic muscle activity, as observed on dynamic EMG, becomes evident. To a certain extent, true spasticity notwithstanding, posture and underlying architecture dictate function.

In children with spastic diplegia, the prevalent postural problems feature inadequacy of trunk flexors as a balance for the extensors; poverty of pelvic mobility and control, often favoring anterior tilt; medial torsion and rotation in the bones and joints of the lower extremities; and persistence of flexion contracture at the hips and knees. These abnormalities result in distribution of nearly 100 percent of body weight onto the medial forefoot. Normally, 60 percent of body weight is carried by the heel. The forefoot is typically aligned in structural varus in the open chain in young children. Therefore, abnormal anterior displacement of heavy load to the medial forefoot forces the foot into pronation.

The position of pronation of the foot structures increases the sagittal-plane pitch of the axes of the talocrural, subtalar, and midtarsal joints. Pronation thus changes the force vectors—and resulting strength—of all the muscles that cross the axes in the foot. The more perpendicular the line of pull to the joint axis, the stronger the force generated. The flexibility of the foot, which results from disruption of congruity in pronation, also permits the muscles to contract to move bones rather than to translate compressive and stabilizing forces from distal to proximal bones (Root et al. 1977; Schenkman 1988).

The calcaneus everts in pronation while the STJ axis rotates medially. The tendon of insertion of the triceps surae group moves lateral to the STJ axis, where it cannot bring about inversion with plantarflexion. The contractile and supinatory strength of the anterior and posterior tibialis muscles is reduced by pronation and enhanced by supination. The insertion of the anterior tibialis moves lateral to the STJ axis in pronation. The posterior tibialis lengthens and loses power. In addition, structural pronation enhances the abduction/

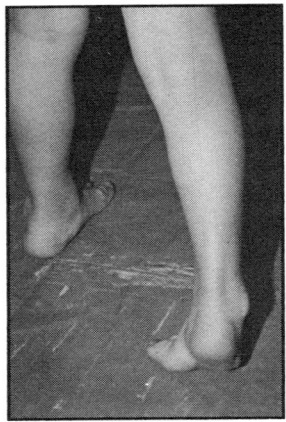

Figure 4.13
Equinovarus deformity (posterior view): Supination with equinus. Note calcaneal inversion, prominent lateral malleolus (displaced posteriorly), forefoot adduction, and plantarflexed first ray.

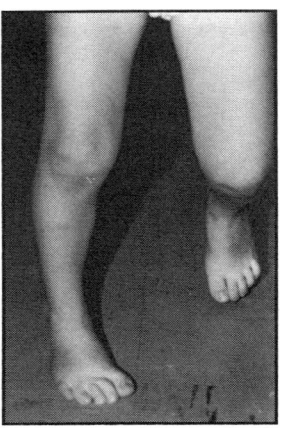

Figure 4.14
Equinovarus: weight rolls to the outer border of the forefoot; floor reaction forces are communicated to the knee joint via the rigid, supinated foot. Forefoot valgus develops.

eversion function of the peroneus longus and long toe extensor muscles, and the flexion power of the long toe flexors.

Therefore, if the muscles of inversion are "quiet" on EMG in the equinovalgus foot, perhaps this quiescence is a consequence of the inability of the muscle to activate across an altered axial pitch, which places the tendon of insertion on the wrong side of, or parallel rather than perpendicular to, the axis of rotation for that muscle (Schenkman 1988).

The biomechanical view would require primary attention to restoring the architecture of the foot before attempting to refine muscle function through surgery or therapeutic exercise. The most revealing evaluation to determine the contribution of true spasticity to equinovalgus deformity might be testing of the dorsal roots with electrical stimulation. This process is currently in use during selective dorsal rhizotomy procedures.

Equinovarus Deformity

Unlike equinovalgus, this deformity is one of hypersupination of the foot combined with limitation of full dorsiflexion mobility (Figures 4.13 and 4.14). Research has revealed that up to 94 percent of the children with congenital spastic hemiplegia eventually reveal equinovarus deformity on the more affected side (Bleck 1987). This deformity, even when functional, is often quite resistant to conservative methods of reduction.

Compensatory pronation commonly occurs in the less affected foot (Jordan et al. 1983).

When most children with congenital hemiplegia begin to walk, they maintain the more affected leg in the primitive position of lateral rotation and abduction. This position may help to clear the forefoot during the swing phase and to avoid stressing the talocrural joint into dorsiflexion in stance (Molnar 1986; Wilson 1987). The foot typically deviates into pronation during this early period. As these children grow older and taller, several factors combine to promote a switch from pronation to supination deviation in the more affected foot, including the following:

• Persistent femoral antetorsion.

• Elevation and retraction of the pelvis.

• Reduction in the proximal femoral anteversion sustained by the original hip lateral rotation contracture.

• Reduction in the width of the base of support.

Equinovarus deformity is associated with compensatory forefoot valgus deformity.

Forefoot valgus—This deformity occurs as a long-term consequence of limited STJ eversion mobility with or without equinus. Forefoot valgus also fosters persistence of hindfoot varus by causing the foot to roll laterally on weight-bearing.

A plantarflexed first ray can falsely suggest that the forefoot is in valgus deformity. This possibility must be identified and ruled out

(Jordan et al. 1983). Long-term associated deformities include hammered toes, forefoot adductus, calcaneal varus, ankle sprains, heavy callus on the plantar first and fifth metatarsal pads and on the base of the fifth metatarsal, unstable gait, and neuralgia (Jordan et al. 1983; Gray 1986; Tiberio 1988).

Hammertoe deformity—With equinovarus deformity, persistent hyperextension at the metatarsophalangeal joints occurs as a compensatory mechanism to achieve clearance of the foot in swing. Hammertoes develop commonly. Usually they involve contracture of the long toe extensors at the MTP and distal interphalangeal joints, as well as flexion contracture of the proximal interphalangeal joints.

Functional Implications of Hypertonus-Induced Deformity

Altered Angle of Gait

The bones within the lower extremity combine with their respective joint alignments to influence the angle of gait. The joints to be considered include the lumbosacral, hip, knee, talocrural, subtalar, midtarsal, tarsometatarsal, and metatarsophalangeal joints. The structural features of the femur, the tibia, the fibula, and the talus must also be evaluated. Collectively or individually, these factors contribute to the angle of progression, which is determined by measuring foot placement relative to the sagittal plane.

Increased Angle of Gait

If the angle of gait exceeds 15 degrees lateral to the sagittal plane, weight is distributed to the medial aspect of the foot in stance in abnormal and stressful proportion. This weight distribution can result in pronation deformity (Root et al. 1977) (Figure 4.15). Contributing factors to an increased angle of progression include problems related to joint mobility or bone structure, such as the following:

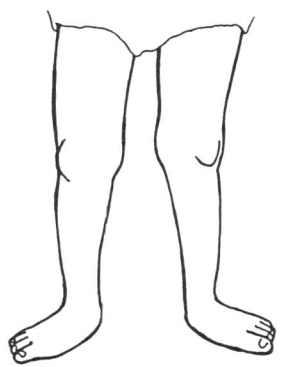

Figure 4.15
Pronation as a consequence of lateral hip rotation contracture, increased angle of gait, and ligamentous laxity.

- The foot may be abnormally abducted by lateral hip rotation contracture (Figures 4.12 and 4.15).

- Persistence of femoral antetorsion can result in compensatory excess tibial lateral torsion, or tibial lateral rotation, or both (Bleck 1982; McCrea 1985; Root et al. 1977; Valmassy 1984; King et al. 1984; Staheli et al. 1985). In this instance, the patellae align medial to the sagittal plane of the leg, the mortice axis is abnormally increased relative to the transcondylar axis at the femur, and the feet align in increased abduction. This malalignment might result from a more successful application of lateral torque forces to the knee and lower leg than to the femoral shaft, both in play positions and in gait.

- Limitation of ankle dorsiflexion mobility might necessitate out-toeing, which functionally shortens the foot by diverting it outward. Forefoot varus deformity eventually increases in response to the lateromedial direction of weight transfer over the forefoot.

- Forefoot abduction with pronation around the MTJ axis can produce an increased angle of gait. In this type of deformity, if the proximal structures orient medially, restoration of the foot structures to a more neutral alignment often results in in-toe gait. The proximal medial torsional and rotational deformities become evident when the pronatory distal compensation is reduced.

- Persistent neonatal forefoot varus deviation can contribute to increased angle of gait. This can happen if progression over the forefoot is facilitated by aligning the transmetatarsal axis closer to the sagittal than to the frontal plane. This type of alignment reduces the need to lower the medial aspect of the forefoot to the ground with forward progression.

Decreased Angle of Gait

The following features of alignment can contribute individually or in combination to a reduced angle of gait, otherwise known as "in-toeing":

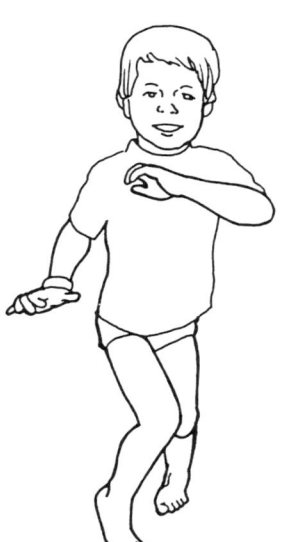

Figure 4.16
Decreased angle of gait—evidence of uncompensated femoral antetorsion, internal (medial) genicular deformity, tibial or talar torsion, or a combination of these.

- A study of 330 children with femoral "anteversion" (and presumably normal tone) determined a significant correlation between in-toeing and the available range of rotation in the extended hip joint. When medial hip rotation exceeds 60 degrees and lateral rotation is limited to 25 degrees or less, femoral anteversion (that is to say, antetorsion) is clinically significant as an influence on in-toeing in gait (Bleck 1982). Uncompensated femoral antetorsion aligns the lower leg and foot in medial rotation under the femur in stance and gait (Figure 4.16).

- In-toeing also results from medial tibiofibular torsion, alone or in combination with rotary laxity in the knee joint (Staheli 1977 (PCNA); Bleck 1982; Hutter et al. 1949; Valmassy 1984; King et al. 1984; McCrea 1985). When the degree of in-toeing varies from step to step, the amount and relative proportions of rotary knee joint mobility is a typical contributing factor. Rotary knee joint motion is a feature of soft tissue adaptations (Valmassy 1984).

- Bleck (1982) reports that unresolved neonatal talar torsion produces medial rotation of the foot under the tibia and fibula, which reduces the angle of gait and produces an appearance of medial tibial torsion. The persisting feature of the talus is the elongated, adducted talar neck, which then articulates with the navicular. Presumably, via the naviculocuboid articulation, the entire foot assumes a medially rotated orientation in keeping with the resulting adduction of the medial pillar. The talar trochlea and body are appropriately aligned within the ankle mortice nearly parallel with the long bisection of the calcaneus. The distinguishing feature in persistent talar torsion is a normal angle of the axis of mortice with an adducted foot (Bleck 1982; Bleck 1987).

- Metatarsus adductus is never normal and, if persistent, initially produces a reduced angle of gait. In time, however, if the deformity is severe enough to cause tripping, compensation to reduce in-toeing occurs in the proximal joints, where lateral rotation occurs to move the toes outward. This combination of problems can result in "skewfoot" deformity, with persistent metatarsus adductus and hindfoot pronation (Agnew 1988).

- Persistence of neonatal adduction of the first ray from the remaining tarsals and metatarsals can also produce in-toeing in gait.

The Equinus Gait Pattern

A review of the biomechanical features of floor reaction force vectors, normal and abnormal, appears in the article by Cerny (1984) on "The Pathomechanics of Stance." Dynamic EMG studies are currently generating new information about muscle action in gait, both normal and abnormal, and are gaining importance in management (Sutherland 1984; DeLuca et al. 1988; Hoffer et al. 1983; Norlin et al. 1986; Perry et al. 1975; Csongradi et al. 1979; Winters et al. 1987; Tylkowski et al. 1988).

In equinus gait (Figure 4.7), the following events of normal gait fail to occur:

- Knee extension at the end of swing, prior to heel strike. This pattern is needed to enhance forward momentum of the body over the opposite stance foot, and to increase step length (Hicks et al. 1988).

- Heel strike.

- Midstance motion of the tibia over the plantigrade foot.

Stride length, stability (as determined by single limb stance duration), and walking velocity are reduced (Norlin et al. 1986; Sutherland 1984). Some children compensate for problems of equilibrium and reduced velocity by replacing ambulation with a modified run (Figure 4.16).

Norlin et al. (1986) conducted a gait study in which 50 ambulatory children with spastic cerebral palsy participated. The study included 28 children with diplegia, 19 with hemiplegia, and three with tetraplegia. Five of these children had undergone surgery at least two years prior to the study. Data collected for the entire group revealed that the study group demonstrated reduced velocity, which does not increase significantly with age, and shorter maximal stride length when compared with a control group. Cadence was comparatively high in the younger children with spasticity but dropped to below normal with an increase in stride duration as the children grew older. The increased duration of stride appears to contribute to the lack of increase in gait velocity with increasing age. Older children with spasticity require a longer time period for each stride, which causes the whole movement to become slower than it was when they were younger.

Considering the children with bilateral involvement, the double support phase was longer than that for the control group. Among those with hemiplegia, the affected and non-affected sides were compared when significant asymmetry was apparent. Compared with the affected side, the non-affected side showed shorter swing, longer single support, prolonged double support, and prolonged total stance phases. Thus the reverse applies to the affected side.

The authors of this study draw the following conclusions:

- Gait deviations in cerebral palsy result from a combination of primary deficit and compensatory mechanisms.
- The variable that most deviates from the control data is stride frequency (cadence), which reveals a decline with increasing age.
- Because we observe reduced ambulatory capability as a lowered velocity, then as a single measurement, velocity is a good indication of gait ability.
- Repeated measurements of gait velocity, stride length, and stride frequency should help describe changes in the gait ability of a patient.

Some form of compensatory motion can usually solve the problem of progressing past the plantarflexed foot: either the knee hyperextends as the child attempts to lower the heel to the ground, with associated hip flexion and anterior pelvic tilt, or the limb is maintained in flexion at the knee and toe-stepping is employed to allow forward progression (McCrea 1985; Perry 1974; Root et al. 1977; Perry 1975; Cerny 1984; Winters et al. 1987).

The Equinovalgus Gait Pattern

When the alignment problems characteristic of equinovalgus are applied to gait, the features of equinus gait correspond to the apropulsive quality of the pronated foot. Persistence of knee flexion in swing and stance phases is accompanied by medial rotary and angular deviation of the lower leg, the knee joint, and the femur. Because femoral torsion typically prevails and the angle of gait is increased by a component of abduction at one or more segments of the foot and lower leg, the lateral rotary excursion during the stance phase fails to appear. The leg remains abnormally medially rotated over the plantarflexed and pronated foot from weight assumption through toe-off.

Lateral weight shifts are usually initiated at the head and upper trunk rather than at the lumbar and sacral segment of the trunk (Perry 1975).

Winters et al. (1987) recently analyzed kinematic data and distinguished four gait patterns among 46 children and young adults with spastic hemiplegia. The four patterns increase in complexity and severity. They include:

- Foot drop in swing with adequate ankle dorsiflexion mobility in stance.
- Static or dynamic contracture of the plantar flexors, with mechanical consequences of floor reaction forces expressed at the knee joint (presumably as hyperextension).

- Stiff-knee gait, which is related to inhibited plantar reflex activity at terminal stance and produces a persistent extension pattern in swing as well.
- Stiff-knee gait with limited hip joint motion.

The authors suggest that surgical lengthening is contraindicated for those in the mildest group.

Equinovarus deformity occurs most often in children with hemiplegia or with profoundly asymmetric diplegia, although it is seen less commonly than equinovalgus in the presence of bilateral involvement. The supinated position of the foot and ankle locks the foot into a rigid lever. This is different from pronation, which unlocks the foot and allows flexibility. When weight is taken on the foot in equinovarus posture, the floor reaction forces can direct the knee laterally with either passive hyperextension or compensatory flexion. The former impedes forward progression. The lateral aspect of the knee joint suffers tensile stresses while the medial knee is abnormally compressed. Proximal to the same foot and knee, the pelvis commonly elevates and retracts (Wilson 1987; Bobath et al. 1976). These pelvic deviations are particularly apparent if a recurvatum tendency occurs in the ipsilateral knee. The typical lack of elongation between the pelvis and ribs on the more-affected hemiplegic side is thus enhanced by the biomechanics at work in the lower extremity (Bly et al. 1980).

Meanwhile, because the STJ does not pronate but rather remains in supination throughout the stance cycle, the metatarsal heads seek the ground via plantarflexion of the first ray and passive eversion around the longitudinal axis of the MTJ (Figure 4.14). Persistence of the resulting forefoot valgus deviation produces a fixed deformity. The rigid valgus forefoot rolls in a medial-to-lateral direction as it seeks full contact with the ground. The roll at the forefoot causes the hindfoot to roll into varus position. In this manner, the valgus forefoot deformity maintains the varus malalignment of the hindfoot.

Problems of Posture, Alignment, and Gait Related to Weakness of Antigravity Musculature and Supporting Tissues

Crouch Posture

Crouch posture appears when the hips, knees, and ankles flex abnormally while the heels remain in contact with the floor during weight-bearing (Figure 4.17). Angles exceeding 30 degrees can occur at the knee and ankle joints (Sutherland 1984; Sutherland et al. 1978). The foot deformity that occurs in crouch posture is known as *calcaneus deformity,* which is the opposite of equinus deformity.

Although crouch posture is seen in children as young as 4 to 6 years of age, this problem often becomes distressing when the child reaches school age and adolescence and encounters multiple difficulties related to deterioration in ambulatory capability. This child is likely to exhibit several functional and alignment problems, including any of the following: (Sutherland 1984; Sutherland et al. 1978; Lotman 1976; Harrington et al. 1983-84; Frost 1971)

- Fatigue
- Deterioration of posture or of ambulatory capability
- Quadriceps weakness or overwork in the lengthened position
- Increased vertical trunk displacement in gait
- Exaggerated arm swing
- Hip flexion contracture
- Medial hip rotation with adduction
- Femoral antetorsion
- Hamstrings contracture
- The onset of knee pain
- Patella alta
- Calcaneus deformity
- Pronation deformity
- Toe clawing
- Pronated cavus foot: high-arched, often with rigid forefoot equinus deformity that topples into pronation, modified by a lack of calcaneal eversion mobility.

The energy expense of knee-flexed ambulation can be devastating. This can be seen in the increased muscular effort and elevated rate of oxygen uptake in children with crouch deformity (Perry et al. 1975; Waters et al. 1985). For example, when the knee is contracted in 25 degrees of flexion, and the weight line passes three inches behind the

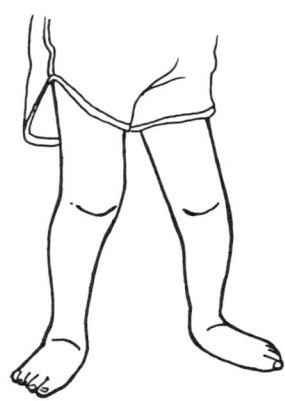

Figure 4.17
Crouch posture: evidence of primary weakness in the ankle plantarflexors. Note pronation, knee flexion, tibial/fibular medial rotation, hip flexion, hip adduction, and medial rotation.

knee axis, compressive work load—that which must be generated by the quadriceps to keep the knee from buckling—amounts to two times body weight (Smith et al. 1986). At angles of 30 to 50 degrees or more, muscle fatigue caused by these enormous stresses can become unmanageable. When there is adequate strength and mobility for proximal and distal compensations, knee flexion of 15 degrees in stance can be tolerated (Perry et al. 1975).

The ankle plantarflexion/knee extension force couple operates in normal gait at the moment in the stance cycle when, at midstance, the center of gravity passes in front of the extended knee. Knee extension is thereafter controlled and maintained by the reverse, eccentric action of the ankle plantarflexors (Sutherland et al. 1978; Harrington et al. 1983-84).

The primary cause of crouch deformity has been identified as weakness in the triceps surae group, particularly the soleus muscle. The lack of stabilizing power (normally affected by reverse action) of the ankle plantar flexors on the tibia allows the tibia to fall too far over the talus and the plantigrade foot in stance. The knee and hip flex in response to the hyperdorsiflexion at the ankle; a secondary deformity of knee flexion and progressive tightness of the hamstrings muscles also develops (Soderberg 1986; Sutherland et al. 1980b; Tachdjian 1985; Sutherland et al. 1978; Cerny 1984).

The center of gravity remains behind the knee joint throughout the stance phase rather than passing anterior to it after midstance. The knee joint remains anterior to the weight line (vertical force vector). Therefore, the knee extensors must work to excess to keep the knees from buckling (Sutherland et al. 1978; Harrington et al. 1983-1984).

Contributing Factors in Crouch Posture

- Surgical intervention undertaken to reduce equinus deformity in the presence of proximal joint contractures (Rang et al. 1986). This appears to be the primary precursor to the development of crouch posture in children with neuromotor impairment (Segal et al. 1987; Sutherland et al. 1978). Segal et al. (1987) define calcaneal gait as the degree of dorsiflexion one standard deviation beyond the mean. They note increased dorsiflexion throughout the stance phase in children who had undergone tendo-Achilles lengthening procedures.

- Overlengthened heel cord tendons. Tendon lengthening does not affect the length of the muscle belly, which remains shortened. Strength is a function of the number of fibers combined with the amount of muscle excursion as is dictated by the overall length of the muscle belly. Therefore, although surgery makes the tendon longer, unless the muscle endures tensile forces that help to stimulate muscle growth, it remains shortened and weak (Rang et al. 1986). The resulting weakness in the plantar flexors often results in overstretch because the necessary extension mobility and control in the hips and/or knees is not available as a counterforce against sinking at the ankles (Bleck 1987; Dillin et al. 1983; Tachdjian 1985; Sutherland et al. 1978). Furthermore, the weakness frequently becomes evident in the form of crouch posture when the child gains body size and weight, as in adolescence.

- Inadequate postoperative distal immobilization. It is likely in some cases that the prescribed time period, consistency of use, and/or design of postoperative orthotic support was inadequate to protect against overstretching of the surgically lengthened ankle triceps surae tendon of insertion.

- Inadequate postoperative therapeutic exercise. When there is adequate mobility at the hip and knee joints, the program of postoperative therapeutic exercise following judiciously undertaken tendo-Achilles lengthenings might have either been omitted or failed in the development of antigravity control and strength in the plantar flexors, the quadriceps, and the hip extensors.

- Overactivity in the hamstrings muscles. Some authors suggest that the limitation of knee extension caused by overuse of the hamstrings is the originating deformity in the development of crouch posture (Harrington et al. 1983-1984). Tylkowski et al. (1988) note prolonged and dysphasic activity of the hamstrings through swing and stance phases in crouch gait.

- Pronation deformity. Pronation facilitates knee flexion and hip flexion and adduction through the rearfoot complex. Problems of pronatory foot alignment therefore enhance the crouch deviations at the ankle, knee, and hip (Jordan et al. 1983).

Hypotonia

Hypotonia induces a gravity-bound approach to movement that is easily discouraged by challenges to dynamic stabilization. Most hypotonic children are weak and favor positional stability, whereby they retain a large base of support. They tend to move primarily on the sagittal plane, and as little as necessary. Ligamentous laxity frequently accompanies generalized hypotonia.

Pelvis—Children with generalized hypotonia typically reveal persistent anterior pelvic tilt in standing, with hyperextension through the lumbar spine, secondary to abdominal weakness (Embrey et al. 1983). As a result of abdominal weakness, the pelvis lacks stabilization from the anterior aspect. In addition, posterolateral hip musculature fails to gain optimum strength (Bly et al. 1980).

Hip—Persistent proximal femoral anteversion (lateral hip rotational position for function) is a common feature of hypotonic stance and gait, as the young child seeks maximum positional stability on a wide base of support. As noted above, a persistently increased angle of gait promotes pronation deformity and gradual loss of ankle dorsiflexion mobility.

Knee—Knee hyperextension and, more severely, genu recurvatum are frequent findings in this population, as the child compensates to distribute body weight around the line of weight-bearing in the presence of increased lumbar lordosis, anterior pelvic tilt, and a retroverted proximal tibial plateau (Wilson 1987; Jordan et al. 1983; Scherzer et al. 1982; Embrey et al. 1983; Bernhardt 1988).

Talocrural joint—Weakness in the triceps surae group might also foster hyperextension at the knee as a passive substitute for active control of the knee and ankle joints by calf musculature and quadriceps.

The following section discusses foot deformity associated with hypotonia: flexible pes planus deformity (pes valgus, hypermobile flat foot).

The Foot in Hypotonia

Flexible pes planus is identified when the longitudinal arch flattens or disappears in standing but reappears off weight-bearing (Giallonardo 1988; Regnauld 1986; Rose et al. 1985; D'Amico 1984; Tachdjian 1985; Bleck et al. 1977; Tax 1985). Ankle mobility is full, and there is no evidence of hypertonus in the plantar flexors. The distinguishing features of this type of "flat foot" include the same components as normal pronation of the foot, expressed to an exaggerated degree (Regnauld 1986; Tachdjian 1985; Bleck et al. 1977; LeLievre 1970; Rose 1962; Tax 1985).

Although few authors refer to the problem of pes planus in the context of pediatric neurologic disorders, the high incidence of this deformity is clinically and empirically evident in this population (Carlson et al. 1979; Rose et al. 1985; Regnauld 1986; Salek 1977). In fact, any child who presents with flat feet should be assessed thoroughly for neurologic deficit (D'Amico 1984; Fixsen 1982). Children with a wide spectrum of neuromotor impairment in which hypotonia and/or ligamentous laxity can be observed may exhibit pes planus. This spectrum includes the problems of attention deficit disorder and learning disability, generalized congenital hypotonia often associated with mental retardation, congenital ataxia, and Down syndrome (Salek 1977; Salek 1981; Fixsen 1982; Shepherd 1980; Connolly 1984; Armstrong et al. 1987).

In preschoolers, the features that distinguish the foot that is abnormally pronated (Figure 4.18) from the immature foot—in which a small measure of weight-bearing pronation is expected (Figure 4.19)—include the following (McCrea 1985; Jordan et al. 1983; Rose et al. 1985; Regnauld 1986; Root et al. 1971; Valmassy 1984):

- Hypermobility of the foot and ankle joints.
- Postural alignment in the legs favors an increased positional base, with evidence of exaggerated equilibrium reactions.
- In relaxed calcaneal stance position, calcaneal valgus relative to the sagittal plane exceeds a value that is derived by subtracting the child's age from the number 7 (Valmassy 1984).
- The forefoot abducts on the hindfoot.
- The first ray dorsiflexes on the navicular.
- The navicular abducts and dorsiflexes on the talar head.
- The weight-bearing footprint taken in stance gait reveals convexity on the medial border with concavity on the lateral border.
- The cuboid abducts and dorsiflexes on the calcaneus.

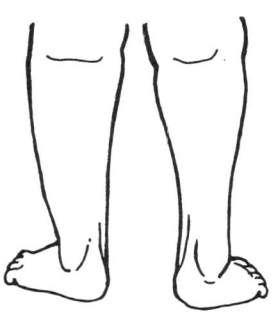

Figure 4.18
Abnormal pronation (posterior view). Pes valgus (pes planus, pronation deformity).

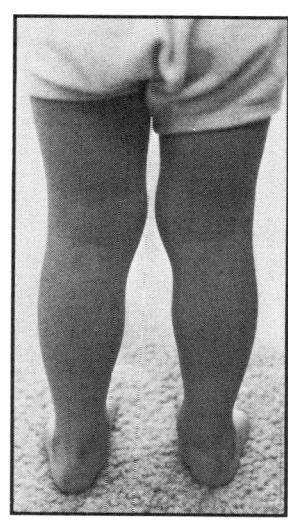

Figure 4.19
Normal relaxed calcaneal stance, less than 5 degrees—age 3 years.

- The long toe extensors convert to evertors of the forefoot; this is caused by the shift in underlying structural alignment.

- The peroneus longus converts from a plantarflexor of the first ray to an abductor of the forefoot.

- The toes flex and deviate laterally, particularly the hallux, which also rotates medially (Rose et al. 1985).

- In weight-bearing, passive hyperextension of the great toe at the MTP joint fails to elicit either or both of two normal effects: elevation of the medial arch and lateral rotation of the tibia and fibula. In more severe deformity, neither effect occurs; in moderate deformity, the tibial rotation component is missing (Rose et al. 1985).

Consistent excursion of the foot into abnormal pronation can impede the modeling into lateral torsion of the more proximal long bones (the suprastructures) by imposing medial torque forces via the closed kinetic chain (Tiberio 1988).

On open-chain examination of the chronically pronated foot, the range of passive calcaneal eversion equals or exceeds that of inversion. This relative mobility indicates laxity in the medial supporting ligaments and shortening of the peroneal tendons and lateral ligaments (Figures 4.20 and 4.21). In relaxed calcaneal stance, calcaneal valgus also exceeds the normal age-appropriate limit (Root et al. 1971; McCrea 1985; Root et al. 1977; Valmassy 1984). Valgus deviation beyond 10 degrees is abnormal at any age. Open-chain evaluation also typically reveals persistence of forefoot varus deformity.

Pronation deformity increases the weight-bearing roentgenographic values of the lateral and dorsal talocalcaneal angles, the lateral talar declination angle and the lateral and talo-first-metatarsal angle (Regnauld 1986; Tachdjian 1985; Bleck et al. 1977; Vanderwilde et al. 1988; McCrea 1985).

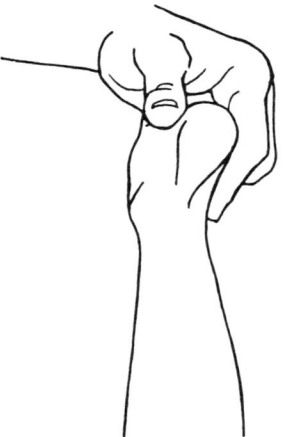

Figure 4.20
Evidence of laxity in the medial and plantar supporting ligaments: calcaneal eversion = 27 degrees . . .

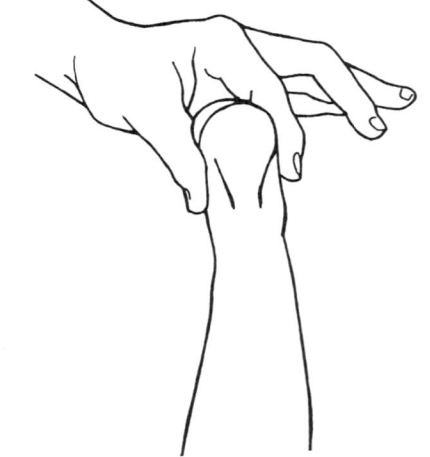

Figure 4.21 . . . and shortening in the lateral ligaments and peroneals: inversion = 4 degrees. Ratio of inversion to eversion = 1:7 vs. normal 2:1 to 4:1. (Figures 4.20 and 4.21 show the left foot.)

Functional Implications of Flexible Pes Planus

During the latter 85 percent of the stance phase within the mature gait cycle, the normal STJ complex moves through neutral (congruent) alignment into supination while the foot assumes and transfers the full body weight (Root et al. 1977; Gray 1986). The assembled structures of the foot convert from a loose adapter to a rigid lever. The lateral assembled pillar bears the body weight through terminal stance to heel-off, as the structures gain maximum congruity. Lateral rotation occurs through the entire lower extremity during this conversion process at the STJ.

The pronated foot remains loose and adaptable throughout the stance phase of gait. The rigid lever function fails to occur and the foot loses its propulsion capability. Terminal contact at toe-off occurs over the medial aspect of the foot, and the medial pillar assumes primary weight-bearing function in stance.

Pronation compromises the function of the muscles that are not normally used to support and stabilize the ankle and the arches of the foot, limiting their endurance (Regnauld 1986; Gray 1986; D'-Amico 1984; Root et al. 1977). Reduction of the degree of pronation is therefore likely to be of significant value as protection for the medial ligaments of the foot and the surrounding musculature from prolonged and abnormal stresses (D'Amico 1984).

Pronation deformity can worsen the faulty weight transfers and postural adjustments associated with neuromotor disorder. As the closed kinetic chain fails to operate effectively, many children demonstrate primitive foot eversion responses to weight shift (Molnar 1985; Molnar 1986; McCrea 1985; Jordan et al. 1983; Salek 1977; Salek 1981; Root et al. 1977; Scherzer et al. 1982; Bleck 1987; Gunsolus et al. 1975) (Figure 4.22). In the presence of hypotonia, ligamentous laxity, or developmental delay, the potential for "spontaneous correction" of pronation is limited by the problems of underdeveloped ligamentous structures, poor proximal antigravity strength and postural control, and compensatory distal stabilizing mechanisms (McCrea 1985; Jordan et al. 1983; Salek 1977; Salek 1981; LeLievre 1970). It is unreasonable to presume, therefore, that the child with neuromotor dysfunction will "outgrow" the pronation deformity.

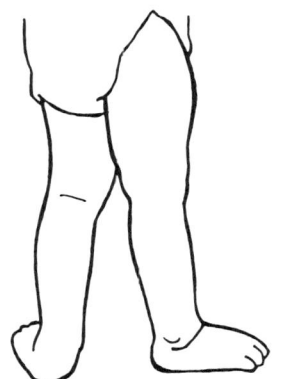

Figure 4.22
Abnormal pronation—lack of closed-chain equilibrium responses to weight shifts.

Summary

Having identified many of the features of alignment and posture that commonly occur in children with hypertonus, hypotonia, and weakness in the triceps surae muscle group, the focus of this chapter has been on problems that arise within the closed chain in stance and in gait.

Chapter 5 will contain some of the history of the development of orthoses as we now know them. The discussion will identify precedents for selection among several splint designs for the pediatric foot and ankle.

References

Agnew, P., DPM. December 8, 1988. Richmond, Virginia. Personal communication.

Armstrong, B. L., J. A. Lewis, and B. D. Cusick. 1987. Speech-language, occupational therapy, and physical therapy evaluation. In *Diagnosis and management of learning disabilities,* edited by F. R. Brown and E. H. Aylward, 79-108. Boston, MA: College-Hill; Little, Brown and Company.

Asher, C. 1975. *Postural variations in childhood.* Boston, MA: Butterworths.

Badell-Ribera, A. 1985. Cerebral palsy: Postural-locomotor prognosis in spastic diplegia. *Archives of Physical Medicine and Rehabilitation* 66:614-619.

Baker, L. D., and L. M. Hill. 1964. Foot alignment in the cerebral palsy patient. *Journal of Bone and Joint Surgery* 46-A(1):1-15.

Bennet, G. C., M. Rang, and D. Jones. 1982. Varus and valgus deformities of the foot in cerebral palsy. *Developmental Medicine and Child Neurology,* 24:499-504.

Bernhardt, D. B. 1988. Prenatal and postnatal growth and development of the foot and ankle. *Physical Therapy* 68(12):1831-1839.

Bleck, E. E. 1982. Developmental orthopaedics. III: Toddlers. *Developmental Medicine and Child Neurology* 24:533-555.

Bleck, E. E. 1987. Orthopaedic management in cerebral palsy. *Clinics in Developmental Medicine, no. 99/100.* Philadelphia, PA: J. B. Lippincott.

Bleck, E. E., and U. J. Berzins. 1977. Conservative management of pes valgus with plantar flexed talus, flexible. *Clinical Orthopaedics and Related Research,* 22:85-92.

Bly, L. 1983. *Components of normal movement during the first year of life and abnormal development.* Monograph. Oak Park, IL: Neurodevelopmental Treatment Association.

Bly, L., and F. Sterne. 1980. *Baby treatment.* Advanced training in neurodevelopmental treatment. New York Hospital, New York: September 22 - October 3; supplemental week, May 3-7, 1981.

Bobath, B., and K. Bobath. 1976. *Motor development and the different types of cerebral palsy.* London: Heinemann Medical Books, Ltd.

Brooks, S. 1985. *Joint mobilization applied to the neurologically involved child.* Lecture notes and instructional materials. Dallas, TX, August 12-16.

Carlson (incorrectly cited as Colson in the journal), J. M., and G. Berglund. 1979. An effective orthotic design for controlling the unstable subtalar joint. *Orthotics and Prosthetics* 33(1):39-49.

Cary, J. M., R. Lusskin, and R. G. Thompson. 1975. Prescription principles. In *Atlas of orthotics,* edited by W. H. Bunch and members of the American Academy of Orthopedic Surgeons, 235-244. St. Louis: C. V. Mosby.

Cerny, K. 1984. Pathomechanics of stance: Clinical concepts for analysis. *Physical Therapy* 64(12):1851-1859.

Connolly, B. H. 1984. Learning disabilities. In *Pediatric neurologic physical therapy,* edited by S. K. Campbell, 317-352. New York: Churchill Livingstone.

Csongradi, J., E. Bleck, and W. F. Ford. 1979. Gait electromyography in normal and spastic children, with special reference to quadriceps femoris and hamstring muscles. *Developmental Medicine and Child Neurology* 21: 738-743.

D'Amico, J. C. 1984. Developmental flatfoot. In *Symposium on podopediatrics—Clinics in podiatry,* edited by J. V. Ganley. Philadelphia, PA: W. B. Saunders Co.

DeLuca, P. A., J. Giachetto, and J. R. Gage. 1988. Gait lab analysis of spastic equinus deformities: A new system of standardized assessment. *Developmental Medicine and Child Neurology* 30(5):16 (Abstract).

Deusinger, R. H. 1984. Biomechanics in clinical practice. *Physical Therapy* 64(12):1860-1868.

Dillin, W., and R. L. Samilson. 1983. Calcaneus deformity in cerebral palsy. *Foot & Ankle* 4(4):167-170.

Embrey, D., J. Endicott, T. Glenn, and D. L. Jaeger. 1983. Developing better postural tone in grade school children. *Clinical Management in Physical Therapy* 3(3):6-10.

Fabry, G., G. D. McEwen, and A. R. Shands. 1973. Torsion of the femur: A follow-up study in normal and abnormal conditions. *Journal of Bone and Joint Surgery* 55-A(8):1726-1738.

Fixsen, J. A. 1982. The foot in childhood. In *The foot and its disorders, 2d ed.,* edited by L. Klenerman, 55-82. Boston, MA: Blackwell Scientific Publications.

Frost, H. M. 1971. Cerebral palsy: The spastic crouch. *Clinical Orthopaedics and Related Research* 80:2-8.

Giallonardo, L. M. 1988. Clinical evaluation of foot and ankle dysfunction. *Physical Therapy* 68(12):1850-1856.

Goldner, J. L. 1982. Foot and ankle deformities in cerebral palsy (static encephalopathy). In *Disorders of the foot, vol. 1,* edited by M. H. Jahss, 282-334. Philadelphia, PA: W. B. Saunders.

Gray, G. W. 1986. *Enhancing clinical skills through biomechanics.* Lecture notes and instructional materials. South Carolina American Physical Therapy Association annual meeting, Charleston, SC, May 17.

Gunsolus, P., C. Welsh, and C. Houser. 1975. Equilibrium reactions in the feet of children with spastic cerebral palsy and of normal children. *Developmental Medicine and Child Neurology* 17:393-409.

Harrington, E. D., R. S. Lin, and J. R. Gage. 1983-84. Use of the anterior floor reaction orthosis in patients with cerebral palsy. *Orthotics and Prosthetics* (Spring):34-42.

Hensinger, R. N., and E. T. Jones. 1982. Developmental orthopaedics. I: The lower limb. *Developmental Medicine and Child Neurology* 24:95-116.

Hicks, R., N. Durinick, and J. R. Gage. 1988. Differentiation of idiopathic toe-walking and cerebral palsy. *Journal of Pediatric Orthopaedics* 8:160-163.

Hoffer, M., and J. Perry. 1983. Pathodynamics of gait alterations in cerebral palsy and the significance of kinetic electromyography in evaluating foot and ankle problems. *Foot & Ankle* 4(3):100-104.

Hutter, C. G., and M. D. Scott. 1949. Tibial torsion. *Journal of Bone and Joint Surgery* 31-A(3):511-518.

Jordan, R. P., J. Cusack, and B. Rosseque. 1983. *Foot function and its relationship to posture in the pediatric patient with cerebral palsy and other neuromuscular disorders.* Lecture notes and instructional materials. Sponsored by the Neurodevelopmental Treatment Association, New York, May 20-22.

King, H. A., and L. T. Staheli. 1984. Torsional problems in cerebral palsy. *Foot & Ankle* 4(4):180-184.

Lehmann, J. F. 1986. Lower limb orthotics. In *Orthotics, etcetera, 3d ed.,* edited by R. B. Redford, 278-351. Baltimore, MD: Williams and Wilkins.

LeLievre, J. 1970. Current concepts and correction in the valgus foot. *Clinical Orthopaedics and Related Research* 70:44-55.

LeVeau, B. F., and D. B. Bernhardt. 1984. Developmental biomechanics: Effect of forces on the growth, development, and maintenance of the human body. *Physical Therapy* 64(12):1874-1881.

Lotman, D. B. 1976. Knee flexion deformity and patella alta in spastic cerebral palsy. *Developmental Medicine and Child Neurology* 18:315-320.

Mann, R. A. 1985. Biomechanics of the foot. In *Atlas of orthotics, 2d ed.,* edited by W. H. Bunch and members of the American Academy of Orthopedic Surgeons, 112-125. St Louis: C. V. Mosby.

McCrea, J. 1985. *Pediatric orthopedics of the lower extremity: An instructional handbook.* Mount Kisco, NY: Futura.

McDonough, M. W. 1984. Angular and axial deformities of the legs of children. In *Symposium on podopediatrics—Clinics in podiatry,* edited by J. V. Ganley, 601-620. Philadelphia, PA: W. B. Saunders.

Molnar, G. E. 1985. Cerebral palsy. In *Pediatric rehabilitation,* edited by G. E. Molnar, 420-467. Baltimore, MD: Williams and Wilkins.

Molnar, G. E. 1986. Orthotic management of children. In *Orthotics, etcetera, 3d ed.,* edited by J. B. Redford, 352-387. Baltimore, MD: Williams and Wilkins.

Norlin, R., and P. Odenrick. 1986. Development of gait in spastic children with cerebral palsy. *Journal of Pediatric Orthopaedics.* 6:674-680.

Perry, J. 1974. Kinesiology of lower extremity bracing. *Clinical Orthopaedics and Related Research* 102:19-31.

Perry, J. 1975. Cerebral palsy gait. In *Orthopedic aspects of cerebral palsy, Clinics in Developmental Medicine, no. 52/53,* edited by R. L. Samilson, 71-89. Philadelphia, PA: J. B. Lippincott.

Perry, J. 1987. Distal rectus femoris transfer. *Developmental Medicine and Child Neurology* 29:153-157

Perry, J., D. Antonelli, and W. Ford. 1975. Analysis of knee joint forces during flexed-knee stance. *Journal of Bone and Joint Surgery* 57-A(7):961-967.

Pitkow, R. B. 1975. External rotation contracture of the extended hip. *Clinical Orthopaedics and Related Research* 110:139-145.

Rang, M., R. Silver, and J. de la Garza. 1986. Cerebral palsy. In *Pediatric orthopaedics, 2d ed.,* edited by W. W. Lovell and R. B. Winter, 345-396. Philadelphia, PA: J. B. Lippincott.

Redford, J. B. 1986. Principles of orthotic devices. In *Orthotics etcetera, 3d ed.* edited by J. B. Redford, 1-20. Baltimore, MD: Williams and Wilkins.

Regnauld, B. 1986. *The foot: Pathology, aetiology, semiology, clinical investigation and therapy.* New York, NY: Springer-Verlag.

Rodgers, M. M. 1988. Dynamic biomechanics of the normal foot and ankle during walking and running. *Physical Therapy* 68(12):1822-1830.

Rodgers, M. M., and P. R. Cavanagh. 1984. Glossary of biomechanical terms, concepts, and units. *Physical Therapy* 64(12):1886-1902.

Root, L. 1984. Varus and valgus foot in cerebral palsy and its management. *Foot & Ankle* 4(4):174-179.

Root, M. L., W. P. Orien, and J. H. Weed. 1977. *Normal and abnormal function of the foot: Clinical biomechanics, vol. 2.* Los Angeles, CA: Clinical Biomechanics Corporation.

Root, M. L., W. P. Orien, J. H. Weed, and R. J. Hughes. 1971. *Biomechanical examination of the foot, vol. 1.* Los Angeles, CA: Clinical Biomechanics Corporation.

Rose, G. K. 1962. Correction of the pronated foot. *Journal of Bone and Joint Surgery* 44-B(3):642-648.

Rose, G. K., E. A. Welton, and T. Marshall. 1985. The diagnosis of flat foot in the child. *Journal of Bone and Joint Surgery* 67-B(1):71-18.

Rosenthal, R. K. 1984. The use of orthotics in foot and ankle problems in cerebral palsy. *Foot & Ankle* 4(4):195-200.

Rosenthal, R. K., S. D. Deutch, W. Miller, W. Schumann, and J. E. Hall. 1975. A fixed-ankle, below-knee orthosis for the management of genu recurvatum in spastic cerebral palsy. *Journal of Bone and Joint Surgery* 57-A(4):545-547.

Salek, B. 1977. *The significance of structural and functional development in the normal foot and therapeutic implications thereof in the child with neuromotor disorder.* Unpublished monograph. Commack, NY: Suffolk Rehabilitation Center.

Salek, B. 1981. *Corrective footwear in young children with neuromuscular disorders.* Lecture notes and instructional materials. Neurodevelopmental Treatment Association, Eastern Region, Philadelphia, November 8.

Schafer, R. C. 1987. *Clinical biomechanics: Musculoskeletal actions and reactions, ed 2.* Baltimore, MD: Williams and Wilkins.

Schenkman, M. 1988. *Taking it a step further.* Lecture notes and instructional material. Indianapolis, IN: November 11-13.

Scherzer, A. L., and I. Tscharnuter. 1982. *Early diagnosis and therapy in cerebral palsy: A primer on infant developmental problems.* New York, NY: Dekker.

Segal, L. S., J. M. Mazur, S. E. Sienko, and M. Mauterer. 1987. Calcaneal gait in spastic diplegia after heel-cord lengthening: A preliminary study with gait analysis. *Developmental Medicine and Child Neurology Supplement 55,* 29(5):5 (Abstract).

Shepherd, R. B. (1980) *Physiotherapy in paediatrics, 2d ed.* London: William Heinemann Medical Books, Ltd.

Silver, R. L., J. de la Garza, and M. Rang. 1985. The myth of muscle balance. *Journal of Bone and Joint Surgery* 67-B(3):432-435.

Skinner, S. R., and D. K. Lester. 1985. Dynamic EMG findings in valgus hindfoot deformity in spastic cerebral palsy. *Developmental Medicine and Child Neurology* 27:107 (Abstract).

Smith, E. M., and R. C. Juvinall. 1986. Mechanics of orthotics. In *Orthotics, etcetera, 3d ed.* edited by J. B. Redford, 21-51. Baltimore, MD: Williams and Wilkins.

Soderberg, G. L. 1986. *Kinesiology: Application to pathological motion.* Baltimore, MD: Williams and Wilkins.

Spencer, A. M., and V. A. Person. 1984. Casting and orthotics for children. In *Symposium on podopediatrics—Clinics in podiatry,* edited by J. V. Ganley, 621-629. Philadelphia, PA: W. B. Saunders Co.

Staheli, L. T. 1977. The prone hip extension test. *Clinical Orthopaedics and Related Research (CORR)* 123:12-15.

Staheli, L. T. 1977. Torsional deformity. *Pediatric Clinics of North America (PCNA)* 24(4):799-811.

Staheli, L. T., D. E. Chew, and M. Corbett. 1987. The longitudinal arch: A survey of 882 feet in normal children and adults. *Journal of Bone and Joint Surgery* 69-A(3):426-428

Staheli, L. T., M. Corbett, W. Craig, and H. King. 1985. Lower-extremity rotational problems in children. *Journal of Bone and Joint Surgery* 67-A: 39-44.

Staheli, L. T., W. R. Duncan, and E. Schaefer. 1968. Growth alterations in the hemiplegic child. *Clinical Orthopaedics and Related Research* 40:205-212.

Sutherland, D. H. 1984. *Gait disorders in childhood and adolescence.* Baltimore, MD: Williams and Wilkins.

Sutherland, D. H., and L. Cooper. 1978. The pathomechanics of progressive crouch gait in spastic diplegia. *Orthopedic Clinics of North America* 9(1):143-154.

Sutherland, D. H., L. Cooper, and D. Daniel. 1980b. The role of the ankle plantar flexors in normal walking. *Journal of Bone and Joint Surgery* 62-A(3):354-363.

Sutherland, D. H., R. Olshen, L. Cooper, and S. L-Y. Woo. 1980a. The development of mature gait. *Journal of Bone and Joint Surgery* 62-A(3):336-353.

Tachdjian, M. 1985. *The child's foot.* Philadelphia, PA: W. B. Saunders.

Tax, H. R. 1985. *Podopediatrics, 2d ed.* Baltimore, MD: Williams and Wilkins.

Tiberio, D. 1988. Pathomechanics of structural foot deformities. *Physical Therapy* 68(12):1840-1849.

Tylkowski, C. M., V. Howell-Garvey, and G. Miller. 1988. The influence of hamstring and hip flexor musculature on crouch gait in spastic cerebral palsy as determined by gait analysis. *Developmental Medicine and Child Neurology* 30(5):14-15 (Abstract).

Valmassy, R. L. 1984. Biomechanical evaluation of the child. In *Symposium on podopediatrics—Clinics in podiatry,* edited by J. V. Ganley, 563-579. Philadelphia, PA: W. B. Saunders.

Vanderwilde, R., L. T. Staheli, D. E. Chew, and V. Malagon. 1988. Measurements on radiographs of the foot in normal infants and children. *Journal of Bone and Joint Surgery* 70-A(3):407-415.

Waters, R. L., and B. R. Lunsford. 1985. Energy expenditure of normal and pathologic gait: Application to orthotic prescription. In *Atlas of orthotics, 2d ed.,* edited by W. H. Bunch and others of the American Academy of Orthopedic Surgeons. St. Louis, MO: C. V. Mosby.

Westin, G. W., and S. Dye. 1983. Conservative management of cerebral palsy in the growing child. *Foot & Ankle* 4(3):160-163.

Wilson, J. M. 1987. Developing ambulation skills. In *Therapeutic exercise in developmental disabilities,* edited by B. H. Connolly and P. C. Montgomery, 83-94. Chattanooga, TN: Chattanooga Corporation, Education Division.

Winters, T. F., J. R. Gage, and R. Hicks. 1987. Gait patterns in spastic hemiplegia in children and young adults. *Journal of Bone and Joint Surgery* 69-A(3):437-441.

Wright, D. G., S. M. Desai, and W. H. Henderson. 1964. Action of the subtalar and ankle-joint complex during the stance phase of walking. *Journal of Bone and Joint Surgery* 46-A:361-464.

Management Guidelines for Using Splints

Objectives for the Reader

- To specify the goals of managing pediatric foot and ankle deformity with splints and orthoses.

- To discuss the indications and limitations of several designs of splints for the foot and ankle, in the context of the history behind—and the clinical indications and functional limitations of—comparable orthoses.

- To explain the advantages and disadvantages of intervening to reduce foot and ankle deformity with splints.

- To differentiate between the design modifications of the stabilizing foot splint (SFS) in terms of specific indications and rationale. These devices include the standard SFS; the SFS with variations such as an extended lateral forefoot wall, a flexible forefoot post, a rigid medial gait extension, or a rigid lateral gait extension; and the supramalleolar design.

- To suggest at least one appropriate splint model for each of the common deformities of the foot and/or ankle in children with neuromotor deficit, including the following: flexible pes planus, functional equinus, equinovalgus, equinovarus, and crouch deformity.

" If the same biomechanical design is used in orthoses, the results are quantifiably similar, even though materials used and the appearances may be different."

—Justis F. Lehmann (1986)

As discussed previously, foot deformity in children with neuromotor disorders reveals evidence of childhood plasticity of bone and soft tissue. Ossification in the bones of the foot is a gradual process, spanning more than 20 years. The soft tissues—including muscle, capsule, and ligament—stretch and shorten, adapting to chronic stresses of postural deviations and muscle power imbalance. These changes in soft tissue status are known as "creep." Laxity in the supporting ligaments, however, may be either the cause or the consequence of prolonged application of deforming forces (Baker et al. 1964; Perry 1975; Bleck 1987; Bunch et al. 1985; Goldner 1982; Deusinger 1984; Root et al. 1977). The current methods of conservative management of foot deformity employ the principle of creep, using external support systems to reverse the process as growth proceeds (LeVeau et al. 1984).

The ideal pediatric management team consists of the therapist, the orthopedist, the orthotist—and in some facilities, the physiatrist and the podiatrist—all of whom have interest and experience in the management of children with central nervous system deficits. Such management is complicated, because individualized compensatory motor patterns require equally customized interventions. Despite the body of knowledge of biomechanics that has accumulated in the past 20 years, we can only anticipate, and not predict, the potential effectiveness of an orthosis. The management team can ascertain its functional impact only after supervised implementation.

Management Considerations

The method of assigning or assuming management roles differs among facilities. Team members who share a common point of view about the importance of meeting specific criteria for alignment and function should be able to agree on who will provide the primary splint fabrication services for the foot and ankle. A trained associate team member who assumes the role of splint maker will allow the physical therapist time to attend to other management matters. For example, an interested and trained orthotist, an orthopedic technician, a physical or occupational therapist, or a therapy assistant or aide might be assigned by the team to assume most of the responsibility of trimming and finishing devices. The mold, however, might be taken by a team that includes the primary physical therapist. The issue is not whether splinting is a function of occupational or physical therapy, but rather whether competent staff members are participating in the effort with the most efficiency of time allocation.

The selection of splints and orthoses frequently requires that the management team consider the broader issues of child development. For instance, the child who demonstrates poor potential for walking might have psychologic and physiologic needs to be met before achieving the upright position (Molnar 1985; Molnar 1986). Standing can be a modality used for the prevention of contractures at the hip and knee and as a means of achieving improved midline orientation (Wilson 1987). Because most infants assume the upright position independently by the age of 10 months, a developmentally appropriate therapeutic intervention offers the infant with neuromotor disorder the opportunity to experience this milestone with a minimum of postural deviation and a maximum of efficiency. Adequate support for the trunk, pelvis, legs, and feet are components of this management goal, and foot splints would likely be indicated.

Historical Perspectives on Current Concepts

Since the late 1960s, when high-temperature, total-contact plastic orthoses became available, the high-top shoe attached to a double-iron short leg brace has been recognized as an unsatisfactory approach to securing the spastic foot and ankle in the plantigrade position (Bleck 1987; Salek 1981; Staheli et al. 1980; Rosenthal 1984). The leather soon deforms under the stress of hypertonic deviations; it takes the shape of the deforming foot and ankle (Figure 5.1). Furthermore, the heel does not remain seated in the shoe (Bleck 1987; Salek 1981; Cailliet 1983; Rosenthal 1984). The role of the shoe as a foundation for the metal uprights is rapidly compromised.

High-temperature thermoplastics such as polypropylene or copolymer blends are commonly used to achieve a molded, total-contact support for the foot and ankle. These materials have a direct influence on joint alignment and function. Total-contact plastic orthoses have, however, also created a host of problems related to skin

Figure 5.1
Breakdown of shoe leather accommodates and reveals deforming forces in the foot and ankle.

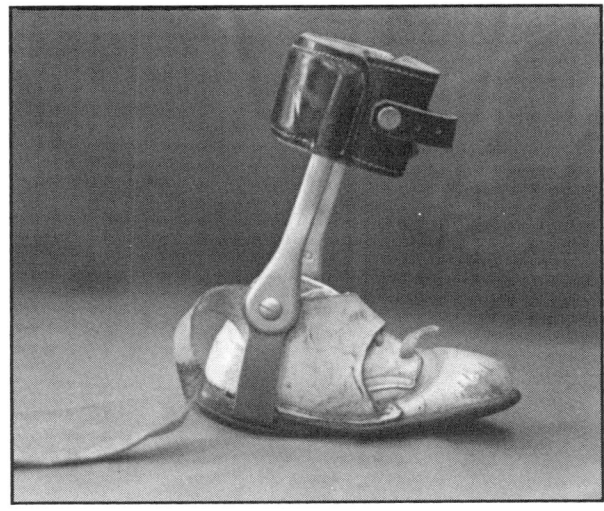

tolerance and associated functional consequences in the free joints. The increasing use and influence of these plastic devices has inspired the development of a biomechanical approach to the design and the implementation of orthotic systems (Perry 1974; Rosenthal 1984; Lehmann 1986; Smith et al. 1986; Harrington et al. 1983-84; McCollough 1985; Meyer 1974; McCollough 1974).

The concept of "bracing" was originally considered to be the shoring up of falling or paralyzed body segments. As thermoplastics have come into use, this concept has shifted to a more dynamic idea of promoting improved functional efficiency (Bunch et al. 1985; Perry 1974; Meyer 1974; McCollough 1974). This new view has, in turn, led to developments in orthoses that provide minimum stabilization while restoring proper structural and biomechanical alignment, as in the now-familiar UCBL shoe insert (McCrea 1985; Root et al. 1977; Jordan et al. 1983; Rosenthal 1984; Lehmann 1986; Meyer 1974; McCollough 1974; Henderson et al. 1967; Bleck et al. 1977; Helfet 1956; Tachdjian 1985). Gait analysis—using video recordings, force plates, and electromyographic (EMG) analysis—offers the greatest potential for gaining insights into factors of mechanical and functional influence.

Goals of Intervention with Lower Extremity Orthoses and Splints

The following principles have been identified in the orthotics literature concerning management of the pediatric population. The priority assigned to the principles varies depending upon the authors cited.

Prevention of Contractures and Deformity

This is the most common purpose for management with orthoses for children with chronic neuromotor impairment. The orthosis ideally protects cartilaginous and soft tissues from the deforming effects of inappropriate weight-bearing and tensile strains (Molnar 1985; Bunch et al. 1985; Fishman et al. 1985; Cary et al. 1975; LeVeau et al. 1984; D'Amico 1984; Redford 1986).

Correction of Deformity

Creep is implemented in the process of correcting foot deformities (LeVeau et al. 1984; Deusinger 1984; Westin et al. 1983; Redford 1986). Casts, splints, and orthoses are used to stabilize bony structures during growth. They also apply corrective forces to the weight-bearing joints over a prolonged period of time and growth (Molnar 1985; LeVeau et al. 1984; Bleck et al. 1977; Westin et al. 1983; D'Amico 1984; Spencer et al. 1984; Harris et al. 1986). Body weight, size, and skin tolerance are limiting factors in this application (Fishman et al. 1985).

Provision of Optimal Joint Alignment

The arrangement of the structures of the foot and ankle dictate the efficiency with which the overlying muscles function. Joint axes must be aligned properly in order to respond appropriately to direction and degree of force applied by muscle and weight-bearing.

In orthotic construction, optimal joint alignment unfortunately is often overlooked. Many high-temperature plastic orthoses are molded around the foot deformity while the child sits with the foot resting on a plank. No attempt is made in this procedure to align the subtalar and midtarsal joints in functional position. There are exceptions, certainly, as is evident in the writings of such authors as Rosenthal (1984), Carlson et al. (1979), and Redford (1986).

Selective, Minimal Restriction of Motion

Without compromising structural support for optimum biomechanical function, an orthosis or splint offers as many normal movement options as possible. For example, the hinged ankle-foot orthosis or splint permits a predetermined range of sagittal plane ankle motion while prohibiting undesirable valgus or varus deviation in the foot. The UCBL shoe insert, the supramalleolar orthosis, and the hinged crouch-control splint are also examples of this principle of selective restriction of motion. (See below for more details regarding these devices.)

Protection of Weak Antigravity Muscles

Weakness occurs either following surgery (Bleck 1987; Bunch et al. 1985; Goldner 1982; Harrington et al. 1983-84), secondary to hypotonia (Salek 1981; Fixsen 1982), or following prolonged disuse of a muscle group. Weakness can lead to overstretch of the muscle tendon and associated connective tissues. Weakness also places abnormally high compensatory demands upon other muscle groups. For example, crouch deformity results from weakness in the triceps surae muscle group. The functional and biomechanical consequences are devastating. (See Chapter 4 for more details regarding crouch deformity.)

Control of Tone and of Tonus-Related Deviations

This purpose has not been substantiated by research. However, clinical evidence shows that attention to structural alignment in the foot promotes an improved balance of muscle power. Maintaining structural alignment also reduces the need to seek stability with compensatory balancing mechanisms that often generate excessive muscle tone (Bunch et al. 1985; Salek 1981; Rosenthal 1984; Zachazewski et al. 1982; Harris et al. 1986; Ford et al. 1986; Jordan 1984).

Enhancement of Experience

Biomechanical support devices help to provide the nonambulatory child with the experience and physiologic benefits of the standing position without deforming the feet in the process. Devices that offer support of the structures of the foot and ankle and equipment that facilitates achievement of the upright posture are included in this context (Molnar 1985; Salek 1981; Levitt 1982).

Attention to Cosmesis and Weight

High-temperature thermoplastics offer a measure of cosmesis and are very light in weight. Splints are equally light, but their typical bulkiness detracts from the goal of optimum cosmesis. With improvements in splint materials that allow increased durability with decreased thickness, cosmesis should improve.

Limitations of Intervention with Splints, Orthoses, and Casts

There are, of course, limitations inherent in all of the procedures described in this chapter, including the following.

Casts, splints, and orthoses cannot directly change torsional deformities in the long bones of the leg. These deformities seem instead to require repeated application of active, muscle-induced tensile forces for reconstruction (McCrea 1985; Bleck 1982). Foot and ankle-foot support systems are often effective, however, in altering the angles of articulation and motion at the hips and knees. Adequate distal support systems relieve in some measure abnormal torque, tensile, and compressive stresses on the proximal bones and joints (McCrea 1985; Jordan et al. 1983; Regnauld 1986) (Figures 5.2 and 5.3).

The role of orthoses and splints is also primarily limited to maintenance of achievable alignment and reduction of functional deformity in children with nonparalytic neuromotor deficit. The skin over the bony prominences is too tender to withstand the conflict between corrective rigid support systems and fixed deformity (Molnar 1985; Molnar 1986; Cary et al. 1975). Splints or orthoses used to gain range at the ankle or foot are generally poorly tolerated; skin breakdown frequently occurs with their use.

Using corrective casts in series is a conservative intervention measure to help regain lost extensibility in muscle and connective tissue at the knee, ankle, and foot. If the casting process fails, surgical correction may have to be considered (Westin et al. 1983; Tardieu et al. 1982; Gritzka et al. 1986; Hoffer et al. 1987; Tardieu et al. 1987).

None of these interventions is adequate as a substitute for a consistent, well-directed therapeutic exercise program. Antigravity strength and control of the trunk and pelvis are essential for the achievement of dynamic balance (Sellers 1988; Riley et al. 1987). No foot support system is sufficient to substitute for such proximal strengthening and organization.

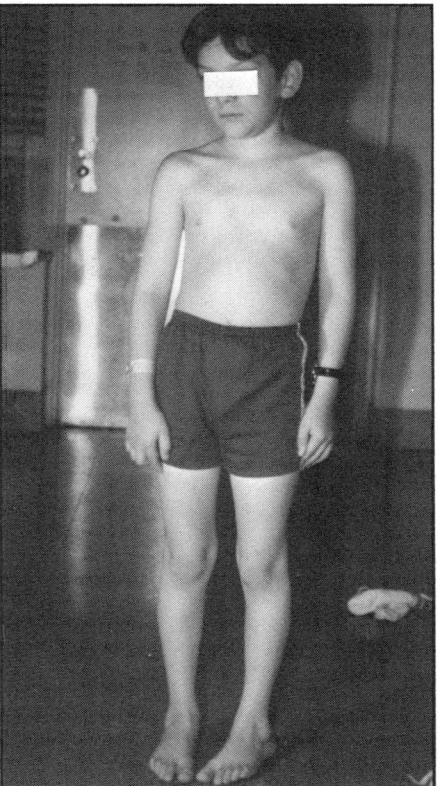

Figure 5.2 Postural deviations, uncorrected.

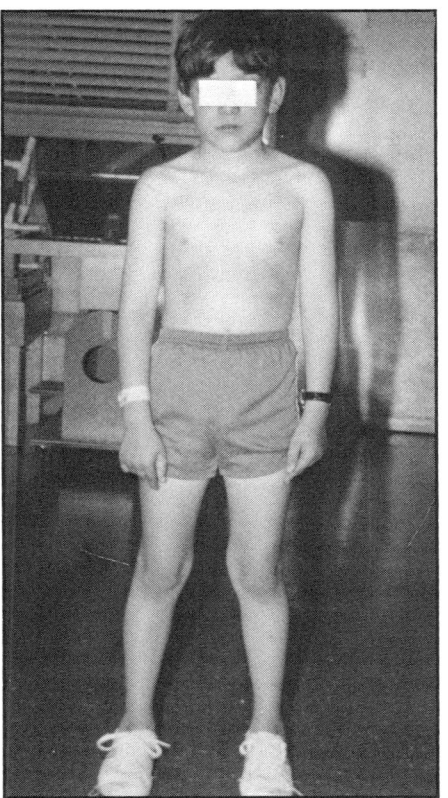

Figure 5.3 Improved joint alignment, using stabilizing foot splints to support the STJ complex. Changes reflect joint realignments rather than structural alterations in the long bones.

Splints: an Alternative to Casts and Orthoses

Orthoses are an established and valuable resource for the effective management of children with neuromotor disorder. Their continued use is predictable as new materials are developed, and the creation of new designs enhances their effectiveness.

It is fitting that the physical therapist should take a direct role in the management of foot deformity, because the therapist is the person most intimately acquainted with the child's weight-bearing capabilities and problems. Compared to all the other team members, the physical therapist devotes the greatest amount of time and attention to the status and function of the foot and lower extremities and is the best informed regarding the child's postural and functional problems as they relate to foot and ankle function. Splinting falls within the domain of the therapist, who typically provides splints for burns and bed rest. More recently, therapists have been using splints for foot and ankle support in stance and gait.

While on staff at Children's Rehabilitation Center (CRC)—recently renamed the Kluge Children's Rehabilitation Center and Research Institute—in Charlottesville, Virginia, I developed these splinting techniques together with Michael Smith, O.T.C. The evolution of these techniques began with a casting program in 1977. In 1980 the staff used Aquaplast-T® (see Appendix 4 for sources), a low-temperature thermoplastic splinting material, to produce ankle-foot splints first for children with myelodysplasia and soon afterward for children with cerebral palsy. Initially we considered these splints as an alternative follow-up system after removing below-knee casts that were used for children with hypertonic cerebral palsy. However, between 1981 and 1985, we produced an increasing variety of splints (Figure 5.4) in staggering numbers for a cerebral palsy caseload that exceeded 650 children. At the same time, we used fewer and fewer casts. Eventually, the splints almost entirely replaced bivalved casts as an intervention. On certain occasions, the splints replaced orthoses, for the reasons discussed below.

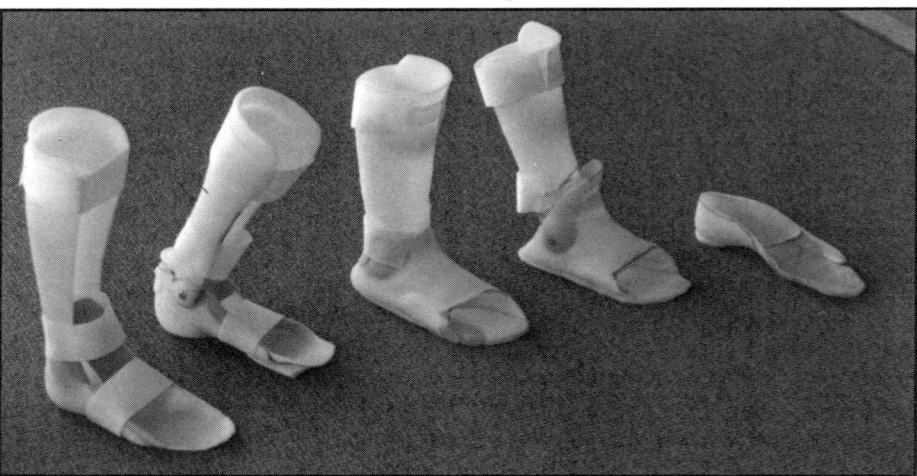

Figure 5.4 Splints of varying design—(left to right) solid and hinged ankle-foot splints; solid and hinged crouch-control splints; modified heel stabilizer with lateral wall and first metatarsal post.

Uses for Lower Extremity Splints

If the circumstances are appropriate, thoughtful and creative use of splints for the foot and ankle can be both a cost-effective and convenient intervention. The variety of splint designs has increased steadily as new applications of biomechanical concepts have been identified and implemented (Figure 5.4).

Lower extremity splints have been used successfully in the following ways:

- As an alternative to expensive orthoses for small children who grow rapidly while exhibiting changes in foot size and alignment.

- As a short-term distal support system during rehabilitation:

    — Following head trauma, in which functional status changes frequently. In the hospital setting, trained clinicians can fabricate and apply splints within one day for use as an aid in rehabilitation. As the patient recovers, changes may occur in tone or functional status. The therapist can expediently accommodate to these changes by modifying the splint design.

    — Following surgical intervention, to enhance distal stability and control. This is often needed after hamstrings lengthening, tendo-Achilles lengthening, or osteotomy. Any evidence of abnormal deviation in the foot structures warrants an attempt to realign them, regardless of the surgical procedure.

    — After the triceps surae group has been weakened surgically. When this has happened, the lengthened muscle tendon should be protected from overstretch with adequate use of a support system. However, most orthoses used for postoperative intervention are discarded for daytime use within six months. One or two splints might suffice for this purpose. Longevity of the device is not a functional requirement for the purposes of short-term postoperative protection. The high cost of high-temperature plastic orthoses can be avoided in these instances.

    — Within the first three to six months following selective dorsal rhizotomy. Children who have experienced selective dorsal rhizotomy frequently exhibit a brief period of significant lower extremity weakness. This is possibly related to confusion in responding to the change in tonus, or it may be related to real weakness in musculature that was previously used only in pathological hypertonic patterns (Fasano et al. 1978; Peacock et al. 1981; Peacock et al. 1982; Ploeger et al. 1987; Irwin-Carruthers et al. 1985; Jordan 1987; Wilson et al. 1988).

In the absence of soft-tissue contracture, prompt application of distal stabilizing splints following rhizotomy aligns the joints of the foot and ankle in proper, functional position for stance. Doing this can facilitate the rehabilitation process by reducing the demand for antigravity strength in the distal musculature (Wilson et al. 1988). Distal stabilization enhances the effort to build strength proximally by reducing the overall workload required to maintain and move in the upright position. Initially either hinged or solid ankle devices would be used, depending on the degree of stabilization required.

Splint support can be reduced gradually by a change of design to less restrictive models. Splint support can be withdrawn as the foot gains stability. The status of the foot and ankle should be monitored frequently and at regular intervals during the first two postoperative years.

- As a prototype or design trial. There are times when a child presents the evaluative team with a perplexing problem of selecting the most efficient or appropriate style of orthosis. Because the orthosis is often costly, any measure of certainty is welcome. In these instances, the team should pretest a proposed orthotic design by first replicating it in a splint. This helps determine the design's functional impact before the orthosis is prescribed. This trial is useful in the management of patients of all ages who require orthotic intervention.

- As an evaluation tool in clinical decision making. By aligning the foot structures in optimum functional position, the management team can observe the influence of foot deformity on a complicated gait deficit. This can take place either with or without computerized gait analysis. The team can then determine a plan of intervention with an appreciation for the proximal compensatory mechanisms that the child has developed in response to foot deformity.

- As interim support. The fabrication of an orthosis can often require a period of two to four weeks or more between molding and delivery. A supportive splint, however, can be provided immediately, during the same clinic visit at which the orthotic prescription was generated and the mold taken. The child thereby receives a needed support system during the interim between molding and delivery. In this way a potential gap in the delivery of care is filled inexpensively.

- As a means of providing a variety of function-specific support systems. The child might require several different devices to meet the needs for support during varying activities. For example, cosmesis, comfort, or minimal weight-bearing demand may warrant the occasional use of a foot support device despite a prevailing need for ankle-foot support or knee control. The low cost of splints helps to facilitate the provision of such management alternatives.

Advantages of Using Splints

Aquaplast-T® was used in the development of all the devices described below, and the advantages and disadvantages of using this particular material are presented. Orfit® is a similar material that is imported from Belgium and sold in the United States at a comparable price. (See Appendix 4 for sources.) It has a few features that are different from Aquaplast-T®. The properties, advantages, and disadvantages of Aquaplast-T® as a splinting material are disclosed below. There may be other splinting materials that have comparable molding properties and fewer disadvantages. Therapists should be conscientious in applying the principles of molding the foot structures to the exploration of any new materials and methods. The following advantages of Aquaplast-T® or Orfit® as a medium have been identified:

- Low cost. Splints often cost only 20 to 25 percent of the price of orthoses of comparable design, including the clinician's time and materials. Replacement requirements caused by a child's growth impose a heavy burden of expense on the family—or the health care provider—which is considerably reduced by using low-cost splints. Many state agencies that provide funding for children with chronic disability cannot afford to allocate funds for more than one pair of orthoses in a year. Children grow more rapidly than that and commonly wear a pair of orthoses long after they no longer fit or support the foot adequately. They often have to discard their ill-fitting orthoses and wait for more funding or their next clinic visit. Splints can usually be made as often as needed through the year without exceeding the cost of one pair of orthoses.

- Chemical/mechanical characteristics. Aquaplast-T® is a modified formula of the original Aquaplast®, which was notoriously sticky when heated and too difficult to use efficiently. A wax coating has been applied to the T formula, which eliminates the stickiness. Both Aquaplast-T® and Orfit® feature the following characteristics:

  — Low-temperature heating, which allows the clinician to mold the device directly on the foot and leg.

  — Rapid setting time, within 3 to 4 minutes.

  — Uniform elasticity, which allows both close contouring to occur with retraction of the material around the limb segment and a relatively even thickness of the finished splints.

  — Transparency while it is warm and setting, which gives the splint-maker a visual cue about readiness for removal.

  — Modifiability with the use of a heat gun, scissors, or utility knife.

  — Capacity for self-bonding, which permits the clinician to post extrinsically if needed with the same material. Extrinsic posting fills the space between the properly aligned splint and the ground. It effectively brings the ground up to the contour of the device to prohibit deviation under loading stresses.

- Simplicity of the fabrication process. Clinicians (including any of the attending team members as well as the orthopedic technician) should receive training in suggested methods of securing optimum, age-specific biomechanical alignment, as well as in the proper use of the splint material. The fabrication of up to five molds of each splint design usually serves as adequate practice before achieving an acceptable level of cosmesis.

- Time. Most splints can be completed and applied within a time period of 20 to 60 minutes each, provided the design is not too complicated. This waiting period compares favorably with the typical wait of weeks for comparable orthoses.

- Creativity and specificity in splint design. The therapist or orthotist can use a knowledge of biomechanics to modify splint designs to address individual problems. The cost-effectiveness of the creative process that uses splint material encourages the evolution of new design concepts. The fit and functional impact of any new design is readily apparent. The clinician can discard failures while retaining the lessons acquired in this process.

- Flexibility. Aquaplast-T® lacks true rigidity after setting. Splints made for the foot typically flare slightly under body weight. Slight excursions of the calcaneus can occur while the splint strains or when the child wears socks of typical thickness.

- Aquaplast-T® is available in colors.

Disadvantages of Using Splints

There are disadvantages, of course, which include the following:

- Bulkiness. In the form available currently, ankle-foot splints and supramalleolar foot splints that are made of Aquaplast-T® of 1/8-inch thickness generally require an increase of up to two shoe sizes over the size that the child ordinarily wears. Larger children and adolescents require a thicker material (3/16-inch thick) to gain adequate structural support from the device. This thickness is feasible in the hospital setting but is often not practical for the child who is in school.

  Orfit's® stiff formula (1/8-inch thick) is slightly stronger than Aquaplast-T®, but it is not as resistant to flexure and torque forces as is the 3/16-inch Aquaplast-T®.

- Shrinkage. Aquaplast-T®, particularly the 3/16-inch thick material, shrinks in the final minutes of setting. Usually the application of a second sock of medium to heavy thickness before molding eliminates this problem.

  Orfit® does not shrink. It is intended for molding directly on the skin. However, children typically wear thick socks and would not be able to fit into many designs of Orfit® splints unless they were molded over a thick sock covered with stockinet. Orfit® material is often used over cotton stockinet even though it bonds with the stockinet during setting. Separating the hardened splint from the stockinet is mildly challenging, but it is possible.

- Durability-related limitations on use. Most ambulatory children can achieve adequate support for the ankle and foot with splints, at least for a period of three to four months, and often longer for small children. If the splint cracks within the first few weeks of implementation, the child may require the durability of high-temperature plastics.

- Meltdown. The feature of low-temperature softening becomes a problem when, having been left in close proximity to any strong source of heat such as a wood stove, fireplace, campfire, radiator, or sunshine through a window at home or in the car, the splint melts and deforms. The therapist should caution all caregivers about this potential problem.

- Flexibility. Most Aquaplast-T® splints for the ankle and foot cannot resist torque forces. Twist can be imposed at the shaft and within the foot piece. Adaptations for strength include the following: adding an anterior overlapping shell to a standard style of ankle-foot splint; forming the device over the dorsum of the foot and ankle (for example, the crouch-control ankle-foot splint); or increasing the thickness of the device by adding an extra layer of material where increased rigidity is needed.

  Orfit's® stiff formula allows less flexing than Aquaplast-T® under stress; it might be a favorable alternative. However, it does not resist torque forces well. The stronger material against torque is Aquaplast-T® in the 3/16-inch thickness.

Problem-Specific Management of Pediatric Foot Deformity

Many of the guidelines proposed in this text logically apply to orthoses as well as to the splints and casts covered in this book. Precedents and perspective on the determination of criteria for specific splint designs is drawn from the history and current uses of a variety of orthoses. The same considerations that apply to the prescribing of an orthosis also apply to selecting from among splint designs. Splints often serve as an adjunct to, rather than a substitute for, well-designed orthoses.

The suggestions for intervention that follow in this chapter are derived from the principles of maintenance of normal, age-appropriate alignment and function of the foot and ankle, combined with several years of clinical experience. It is best for any clinician to modify procedures and rationale as new concepts and new materials are encountered. Ongoing clinical experience also helps to shape the process of modification indefinitely, as long as there is room for improvement.

Splints are first discussed within the context of the common problems of foot deformity in children with neuromotor disorder, beginning with flexible pes valgus, which is (with the exception of pure equinus deformity) the least complicated. As the management principles for pes valgus are discussed, the clinician should keep in mind that many of the same principles and concerns apply also to the problems of equinovalgus and the type of crouch deformity in which pronation of the foot is a component.

Principles of Aligning the Pediatric Foot for Weight-Bearing Function

Valmassy (1984) states that most children reveal a varus deviation of the STJ and the MTJ when the foot structures are aligned in neutral (congruent) position. He suggests that the goal of intervening to reduce abnormal pronation in children is not to achieve neutral alignment in standing—which, because normal children stand in diminishing degrees of pronation, would be abnormal—but to align the calcaneus in vertical position. Gray (1986) states that the calcaneus is most stable when both plantar condyles (or tubercles) are on the ground. Tiberio (1988) suggests that the plantar condyles are essentially plantigrade when the calcaneus is aligned within 3 degrees of the sagittal plane.

If we consider the relaxed calcaneal stance angle in terms of a diminishing value—from 6 degrees of valgus at age 1 year to 2 degrees at age 5 years, and thereafter falling within 2 degrees of the sagittal plane into either varus or valgus—a question arises about molding the calcaneus for stance in young children. I usually respond to these issues by concurring with Valmassy (1984). Generally, I mold for splints with the calcaneus aligned in midposition, or 2 degrees medial to the sagittal plane, for the following reasons:

- The splint is molded over a sock of a thickness that the child typically wears, plus a layer of stockinet.
- The splint material is slightly flexible under body weight, particularly in the SFS designs.
- The very young child's foot is often covered with fatty tissue around the heel.

The three factors discussed above create space, which allows the calcaneus to deviate a few degrees into valgus under loading. (This space is created because of the splint's flexibility, or by the movement of the calcaneus within the skin cover, or by both). For example, a 3-year-old child should have up to 4 degrees of calcaneal valgus excursion capability in the splint. (The number 7 minus 3 equals 4.) Careful examination of the standing calcaneus, using a gravity-driven angle finder (see Appendix 4 for sources), reveals that 4 degrees of calcaneal valgus is nearly indiscernible to the naked eye. MRI or radiographs would disclose the true amount of excursion that occurs. (However, in my experience, most physicians are reluctant either to expose children to radiation or to impose the cost of such studies on those who provide the children's financial support.)

Functional calcaneal midstance position—When molding the subtalar joint for a foot splint for a young child, it is important to remember that the splint must take account of any existing deviation of the distal third of the lower leg, which is usually a consequence of medial rotation deformity at the knee joint. Therefore, the vertical bisection of the distal third of the lower leg should be measured with the angle finder *while the child's calcaneus is maintained on the sagittal plane.* This assessment should be done in standing position, using passive rotation of the leg while the foot is loaded. The resulting value is the child's functional calcaneal midstance position.

In molding the splint with the child in prone position, the posterior distal bisection of the lower leg is tilted medially on the frontal plane—toward the other leg—the same number of degrees as was determined in functional calcaneal midstance position. The calcaneus is held on the sagittal plane.

D'Amico (1984) often tilts the calcaneus into 2 degrees of varus when posting orthoses for management of developmental flatfoot in children. This calcaneal post can be accomplished by tilting the lower leg 2 degrees less at molding.

Forefoot varus deformity—Among children with neuromotor deficit, forefoot varus deformity is often excessive for the child's age. The deformity may resist expedient correction by a combined intervention using STJ stabilization with an SFS and therapeutic mobilization of the MTJ and first ray. In this circumstance, the mature foot might be managed more adequately with a flexible, wedge-shaped extension of the plantar surface of the SFS under the medial three or four metatarsal heads. The wedge inclines gradually toward the medial side of the foot. It is made of high-density foam padding material. The ground is therefore effectively raised toward the inverted metatarsal heads while the calcaneus is supported in functional midposition. The forefoot is effectively prevented from pronating abnormally to contact the ground and thus from bringing the hindfoot along with it into pronation. However, forefoot varus posting is not appropriate for all children, and the degree of support that is considered appropriate is a matter of debate.

To Post, or Not to Post?

Children with normal neuromotor function begin life with severe forefoot varus deformity averaging approximately 15 degrees, which reduces to less than 10 degrees at age 1 year. By age 4 years, the foot structures become fully capable of conversion to a rigid lever of propulsion. Most children achieve maturity in the lower extremity musculoskeletal developmental parameters during their first six to eight years of life. For some children, the developmental process of modeling of the foot structures continues into adolescence (D'Amico 1984).

Posting the forefoot in varus becomes an issue of whether or not to interfere with the potential for modeling into normal alignment at the forefoot. Pronation around the MTJ longitudinal axis is needed to help gain the perpendicular relationship between the calcaneus and the metatarsal heads and to improve the intrinsic mechanical balance of the foot for weight-bearing. The first ray must plantarflex and evert to contribute to the reduction of varus. Valmassy (1984) suggests that forefoot varus does not resolve and recommends posting in children. D'Amico (1984) and Spencer et al. (1984) disagree with Valmassy and urge caution in neutralizing structural forefoot deficiencies by posting in children under age 10 years.

This discussion concerning forefoot posting occurs nowhere in the literature in reference to children with neuromotor deficit, including those with hypotonia, known ligamentous laxity, and/or other problems of regulation of tonus and sensorimotor organization. However, open-chain assessment of the foot structures in these children often reveals persistence of significant structural forefoot varus deformity that may be increased by pronatory weight-bearing forces. Open-chain assessment also often reveals abnormal neutral subtalar joint alignment in varus.

What should the clinician do about forefoot varus in these children? The modeling forces evident in children without neuromotor deficit are not available to these children, whose postural control mechanisms are either aberrant or underdeveloped. Until clinical research is undertaken using gait analysis, roentgenographic findings and long-term (that is, ten years) observation of specific alignment parameters, the clinician must proceed to intervene with informed judgment and close and precise clinical observation and assessment methods. The rule to be applied here is this: Do not post the forefoot in children under age 3 years. If other measures fail for children between 3 and 10 years of age, proceed to post the forefoot with reluctance, and with a material that will compress within weeks of wear. Continue mobilization efforts. Reevaluate the foot at frequent and regular intervals. Reduce the height of the forefoot post as soon as it is superfluous. Changes in forefoot/hindfoot alignment in congruity will signal that it is time to reduce the height of the post. The goal is the achievement of active and consistent plantarflexion of the medial rays and a stable hindfoot.

Management of Flexible Foot Deformities Using the Stabilizing Foot Splint (SFS)

History and Rationale

Outside of surgery, the path to securing adequate protection for the structures of the foot in children with neuromotor deficit is littered with various combinations of "corrective shoes," high-topped "orthopedic" shoes, heel/sole wedges, "arch supports," scaphoid pads, and navicular pads. All of these products have been scrutinized and discarded by many clinicians as ineffective (Bleck et al. 1977; Salek 1981; Bleck 1987; Carlson et al. 1979; Rose 1962; Staheli et al. 1980).

In the late 1950s, the principles of application of floor reaction forces to counteract valgus deviation of the calcaneus were applied in the development of the Helfet heel seat and the Schwartz meniscus (Helfet 1956; LeLievre 1970; Rose 1962; Bleck et al. 1977). In 1967, Henderson and Campbell presented their UCBL (University of California Biomechanics Laboratory) shoe insert. The UCBL shoe insert is rigid, deeper than the meniscus, and, if molded correctly, grips the calcaneus closely, particularly on the medial aspect (Carlson et al. 1979). The plantar contact surface under the heel is flattened. In weight-bearing, the flat plantar surface lowers into full contact with the ground. At the same time, the medial and lateral walls of the insert grip the calcaneus, prohibiting it from rolling into abnormal valgus. The distal end of this insert projects under the plantar surface of the foot, curving into the normal contour of the longitudinal arch; it ends proximal and adjacent to the heads of the metatarsal. The UCBL shoe insert is usually made of rigid, high-temperature thermoplastics (Henderson et al. 1967).

Developments in the application of principles developed through biomechanical engineering to the field of orthotics have produced for the able-bodied population a rapidly growing industry: foot orthoses and "sporthotics" that use a minimum of materials to achieve the ideal hindfoot/forefoot relationship under a variety of functional conditions (Huber 1985; Franco 1987; Lockard 1988). For the motor-impaired child, however, these devices often seem to ask too much of the postural control mechanism.

In 1965, Berzins undertook a 10-year prospective study of the effectiveness of the Helfet heel seat and the UCBL shoe insert in the management of flexible pes valgus (apparently in children with normal tone) (Bleck et al. 1977). The mean age of the 71 children in the study group was 4.7 years. The mean duration of orthotic use was 14.5 months. The overall failure rate averaged 20 percent. The remaining 80 percent showed either improvement or correction of talar plantarflexion, the latter to within the authors' accepted maximum of 35 degrees.

By 1977, Berzins and Bleck had determined that correction of pes valgus foot deformity was significantly greater under two conditions:

- When the devices were initially used to treat children younger than 3 years (although they were effective when initiated up to the age of 8 years).
- When the devices were implemented for longer durations, comparing interventions lasting 6 months or less with those that spanned between 24 and 46 months.

The children who were considered in these studies apparently did not demonstrate neuromotor dysfunction in association with their pronation deformity. Most likely, these children brought adequate postural adjustment skills to the process of achieving deformity correction.

Several other authors report excellent results with the same or similar foot orthoses Carlson et al. 1979; Rose 1962; Rosenthal 1984; D'Amico 1984; Spencer et al. 1984; Lockard 1988; Cailliet 1983; Franco 1987; Huber 1985; Gray 1986). Huber (1985) suggests that alignment of the calcaneus is critical in evaluating a neurologically impaired client. He warns that slight deviation into valgus (5 to 8 degrees) appears to precipitate pes planus deformity in adults. Progressive genu valgum is then seen occasionally. Carlson et al. (1979) note the high incidence of STJ instability in children with cerebral palsy and recommend intervening with the UCBL shoe insert when control of ankle motions or alignment is not indicated. They urge careful attention, while taking the mold, to supporting the STJ via the calcaneal inclination and the sustentaculum tali. Rosenthal (1984) also advises the use of the foot orthosis (UCBL shoe insert)—modified to meet the needs for support or alignment—for cerebral palsied children with problems of pes valgus, pes varus, and metatarsus adductus. Lockard (1988) offers references citing the potential benefit of using "heel stabilizers and shoe inserts" for neurologically impaired patients who reveal pes planovalgus due to ligament laxity or hypotonia.

The following foot splint designs are derived from the design of the UCBL shoe insert. They are suggested for use in managing mild to moderate pronation deformity of varying degrees in children with neuromotor impairment. Using the standard stabilizing foot splint

(SFS) as an intervention for equinus and equinus-related problems is not effective, because heel contact is limited in equinus deformities.

The Stabilizing Foot Splint (SFS)

The stabilizing foot splint (SFS) implements the same concepts as the UCBL shoe insert: it closely conforms to the structures of the hindfoot and lesser tarsus. It also uses floor reaction forces in weight-bearing to stabilize the calcaneus against deviating into abnormal valgus position (Figures 5.5, 5.6, and 5.7).

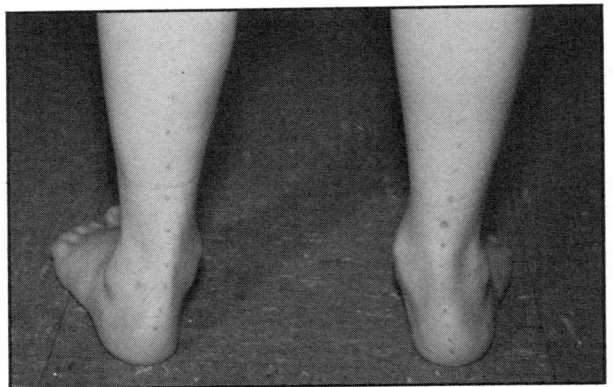

Figure 5.5 Before applying stabilizing foot splints (SFS).

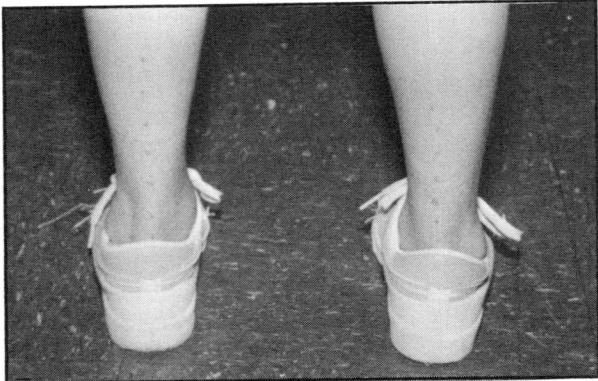

Figure 5.6 After applying SFS. Note apparent reduction of calcaneal valgus deviation. Lateral malleoli are more prominent and displaced more posteriorly, indicating tibiofibular lateral rotation.

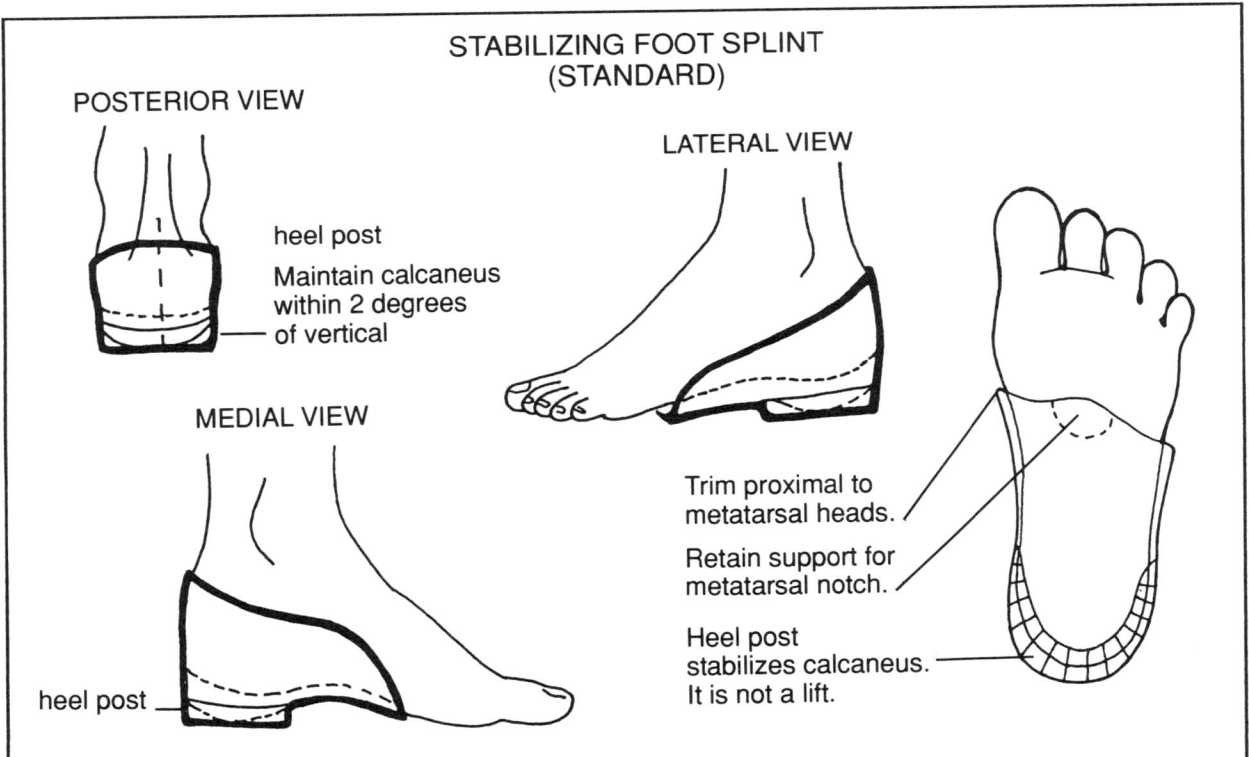

STABILIZING FOOT SPLINT
(STANDARD)

POSTERIOR VIEW

heel post
Maintain calcaneus within 2 degrees of vertical

LATERAL VIEW

MEDIAL VIEW

heel post

Trim proximal to metatarsal heads.

Retain support for metatarsal notch.

Heel post stabilizes calcaneus. It is not a lift.

Figure 5.7

Among the differences between the SFS and the UCBL is the relative flexibility of the Aquaplast-T® splint material compared to the rigid shoe insert. Depending upon the weight of the child, the splint calls upon the heel box of the shoe to assist in applying the needed floor reaction forces to the hindfoot. (Orfit® stiff splint material is more rigid than Aquaplast-T® in 1/8-inch thickness.) Also, the SFS is made to cup the heel, which is then stabilized by posting between the aligned heel and ground with the same splint material. (See Chapter 7 for more on posting.) The result is a splint that is significantly more stable as a freestanding structure than is the UCBL insert. Furthermore, flexible forefoot posts are sometimes added to the SFS for the older child, usually by adding a dense foam and moleskin extension to the anterior edge of the device. The UCBL insert does not feature a forefoot post.

The heavier the child, the more significant becomes the feature of flexibility, as the walls of the SFS models made of Aquaplast-T®, trimmed below the malleoli, spread under the child's weight. (The Orfit® stabilizer is less flexible.) Flexibility can work to the child's advantage, however, because if the foot structures grow more rigid with age, tolerance for rigid support can wane (Jordan et al. 1983). The child's tolerance determines continued use of this design.

Modifying the SFS Design

Enhancing Supportive Features

Because children with neuromotor impairment demonstrate difficulty both in executing adequate weight shifts and in adjusting to postural changes, the basic SFS design often requires additional structural features to maintain alignment in the foot. Such modifications include the following, in order of increasing degree:

Forefoot varus post—As discussed previously, the clinician should be reluctant to post the varus forefoot in children between ages 3 and 10. If it must be done, the clinician should use crushable dense foam materials such as Plastazote®. (See Appendix 4 for sources.) The height of the post is kept to the minimum needed to prevent pronatory hindfoot compensation.

To calculate the angle at which to build the forefoot post, I recommend using the following process:

1. Measure the distal lower leg varum in calcaneal midposition in standing position.
2. Measure the STJ neutral position.
3. Lock the foot structures in congruity.
4. Measure the congruous forefoot/transverse plane angle.
5. Subtract the calcaneal value from the forefoot value, as would occur in aligning the calcaneus at 0 degrees in midstance.
6. Subtract the value for midstance lower leg varum.
7. The resulting figure equals the number of degrees remaining through which the forefoot must pronate—or the first ray must plantarflex—to contact the ground.

If the post is made of a material that will slowly "bottom out" or flatten under loading, a gradual modeling process might proceed if there is adequate hindfoot stabilization. In the older child or adolescent, if the flattening of the varus post induces abnormal pronatory compensation at the hindfoot and discomfort due to shear forces, replace the post with PPT® padding (see Appendix 4 for sources) (Figure 5.8).

Medial gait extension modification for out-toeing—An interesting consequence of extending a rigid forefoot post under the first metatarsal head and toe is an alteration in the angle of gait, sometimes combined with a reduction in toe-walking (Jordan 1984). If a low medial wall is retained beside the first metatarsal extension, the splint does not bend on the sagittal plane (Figure 5.9). The child who typically walks with an increased angle of gait experiences a stiff obstruction to forward progression in the first metatarsal post. The lateral forefoot is unencumbered, however, though it is supported on 1/8-inch thickness of PPT® and moleskin to level the metatarsal heads while it yields to the forces of forward movement. Thus the child who out-toes excessively prefers to walk in the splint by rolling off the lateral aspect of the posted forefoot rather than the medial. The child must reduce the angle of gait in order to do this.

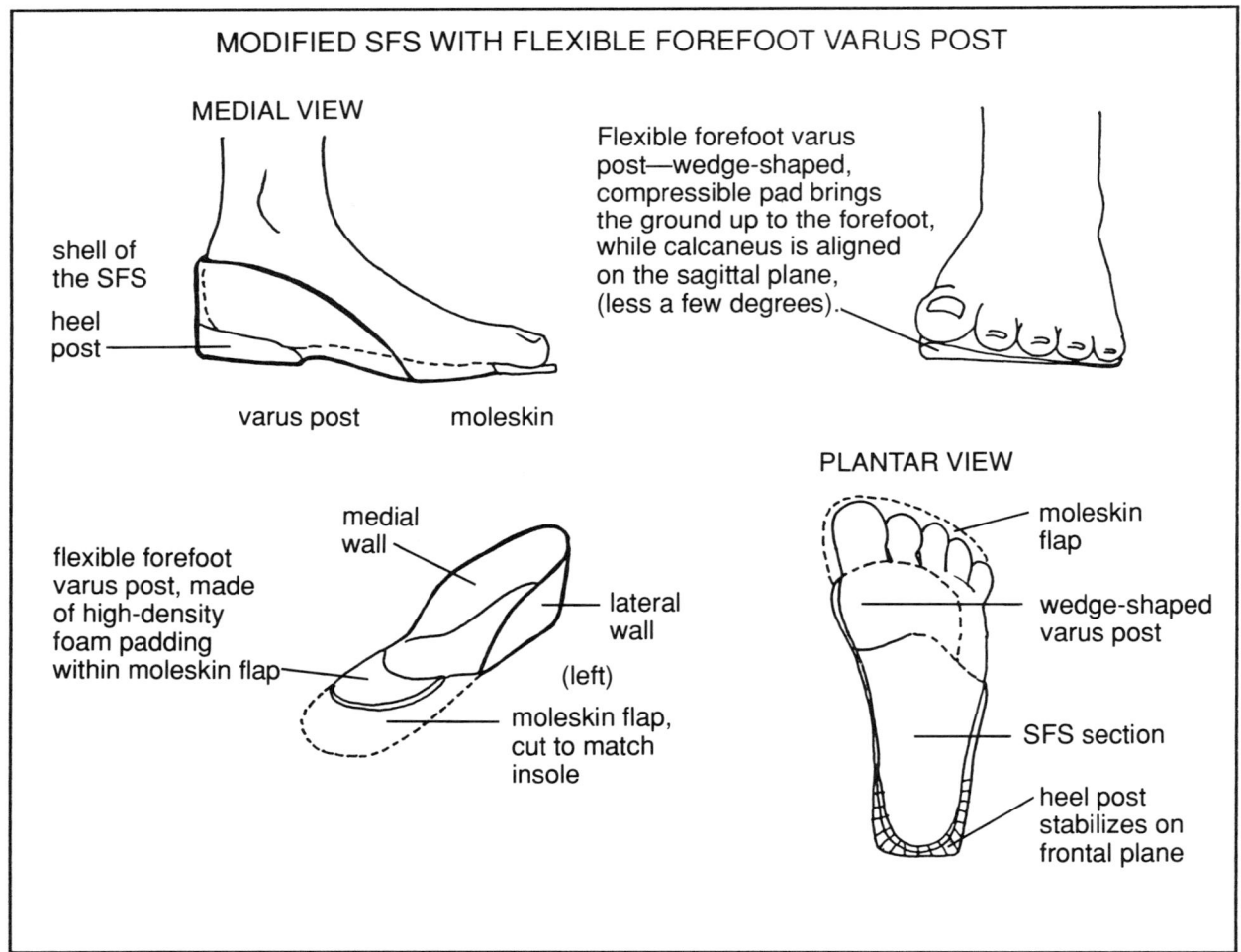

MODIFIED SFS WITH FLEXIBLE FOREFOOT VARUS POST

MEDIAL VIEW

Flexible forefoot varus post—wedge-shaped, compressible pad brings the ground up to the forefoot, while calcaneus is aligned on the sagittal plane, (less a few degrees).

shell of the SFS

heel post

varus post   moleskin

PLANTAR VIEW

flexible forefoot varus post, made of high-density foam padding within moleskin flap

medial wall

lateral wall

(left)

moleskin flap, cut to match insole

moleskin flap

wedge-shaped varus post

SFS section

heel post stabilizes on frontal plane

Figure 5.8

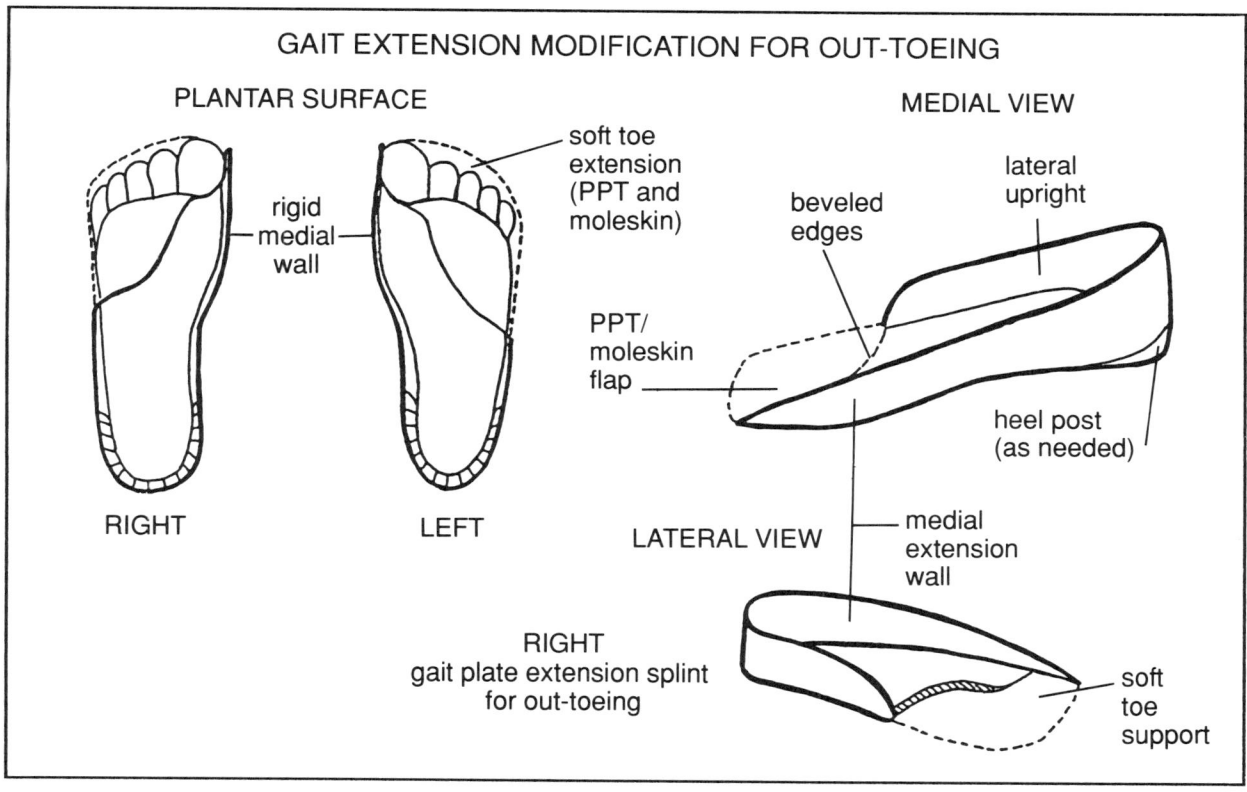

Figure 5.9

Use of the medial gait extension splint requires the availability of a full range of rotary mobility at the hip joint. The child must be young, with ample modeling capability remaining in the long bones of the lower extremity (Spencer et al. 1984). In the child who is 8 years of age or older, increased structural femoral antetorsion with compensatory lateral torsion in the lower leg is not likely to resolve with prolonged use of the medial gait extension splint. Instead, the entire leg simply rotates medially with the foot, changing (but not necessarily improving) the strains imposed on the weight-bearing joints. Perhaps a minimal medial gait extension helps prevent a progressive increase in the angle of gait for the school-age child. Research is needed to explore such questions.

Lateral gait extension modification for in-toeing—The child who in-toes as a result of excessive medial rotary mobility in the knee joint can be encouraged to increase the angle of gait. The child should wear a stabilizing foot splint that aligns the hindfoot and extends a flat, rigid post under and beside the lateral aspect of the forefoot. The extension is trimmed on a diagonal, from a point proximal to the first metatarsal head to a point distal to the fifth toe (Jordan 1984). The plantar edge is bevelled for comfort. Like the medial gait extension, the lateral extension is reinforced with a low lateral wall that prohibits the extension from bending on the sagittal plane (Figure 5.10).

The child who wears the lateral gait extension splint adducts the foot in the stance phase of gait and encounters a stiff resistance to progression forward, which is imposed by the rigid lateral extension.

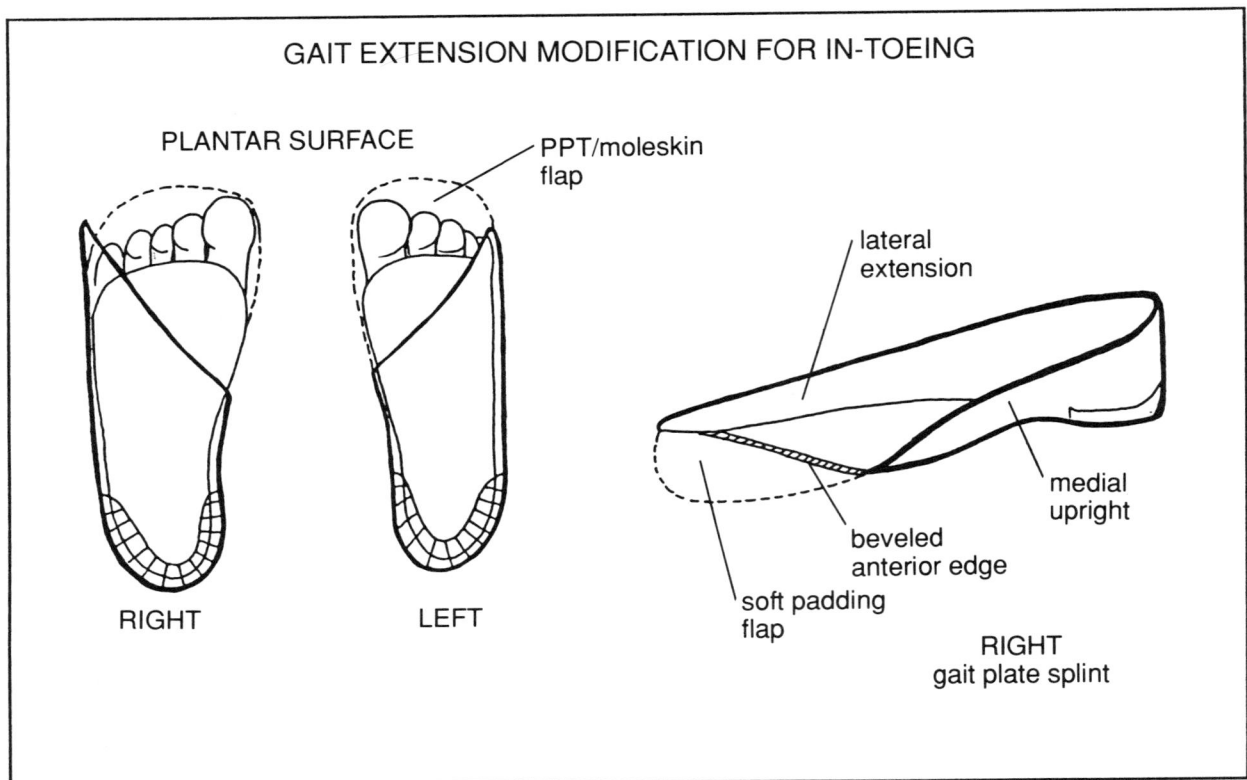

GAIT EXTENSION MODIFICATION FOR IN-TOEING

PLANTAR SURFACE

PPT/moleskin flap

lateral extension

medial upright

beveled anterior edge

soft padding flap

RIGHT

LEFT

RIGHT gait plate splint

Figure 5.10

The medial forefoot is supported on a 1/8-inch thickness of PPT® padding and moleskin, and extends under stress with forward progression. Thus, the child adjusts the angle of gait outward for a more fluid forward progression over the medial forefoot and toes. Spencer et al. (1984) state that a gait extension for in-toeing may be used between the ages of 2 and 10-12 years.

Lateral forefoot abduction block—This modification is an extension of the lateral wall of the SFS to the end of the fifth toe. The extension is useful if forefoot abduction is a significant feature of pronation, and if the toe area of the shoe is rounded and roomy (Figure 5.11). This feature can be combined with the flexible first metatarsal post, if rigid forefoot varus has been identified. (See Figure 5.4, the splint on the right.)

First metatarsal post—The hypermobile first ray can be managed with a relatively rigid post, formed with a beveled extension of the floor of the SFS, that simulates the stabilizing function of the peroneus longus by protecting the first ray from dorsiflexing past neutral position. Any accompanying varus deformity in the remaining forefoot would also be posted accordingly. The clinician can manage a significant shortening of the first metatarsal (Morton's foot) by posting under the first metatarsal head with a flexible material. The post reduces the time needed for the short first metatarsal head to make full contact with the ground, because the ground is in effect elevated. The first ray is then functionally lengthened by the post (Jordan et al. 1983; Gray 1986).

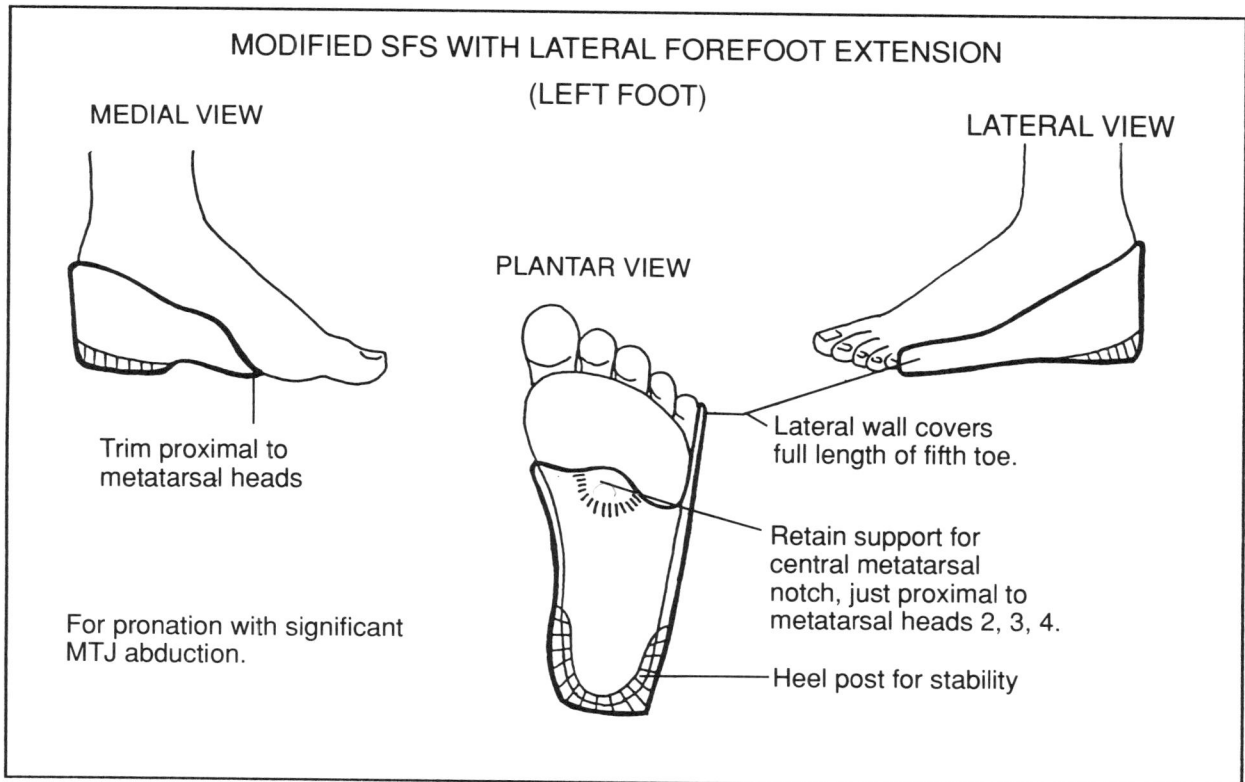

MODIFIED SFS WITH LATERAL FOREFOOT EXTENSION
(LEFT FOOT)

MEDIAL VIEW

LATERAL VIEW

PLANTAR VIEW

Trim proximal to
metatarsal heads

For pronation with significant
MTJ abduction.

Lateral wall covers
full length of fifth toe.

Retain support for
central metatarsal
notch, just proximal to
metatarsal heads 2, 3, 4.

Heel post for stability

Figure 5.11

Dorsal and malleolar extensions—Nancy Hylton developed this design, known now as a dynamic foot orthosis, or the "supramalleolar" orthosis. The entire foot, including the toes, is supported. The medial and lateral walls extend proximally to cover the malleoli and most of the dorsal surface of the foot (Figure 5.12). The effect is one of an ectoskeleton that secures the hindfoot and forefoot in the desired alignment. The heel cord is excluded from coverage by the splint material. A narrow channel of space between the malleoli and proximal to the calcaneus allows a measure of sagittal plane ankle motion. The supramalleolar orthosis is typically made of polypropylene pulled nearly paper-thin over a positive plaster mold (Hylton et al. 1988). The device gains rigidity when straps are added at the midfoot and/or the malleoli and a shoe is applied. Making the supramalleolar AFO with 1/8-inch splinting material produces a bulkier version; 1/16-inch splinting material has been used successfully to fabricate the SMS for small children.

Hylton advocates use of this design for children with equinus-related foot deformity as well as for those with pes valgus. In the presence of spasticity, contours and recesses are molded into the plantar surface of the device, using a plaster footboard (Figure 5.13). For further information regarding the supramalleolar AFO, the clinician may contact N. Hylton at the Children's Therapy Center, Kent, WA 98031.

The SFS modifications described above are derived from biomechanical principles and the experience of several clinicians. Together with the standard SFS, their comparative effectiveness is not yet

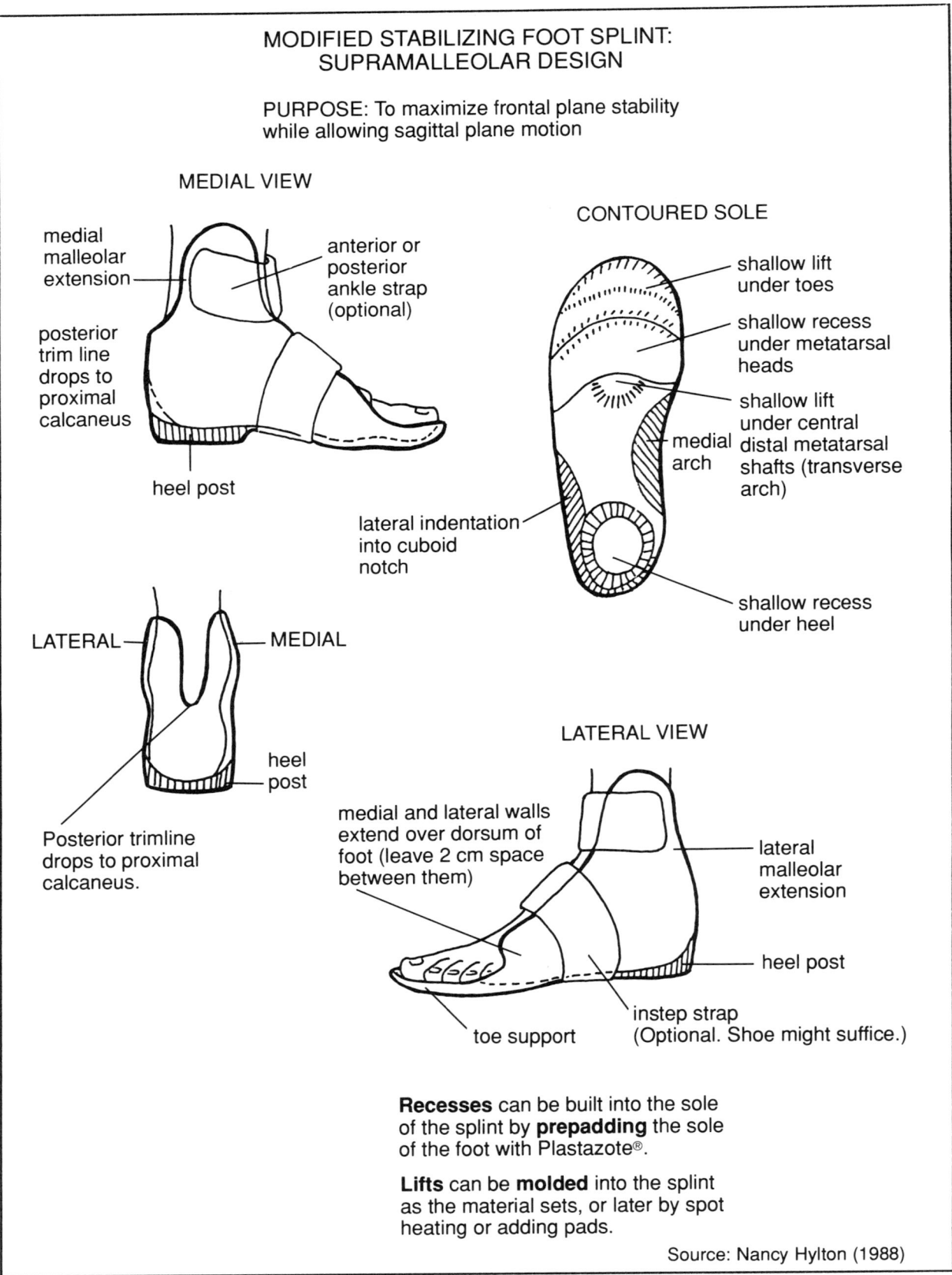

MODIFIED STABILIZING FOOT SPLINT:
SUPRAMALLEOLAR DESIGN

PURPOSE: To maximize frontal plane stability
while allowing sagittal plane motion

MEDIAL VIEW

medial
malleolar
extension

anterior or
posterior
ankle strap
(optional)

posterior
trim line
drops to
proximal
calcaneus

heel post

CONTOURED SOLE

shallow lift
under toes

shallow recess
under metatarsal
heads

shallow lift
under central
distal metatarsal
shafts (transverse
arch)

medial
arch

lateral indentation
into cuboid
notch

shallow recess
under heel

LATERAL   MEDIAL

heel
post

Posterior trimline
drops to proximal
calcaneus.

LATERAL VIEW

medial and lateral walls
extend over dorsum of
foot (leave 2 cm space
between them)

lateral
malleolar
extension

heel post

toe support

instep strap
(Optional. Shoe might suffice.)

Recesses can be built into the sole
of the splint by **prepadding** the sole
of the foot with Plastazote®.

Lifts can be **molded** into the splint
as the material sets, or later by spot
heating or adding pads.

Source: Nancy Hylton (1988)

Figure 5.12

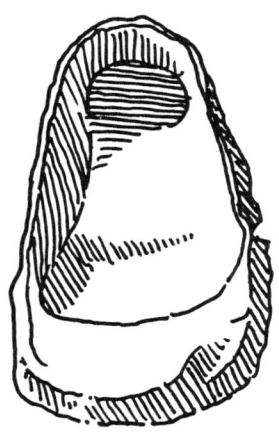

Figure 5.13
Plywood and plaster footboard, used during molding for a dynamic ankle foot orthosis (AFO) to impress contours into the floor of the devices.

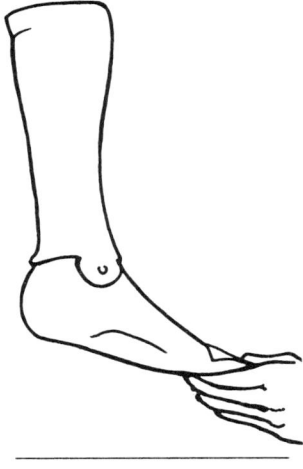

Figure 5.14
Hinged ankle-foot splint with plantarflexion stop reduced to allow sagittal plane motion.

quantified by clinical research. Among other considerations, radiologic assessment is necessary to calculate the talar angle of plantarflexion and the lateral and dorsal talocalcaneal angles before and after intervening with splints. Radiologic assessment would also help to compare these findings to existing normative values for these angles.

In cases in which the standard SFS fails to align the foot structures effectively, prolonged reddening occurs in the skin covering the navicular and the lateral-anterior border of the foot. This indicates that excessive pressure has been endured. By modifying the design of the standard SFS by one of the above methods, the pressure can be relieved in both areas of the foot. If these design modifications do not adequately relieve abnormal pressure, another measure is available: a modified hinged ankle-foot splint.

Maximizing Control of Pronation— The Modified Hinged Ankle-Foot Splint (HAFS)

For the more severe problems of flexible pes valgus, some authors suggest using the solid ankle-foot orthosis, adding a medial tibial flange to the shaft section. The design of the flange assists in preventing medial tibial rotation as a function of pronation. The principle involves the application of a lateral rotation force to the tibia as a means of using proximal support to maintain the desired angle of the transmalleolar axis, and thus of the talus in the ankle mortice (Child Prosthetic and Orthotic Studies 1981). However, because frontal plane instability is the primary problem, the restriction imposed on sagittal plane ankle motion by a solid ankle-foot orthosis is an unnecessary limitation. Nevertheless, the valgus deformity might be too severe to be managed adequately by the floor reaction forces imposed by a foot device.

When the posted and modified SFS fails to achieve realignment, the support system can include the lower leg shaft to anchor the stabilizer above the ankle. In order to avoid restricting desired ankle motion, a hinged ankle-foot splint (HAFS) with the posterior overlap stop adjusted to allow full plantarflexion is an effective intervention. This modification gains frontal plane stability for the STJ complex without prohibiting sagittal plane motion at the ankle (Figure 5.14). The splint typically maintains the hindfoot and forefoot in perpendicular alignment, incorporating any existing distal lower leg varum noted in calcaneal midposition. It should be trimmed according to the need for structural support.

The HAFS is molded over two thick socks and double-thick pads on the malleoli. The splint is worn over one sock, with half the malleolar padding replaced. As a result, the foot section offers a small measure of room for growth and for movement of the foot structures into pronation and supination within the plantigrade shell of the foot piece. This device seems to be comfortable for the patient; the hinged ankle joint allows some freedom of motion while the abundant contact area distributes pressure over a broad surface. The modified HAFS, though usually needed temporarily, should be used consistently (particularly through a period of rapid growth) to protect the medial ligaments of the foot and ankle from strain imposed by abnormal weight-bearing stresses.

Minimizing Supportive Features

Progress in reducing valgus deformity requires continual modification of the support system to allow optimum freedom of movement and adequate opportunity for modeling without compromising the gains made in alignment. For the mild deformity, an interim or evaluative measure that falls between the SFS and a high-temperature thermoplastic or leather orthosis is a low-cut modification of the SFS, which merely cups the plantar surface of the hindfoot and midfoot. This modification is adapted with a moleskin forefoot flap and inserted in lieu of the insole in a stable walking or running shoe. The insert is custom-contoured to the child's foot while maintaining the calcaneus in functional midposition or 2 degrees of varus. Older children might require thin foam padding on the contact surface, such as 1/16-inch thickness PPT® and moleskin, because of the texture and firmness of the splint material.

Another variation of the minimal SFS is a footplate, made of two or three layers of fiber glass cast tape, wetted and applied to the contours of a plaster footboard, such as the one shown in Figure 5.15. When the cast tape hardens, the outer border is trimmed to match the insole of the shoe. It is then covered with padded moleskin, such as Softskin® or Molestick®. (See Appendix 4 for sources.) The footplate is then inserted into the shoe to replace the insole. Some footplates partially cup the calcaneus; others are posted in 2 degrees calcaneus varus; and others maintain shallow walls beside the more distal foot structures.

The footplate is used to offer children with minimal sensorimotor dysfunction, ataxia, and extrapyramidal involvement increased tactile and proprioceptive input from the foot. The contours of the

Figure 5.15
Plaster footboard mold for footplates. Leave metatarsal heads and toes unposted.

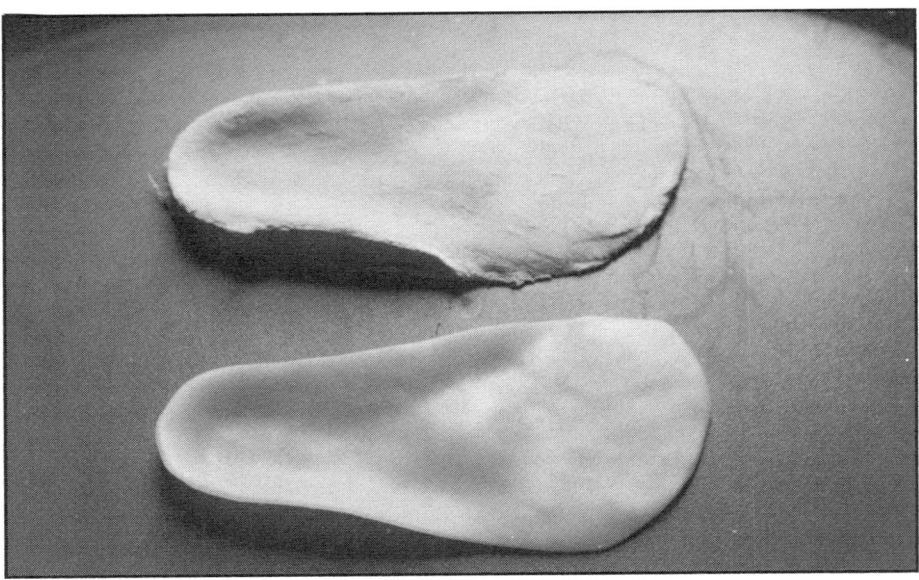

footplate match or exaggerate those of the child's foot at the proximal medial and lateral longitudinal arches and the notch just proximal to metatarsal heads #2 and #3. The raised points purportedly act as sensory cues to help the child find a midline plantigrade orientation for the foot (Coram 1989). No objective evidence regarding the validity of these claims or processes has been obtained. Clinical observation, however, supports their continued use.

Indications for Using the SFS

The SFS represents a range of devices that have been modified in numerous ways. These devices have the primary purpose of regaining proper alignment in the subtalar and midtarsal joints. Clinical indications for selecting among the SFS designs and the modified HAFS include the following:

- Flexible pes planus. Foot structures align normally off weight-bearing and flatten with weight-bearing. Relaxed calcaneal stance deviation exceeds the age-appropriate norm for valgus. The clinician can determine this norm by subtracting the child's age from the number 7 (Valmassy 1984).

- Generalized hypotonia. Signs include persistent flexible lumbar kyphosis in sitting; droopy shoulders; lordosis and knee hyperextension in standing; excessive foot pronation; and evidence of sluggish equilibrium responses.

- Ligamentous laxity. Hypermobility of the joints of the foot indicates a lack of integrity in the supporting structures. Generalized laxity can be confirmed by assessing the wrists, elbows, and fingers for laxity or hypermobility, particularly into extension.

- Calcaneal varus deviation. Although the newborn infant reveals calcaneal varus off weight-bearing, this deviation in relaxed calcaneal stance position is abnormal prior to the age of 7 years. It is also abnormal if it is greater than 2 degrees at 7 years of age and older (Root et al. 1971). For adequate reduction by an SFS, this deformity must be flexible and correctable to 4-6 degrees of calcaneal eversion off weight-bearing. Otherwise, if the deformity is osseus, a soft varus post might be needed to provide the rigid, supinated foot with shock absorption capability within its limited range of motion in early stance in gait. If mobility limitation is the result of soft tissue contracture, serial casting may be an effective means of gaining range into calcaneal eversion.

Varus deformity without an equinus component is rare in children with cerebral palsy who take weight in the standing position. In children with head trauma, however, heel varus often develops as a sequela to equinovarus posturing late in the rehabilitation process. In this case, the posterior tibialis gains a mechanical advantage for supinating the foot further, while the peroneal muscles lose in the resulting imbalance of power. Varus deviation in the STJ and MTJ often persists through swing and stance phases of gait. The STJ is unstable in supination that occurs too soon in stance. The risk of sprain to the talofibular ligaments is adequate reason to provide stabilization to the foot to center the weight-bearing calcaneus in up to 2 degrees of valgus for children age 5 and older. With adequate calcaneal eversion mobility, SFS is often suitable to this purpose, at least as an investigative procedure to determine the feasibility of intervening below the ankle joint.

- Evaluative intervention. Rather than prescribe an orthosis, the application of a foot splint (modified according to the severity of the deformity) can help the team determine readiness for reducing equinus control by lowering or eliminating the shaft section of an ankle-foot device.

- Post-surgical support for the foot structures—following selective dorsal rhizotomy or soft-tissue surgery.

- Potential deformity. If an infant as young as 10 months of age is physiologically and developmentally ready for standing but reveals significant pronation deformity or ligamentous laxity in weight-bearing positions, the foot should be protected from the consequences of creep (D'Amico 1984; Spencer et al. 1984). Infants may be adequately managed using splint material of 1/16-inch thickness, because it is slightly more flexible than the thicker materials. The fat pad is accommodated in the device, which is worn in a stable shoe. The SFS or footplate provides stabilization for the foot, so the child does not require an expensive shoe. Furthermore, the SFS fits into most shoes without increasing the size.

Contraindications for Using the SFS

- Fixed contracture of peroneals, lateral ligaments, triceps surae muscle group, or posterior tibialis. Unless passive, unresisted mobility into full correction is available at the STJ, the skin on the navicular tuberosity will lose in the battle for control between the peroneals and the SFS.

- Significant functional equinus deformity that affects the knee joint or imposes toe-drop or dragging in swing phase.

- Congenital vertical talus deformity.

- Osseous cavus deformity.

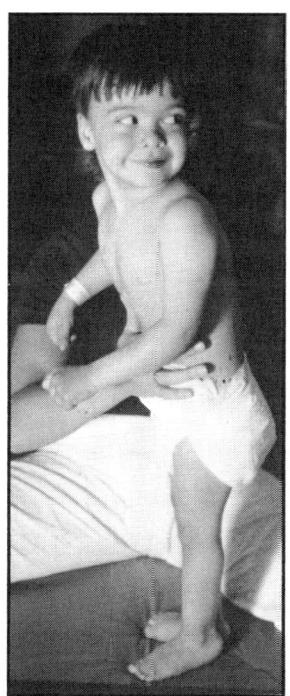

Figure 5.16
Equinovalgus deformity: toe-standing combined with pronation. Hip flexion and/or knee hyperextension occur with the effort to achieve a plantigrade foot.

Managing Functional Equinus with Splints—Hinged, Solid, and Supramalleolar

The two most common postural and functional deviations observed in the hypertonic ankle and foot are reviewed below, along with principles of intervention with splints of varying design.

Equinovalgus

As described in Chapter 4, equinovalgus deformity combines pronation of the foot with limitation of mobility into ankle dorsiflexion (Figure 5.16).

General features of correction of equinovalgus—Despite the obvious evidence of hypertonus and limitation of ankle dorsiflexion mobility, the first area of concern remains the protection of the integrity of the medial and plantar ligaments supporting the STJ and the MTJ (Jordan et al. 1983). Relative to foot alignment, a well-built ankle-foot device achieves the following goals (Figures 5.17, 5.18, and 5.19):

- To prohibit any excursion of the calcaneus into an abnormal degree of eversion, while allowing for any residual distal varum noted in standing in calcaneal midposition within the shaft piece (Figure 5.20).

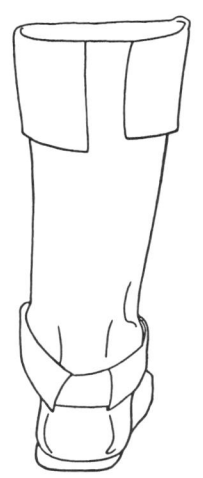

Figure 5.17
Well-built AFS/AFO prohibits abnormal frontal plane deviation of the calcaneus . . .

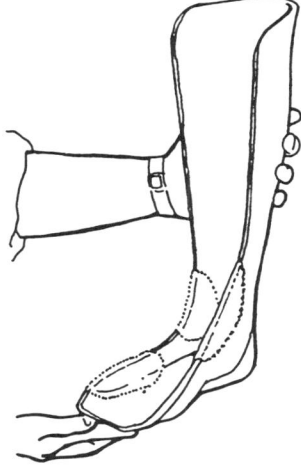

Figure 5.18
. . . and supports the ankle, the STJ, and the longitudinal arch in age-appropriate alignment and, if necessary, blocks forefoot abduction.

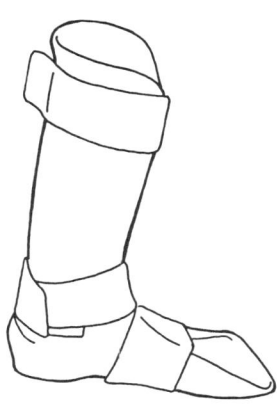

Figure 5.19
SAFS with 5 degrees of dorsiflexion for knee hyperextension control.

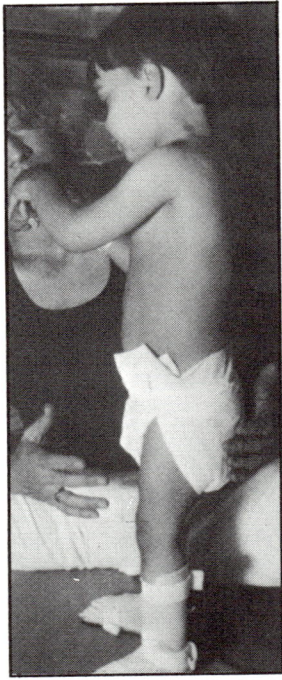

Figure 5.20
With SAFS applied, equinovalgus and knee hyperextension deformities are reduced. (Compare with Figure 5.16.) Stability in standing is enhanced by restoring ankle/STJ/MTJ alignment.

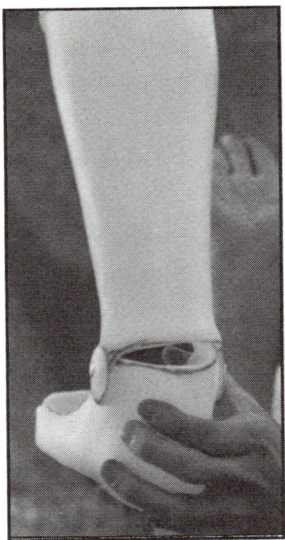

Figure 5.21
Hinged ankle-foot splint (HAFS).

- To prevent the forefoot from deviating into an abnormal degree of abduction with dorsiflexion around the oblique axis of the MTJ (Figure 5.21).
- To provide a shell for the foot that is stable in stance, so the surface under the plantar aspect of the metatarsal heads is perpendicular to the calcaneal vertical bisection.
- To prohibit hindfoot pronation related to abnormal forefoot varus by posting if necessary under the medial metatarsal heads with padding of variable density. (See the discussion of forefoot posting, above.)
- To maintain the age-appropriate dome produced by the medial and lateral longitudinal arches and the transverse arch (Jordan et al. 1983; Rosenthal 1984; Schafer 1987; Hylton et al. 1988).
- To assure adequate toe clearance in swing for safety in gait.
- To prevent abnormal talocrural plantarflexion in stance.

Only after the structures of the foot have been aligned should the clinician attempt to secure a desired ankle position (McCrea 1985; Jordan et al. 1983; Jordan 1984).

Equinovarus

The combination of equinus with supination of the foot constitutes equinovarus deformity, which occurs most commonly, though not exclusively, in children with hemiplegia.

General features of correction of equinovarus—If the deviating foot structures can be passively realigned, a well-built ankle-foot device for managing functional equinovarus deformity achieves the following goals:

- To return the calcaneus to midposition up to 2 degrees of valgus.
- To prevent the talus from abnormally dorsiflexing and abducting.
- To prohibit the forefoot and first ray from abnormally plantarflexing and adducting.
- To provide adequate toe clearance for safety in swing.
- To prohibit abnormal talocrural plantarflexion in stance.

If the equinovarus deformity is fixed (permanent and unyielding to manipulation), a series of casts may be applied as the initial means of regaining mobility into dorsiflexion with pronation before opting for surgical intervention (Westin et al. 1983; Hylton et al 1988). Above-knee casting may be necessary to address any limitation at either the hamstrings or the proximal gastrocnemius, or both (Westin et al. 1983). (See Chapter 6 for management guidelines for static soft tissue contracture.)

The attributes and limitations of ankle-foot devices, both solid and hinged, are discussed next. The focus is on splints as an alternative intervention to orthoses.

The development of the total-contact, hinged AFO has given the management team a new dimension to consider in prescribing orthoses. Each type of AFO—whether solid or hinged—offers benefits and drawbacks, and its functional effectiveness should be carefully evaluated. The availability of low-cost, easily replaceable splints that can replicate the influences of solid and hinged devices is an added advantage during this period of exploration of the limits and possibilities of dynamic total contact support systems. The proposed orthosis can be made first as a splint and modified as needed for optimum functional influence; then, if needed, it can be replicated in polypropylene.

Solid Ankle-Foot Devices

History and Structural Features of the AFO

The solid-ankle, total-contact ankle-foot orthosis (AFO) has become a standard prescription for the child with problems related to functional equinus deformity (Molnar 1986; Rosenthal 1984; Staros et al. 1975; Bunch et al. 1985; Fishman et al. 1985). Roentgenographic studies of foot structures have determined the effectiveness of building corrective alignment features for the joints of the foot into the AFO. Results reveal significant reduction of abnormally high talar plantarflexion and the dorsal talocalcaneal angles (Rosenthal 1984). However, such corrective features are not evident in many AFOs. Rather the floor is often flattened and trimmed proximal to the toes; pronation deformity is frequently evident in the structure. The ankle is usually set at 90 degrees.

Harris et al. (1986) undertook a single-subject study involving polypropylene "inhibitive ankle-foot orthoses" (or splints, as the authors also refer to them), both a supramalleolar style and standard AFO. Plaster molds for these devices were taken using a contoured plaster footboard pressed against the plantar aspect of the foot, the way Hylton recommends (Hylton et al. 1988) (Figure 5.13). Both malleoli are encased by each orthosis, purportedly for maximum frontal plane stability; the toes are fully supported by the floor of the foot section; the longitudinal arches are supported; the lateral aspect of the foot section forms a straight line from heel to toe; and the medial and lateral walls of the foot section are deep. (A hallux adductor strap is evident in each device as well.) The study revealed a significant gain in standing balance in the child when he wore the splints compared to his performance without them.

The Solid Ankle-Foot Splint (SAFS)

If the SAFS is to be used for functional weight-bearing rather than night splinting, it is constructed to maintain the calcaneus in functional midposition. The floor under the metatarsal heads is plantigrade. The malleoli are encased and padded. The ankle is usually positioned in slight dorsiflexion (2 to 5 degrees) in the SAFS. This helps to simulate the normal position of the ankle in standing and to facilitate a functional rather than hyperextended knee position (McCrea 1985; Perry 1974). The medial and lateral longitudinal arches and the transverse arch are molded into the floor of the SAFS (Figure 5.18). The posterior calcaneus is defined during molding on the proximal, medial, and lateral aspects. The existing relationship between the closed-chain calcaneal midposition and the distal lower leg is replicated during molding, or reduced by 2 degrees.

Functional Considerations Regarding Solid-Ankle Devices

For the ambulatory child with functional equinus deformity, the solid ankle-foot device provides the otherwise absent functions of the anterior tibialis in swing and at heel strike. It also acts as a stabilizing force on the tibia during stance, while it prohibits unwanted (as well as desirable) plantarflexion (Lehmann 1986; Rosenthal 1984; Bunch et al. 1985; Perry 1974).

The solid device, however, prohibits the normal excursion of the tibia forward over the plantigrade foot during postural transitions, such as squatting and rising to standing from a sitting position. In gait, the normal 10 to 15 degrees of motion of the tibia over the plantigrade foot after midstance is also prohibited by the solid ankle. Furthermore, the ankle joint normally plantarflexes 20 degrees at heel-off and immediately following heel strike. This plantarflexion is also blocked from occurring in the solid AFO or AFS, resulting in early heel rise. For these reasons, the limitations of ankle motion imposed by the solid device compete with the advantages in the child who is active and ambulatory and able to manage a greater degree of motion at the ankle.

For the severely involved spastic child, for whom the prognosis for ambulation is guarded but daily standing is desirable for physiologic reasons (respiration, digestion), the structures of the foot and the position of the ankle can be effectively protected while they bear weight by applying solid-ankle devices.

When molded properly (so the optimal biomechanical alignment of the joints of the foot is achieved and maintained in the device), the SAFS can be helpful as an intervention to protect the tissues of the foot and ankle against creep. The SAFS also promotes optimal standing. When knee hyperextension occurs in association with equinus, the ankle joint of the SAFS is set at 5 degrees of dorsiflexion (compare Figures 5.16 and 5.20).

The solid-ankle device can also be applied as a short-term measure to mimic the coactivation of muscles at the ankle that occurs normally in the first months of independent walking.

Finally, this is the simplest splint design to use for night splinting to maintain extensibility of the ankle plantarflexors and surrounding connective tissues. The night splint for managing equinovalgus should be molded with the foot structures aligned in neutral (congruent) position. The amount of dorsiflexion is then determined by finding the angle of minimum resistance to passive stretch and setting the splint slightly beyond that angle (Tardieu et al. 1988).

Of course, at the time the clinician molds a night splint for functional equinovarus deformity, setting the foot structures in true neutral alignment would promote permanent shortening of the posterior tibialis and the long toe flexors. Common sense dictates that the night splint for this deformity should be molded to maintain the calcaneus in up to 5 degrees of eversion with talocrural dorsiflexion. In addition, the MTJ oblique axis should be dorsiflexed and abducted, slightly beyond the point of minimal resistance to stretch, and the first ray should be gently dorsiflexed.

Indications for the Solid Ankle-Foot Splint (SAFS)

- Equinus deformity is functional, which allows full passive mobility with minimal resistance off weight-bearing.

- Functional equinus imposes a hyperextension force upon the knee joint in standing.

- Gross motor level approximates 6 months or below. The child does not spontaneously pull to stand or play in self-supported standing position, nor is the child preambulatory yet. For this child, or one in whom preambulatory skills are emerging, loosening the proximal strap helps achieve the ankle dorsiflexion mobility that is adequate for facilitated transitions to standing from sitting or kneeling.

- Foot and ankle deformity is evident in physiologic standing. Protection of the alignment of weight-bearing foot and ankle structures is needed. (Here, STJ neutral position is feasible for structural integrity without walking.)

- Short-term stabilization of the foot and ankle is desirable during rehabilitation following head injury.

- Postoperative support for the foot and ankle—particularly after tendo-Achilles lengthening—is necessary for up to six months to protect the lengthened tissues from overstretch as they heal. (Strengthening of triceps surae should be a focus of treatment out of splints.)

- Sagittal-plane ankle-joint stabilization is required immediately following selective dorsal rhizotomy.

- Recurrence of equinus with bone growth is probable. The SAFS, used for night splinting, sets the ankle joint at an angle that applies slight elongation to the appropriate musculature (Tardieu et al. 1988).

- Because the ankle is fixed near 90 degrees in the SAFS, sleeping postures should be adjusted to minimize any unnecessary torque forces imposed on the knee joint by rotation of the lower leg. Position the child in side-lying position, separating the feet with a pillow. Or slide the child in prone position to the end of the mattress; allow only the splinted feet to hang off the mattress.

- Evaluation is needed in order to ascertain tolerance for and functional impact of a solid ankle device prior to submitting an orthotic prescription.

In all of these applications, a bivalved (or "two-shelled") SAFS might be helpful. This is so particularly if torque forces are evident and flexibility within the device works against the child's functional ability in standing. The clinician can make the bivalved device by adding an anterior shell of splint material to the splinted foot and ankle and extending the straps to enclose both sections of the device.

The child might not need the SAFS throughout the waking day, unless deforming postures of the feet and ankles are apparent in sitting, prone, and supine positions. The SAFS is primarily a positional aid to protect the foot and ankle from experiencing the forces of deformity in weight-bearing positions.

Contraindications for using the SAFS include static contracture of ankle plantar flexors, supinators, and/or evertors.

Hinged Ankle-Foot Devices

History and Rationale

The concept of applying a hinge at the ankle is long-standing (Lehmann 1986; Staros et al. 1975; Fishman et al. 1985). Most hinged devices that were developed prior to the total contact plastic hinged AFO with a posterior contact stop relied on a sturdy shoe as the base. Anterior, posterior, and spring-loaded stops and pinstops were incorporated into the ankle joint set into metal uprights, which were then attached to the shoe with stirrups. Another precursor to the current hinged orthosis is the plastic molded shoe insert attached to standard bilateral metal uprights (Dolan et al. 1969).

Structural Features

Both the total-contact hinged ankle-foot orthosis (HAFO) and splint feature a plantarflexion stop that prohibits a predetermined angle of plantarflexion by simple contact between the posterior aspects of the shaft and foot sections. The contact angle can also be set to allow plantarflexion. Unless modified with anterior contact stops, the hinge permits free ankle dorsiflexion. The foot section is carefully molded to support the structures of the foot in optimum, age-appropriate alignment within a plantigrade shell.

The originator of the HAFO remains unknown and the main source of literature is advertisements for the sale of prefabricated models. However, Carlson (1987) reports having modified the ankle joint location and hardware on the plastic overlap style sometime during the 1970s. The new design featured a single pull of plastic material over the mold, with a double flexure component in the joint. The flexure modification reduces problems of breakage caused by material fatigue, torsion, and buckling during strenuous activities such as ball play. The single-pull design omits the overlap of shaft and foot pieces when rigid plastics are used in fabrication.

Carlson (1985-86) further reports that over 25 percent of the ankle-foot orthoses (AFOs) provided at Gillette Children's Hospital now use the double flexure type of ankle joint. Several hundred of these AFOs have been distributed at Gillette; the primary application has been in the areas of cerebral palsy and postoperative orthotic management of resistant clubfoot deformities.

Functional Considerations for the Hinged Devices

The hinged AFO (or for smaller children, the HAFS) is an excellent choice for intervention in the case of an ambulatory hemiplegic child with equinus-related foot deformity. However, for reasons related both to fatigability of the material under torque forces and to functional considerations, the clinician does not fabricate the ankle joint within the splint to replicate the anatomical axis of mortice. The location of the lateral hinge is altered; this places it anterior and proximal to the anatomical peak of the lateral malleolus. The result is that the axis of the device falls on the transverse plane and on (or rotated slightly medial to) the frontal plane. This adjustment allows the shaft piece to advance forward over the plantigrade foot piece during stance, at a normal angle of gait, with minimum torque on the hinge joints.

In normal gait, the foot and ankle interact in subtle rotary adjustments to weight assumption and progression over the foot. However, the normal angle of gait is close to the sagittal plane (0-10 degrees) after infancy. At the same time, the axis of mortice increases to 20-30 degrees lateral to the frontal plane by school age. Eversion and abduction of the foot accompany ankle dorsiflexion across the true ankle joint axis. At initial loading, while the foot pronates and the ankle dorsiflexes, the ankle joint axis rotates medially and thus reduces approximately 4 to 10 degrees. Thereafter, the foot rotates into supination after midstance while the ankle continues to dorsiflex over the loaded foot. Thus, ankle dorsiflexion does not occur across the true axis of mortice at any time in gait. If dorsiflexion took place across the true, laterally pitched axis of mortice, the foot would have to be adducted up to 20 degrees in order for the lower limb to advance on the sagittal plane.

Because the splint secures the foot and ankle in a way that limits its abnormal pronatory and supinatory excursions around a functional midposition in stance, the clinician must build the splint to accommodate and facilitate the normal, near-sagittal-plane angle of progression. Placing the lateral axis of the hinged splint on or anterior to the frontal plane of the ankle joint permits smooth progression forward over the loaded foot in its normal angle of gait. Within the splint, which is molded over two thick socks and thick malleolar pads, room is available for subtle rotary deviations of the leg and foot structures.

Limitations of the Hinged Devices

Clinical experience indicates the necessity for careful evaluation of the diplegic child with functional equinus deformity. Such a child requires close monitoring to determine the influences on stance and gait of the angle at which the overlap stop prohibits plantarflexion. The clinician must also determine the need for extra positional support against dorsiflexing.

On posture—In some children with diplegia, the prohibition of hypertonic ankle plantarflexion reveals evidence that the triceps surae muscle group is actually weak. There may also be laxity in the ligaments that has been masked by hypertonus (Huber 1985). In addition, the child may be uncertain about the proper use of the triceps surae group to stabilize the tibia in plantigrade standing (Figure 5.22). If crouch posture appears, the supporting angles of knee and ankle flexion increase. When this problem occurs, adding an anterior shell to block the motion of dorsiflexion may prevent the development of crouch posture (Figure 5.23). The shell provides

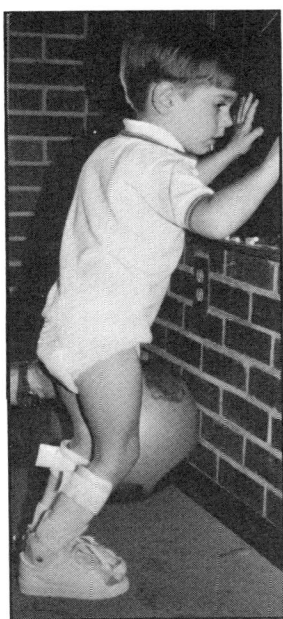

Figure 5.22
HAFS applied: with foot structures aligned, some children reveal inadequate control of the triceps surae muscle group; ankles and knees flex.

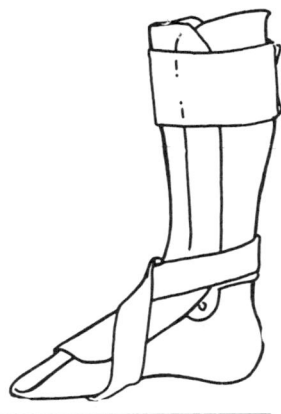

Figure 5.23
HAFS modification-A:
Use an anterior shell,
formed over the
HAFS, to block
excursion beyond a
desired angle of
dorsiflexion.Remove
the shell as strength
and control of the
ankle improve.

external stability that serves the same functional purpose as coactivation at the ankle (Figure 5.24). The stabilized ankle is used in the interim. During this period, the triceps surae group, quadriceps, and hip stabilization musculature can develop strength and control through consistent, functional, therapeutic exercise.

Gillette's orthotic team has also added a simple dorsiflexion stop by fastening a strip of strong Dacron® tether (strap) to the posterior aspect of the articulation. The length of this straps allows a preset degree of dorsiflexion (Carlson 1987). This idea has limited application for hinged Aquaplast® splints because of the flexibility of the splinting material under stress. It may be entirely adequate, however, for preschoolers. Some clinicians suggest combining an elastic strap with a non-stretch strap to allow the recoil properties of the elastic to aid the return to plantarflexion while the non-elastic strap prohibits dorsiflexion at the end point of excursion (Figure 5.25). The modification is likely to be ineffective in the presence of fixed or functional knee flexion contracture.

Ronald Gingras (Chief of Prosthetics and Orthotics at the Shriner's Hospital in Tampa, Florida) has designed a cone-shaped dorsiflexion stop that is located within the hinge. This stop controls the degree of plantarflexion and dorsiflexion without requiring the addition of a posterior stop strap. This type of modification can be added to the hinge on the HAFS by building small bars, using splint material, on the foot piece and shaft piece anterior to the hinge. When the bars contact each other, further dorsiflexion is prohibited (Coram 1989).

Figure 5.24
HAFS with anterior
shell applied.
(Compare with
Figure 5.22.) This is a
temporary measure,
to be used as a
training aid.

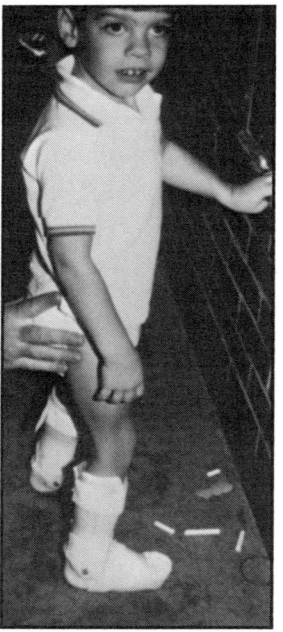

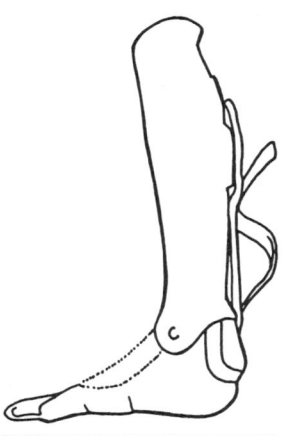

Figure 5.25
HAFS modification-B:
Add stop straps—
elastic and nonelastic
combined—to reduce
excursion into
dorsiflexion.

On gait—Because the hinged ankle-foot device is usually set to prohibit plantarflexion beyond a desired angle (for example, 0-5 degrees of dorsiflexion), the normal ankle plantarflexion that immediately follows heel strike is also prohibited. This results in the foot and knee operating as a unit at that moment in the gait cycle. As the foot lowers to the ground after heel strike, the knee, which lacks disassociation from the ankle and foot, flexes simultaneously. This ankle-knee connection may actually serve to promote the crouching that is sometimes seen in diplegic children with hinged devices.

In addition, the normal motion of 20 degrees of plantarflexion at the end of stance is blocked by the plantarflexion stop. The result is a slightly premature moment of heel-off, which can reduce overall stride length. The triceps surae group can become weakened and atrophy as a result of prolonged prohibition of normal plantarflexion at push-off.

The first thing the clinician must do in order to intervene in the problems related to prohibiting ankle plantarflexion in gait is to assess and prioritize the prevailing influences on gait. Compared to toe-stepping, these are finer points of gait for a child with moderate spastic diplegia or quadriplegia. The need to retrain away from toe-stepping may require a period of consistent refusal to allow the equinus pattern to be expressed. In this case, the tradeoffs are worth the time spent in retraining, because the child gains a proprioceptive memory for more normal weight distribution on the hindfoot in early stance (Selby 1988).

The clinician can gradually increase the available angle of plantarflexion by shaving the proximal edge of the posterior aspect of the foot piece. This results in the further plantarflexion of the ankle joint within the device before the foot piece encounters the stop on the shaft piece. The gradual granting of plantarflexion can offer the child the opportunity to adapt to the added motion in small increments while retaining toe-clearance in swing, and without resorting to the original equinus gait pattern. A separate, more dorsiflexed splint should be worn at night to maintain extensibility in the muscle and connective tissues (Tardieu et al. 1988; Baumann et al. 1986).

Two different mechanisms influence the angle of gait:

- Adjustment of the location of the axis of mortice in the splint by moving the lateral hinge anteriorly or posteriorly to align the foot position in relative abduction or adduction under the leg during stance.

- Maintenance of a vertical wall and a flattened floor on the medial or lateral aspect of the forefoot section of the splint, which creates a rigid resistance to bending on weight-bearing. The wall on the opposite side is carved off, retaining only the floor of the forefoot section. This side bends under stress. With the mobility that is available in the proximal soft tissue structures, a lateral rigid forefoot wall might resist in-toeing, and a medial rigid wall might resist out-toeing.

A commonly made error in molding splints for the foot is dorsiflexing the lateral toes and adjacent metatarsal heads as the splint material hardens. The result is an upward sweep at the lateral forefoot, which serves as a gait extension mechanism that *encourages* in-toe gait.

Finally, the hinged device can be replaced by a high-cut foot splint (SMS), along the lines of the supramalleolar orthosis. This is feasible when the available stability at the foot allows the child to make an efficient postural adjustment at the knees and hips. The clinician can modify the SMS by adding anterior and/or posterior straps proximal to the malleoli, if necessary.

The advantage of exploring these and other still undiscovered possibilities with splints is two-fold: low cost and expedience.

Indications for Using the Hinged Ankle-Foot Splint (HAFS)

The functional equinus may be evident and passive mobility into 5 degrees of dorsiflexion (with minimal resistance) may be available while the foot structures are congruent. In these cases, any of the following conditions would be likely to generate a prescription for a HAFS.

- Emerging preambulatory skills are a focus of the management program. The HAFS would be applied as needed to stabilize the plantigrade foot on the frontal plane during postural transitions, while prohibiting habitual thrusting into equinus.

- Independent, unassisted ambulation features toe-drop in swing and reduced heel contact in stance. Provided that the range, strength, and timing of knee extension are adequate, the HAFS with a posterior stop provides the opportunity for heel strike. The hinged ankle also allows prolonged plantigrade foot support after midstance to terminal stance.

Contraindications for Using the HAFS

- Fixed contracture of ankle plantar flexors, supinators, and/or pronators allows less than 5 degrees of dorsiflexion beyond neutral, with the foot structures in congruent alignment (McCrea 1985; Root et al. 1977).

- Strong resistance to passive ankle dorsiflexion is evident throughout the available range.

- Contracture of the hamstrings limits the popliteal angle to a value greater than 30 degrees.

- Moderate to severe crouch deformity is evident in stance. (See Managing Crouch Deformity with Splints, below.)

- Proximal stability is inadequate for active stabilization. Some ambulatory children with neuromotor impairment lose postural control with a free ankle. These children require the increased stability of a solid ankle until they gain proximal strength, or perhaps a hindfoot alignment, set at STJ neutral position to gain optimum architectural support internally.

Managing Problems Associated with Equinus Deformity

Knee Hyperextension

Rosenthal et al. (1975) determined that setting the ankle at 5 degrees of dorsiflexion in a solid, below-knee orthosis can effectively reduce the problem of genu recurvatum related to equinus in children with cerebral palsy. The principle of floor reaction forces that result from weight-bearing are applied in this design. Like a modern ski boot, a forward moment of force is directed to the posterior proximal tibia in stance; this causes the knee to buckle into slight flexion (Lehmann 1986; Cary et al. 1975; Rosenthal 1984; Perry 1974; Rosenthal et al. 1975). It is best to apply this principle when genu recurvatum measures less than 10-15 degrees (Cary et al. 1975). However, the dorsiflexed ankle does impose a functional compromise. Ankle plantarflexion, after heel strike and after midstance, is prohibited in order to gain control at the knee.

With recent advances in splinting and orthotics, this tradeoff has become less necessary. The Swedish knee cage and the finger splint for swan-neck deformity have inspired the development of a knee hyperextension splint (Figure 5.26). It is a simple device: the splint is molded over the anterior aspect of the knee joint while it is maintained in 40-45 degrees of flexion (Figure 5.27). A hole is cut in the center and straps are added in such a way that they avoid compressing the knee joint. The strap, heavily padded to protect the popliteal space from abnormal pressure, weaves from back to front inside the side panels of the splint. It attaches by folding the remaining ends out to close on Sabregrip® or Velcro® strips (Figure 5.28). (See Appendix 4 for sources.)

Figure 5.26
Knee hyperextension splint.

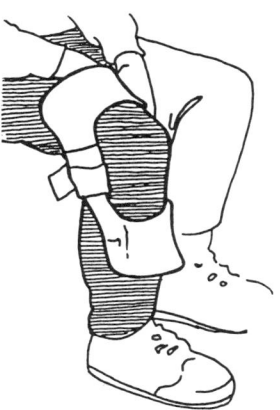

Figure 5.27
Mold over thick pants, or padding, with knee in 30-45 degrees of flexion. Fold side panels for strength.

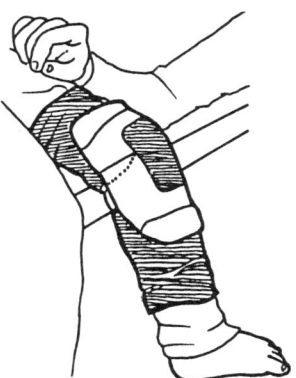

The straps are adjusted in tightness to prohibit the knee joint from hyperextending (Figures 5.29, 5.30, and 5.31). The proximal and distal anterior panels combine with the posterior padded strap to form a 3-point loading system. The inner surfaces of the splint are padded with adhesive-backed foam, both for comfort and to minimize slipping.

The knee hyperextension splint offers the team a specific management alternative for the knee joint, as well as the opportunity to consider the management of the ankle and foot as a separate, rather than a connected, issue. The notion of allowing the ankle to plantarflex up to 20 degrees, or freely, can now be evaluated in combination with the knee splint. The more minimal foot-support systems might suffice. If not, a hinge and shaft can be added. This arrangement will first allow plantarflexion and, if needed, will raise the

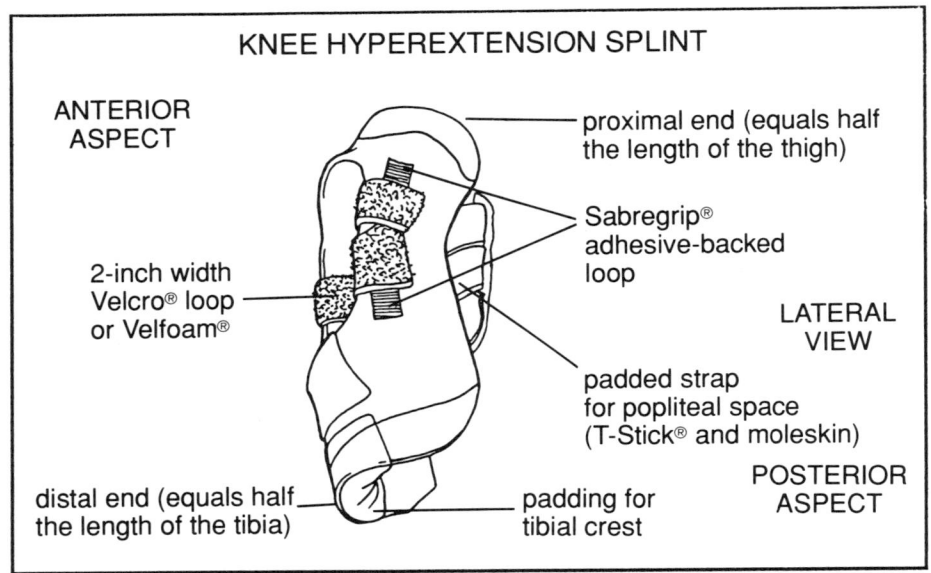

KNEE HYPEREXTENSION SPLINT

ANTERIOR
ASPECT

proximal end (equals half
the length of the thigh)

Sabregrip®
adhesive-backed
loop

2-inch width
Velcro® loop
or Velfoam®

LATERAL
VIEW

padded strap
for popliteal space
(T-Stick® and moleskin)

distal end (equals half
the length of the tibia)

padding for
tibial crest

POSTERIOR
ASPECT

Figure 5.28

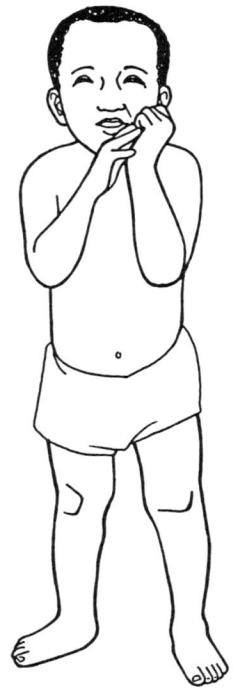

Figure 5.29
Right knee
hyperextension,
associated with
equinus deformity.

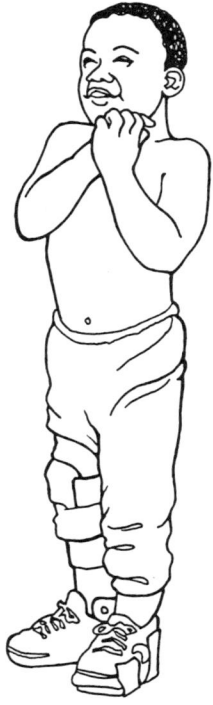

Figure 5.30
Right knee
hyperextension,
corrected using knee
hyperextension splint,
combined with HAFS
with 10-degree plan-
tarflexion stop. (Note
lift added to left shoe
to level the pelvis.)

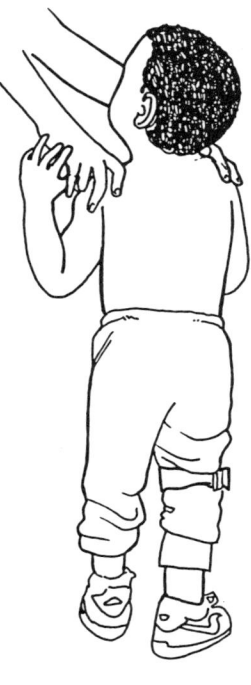

Figure 5.31
Corrected right knee
hyperextension,
posterior view.
Velfoam® strap is
padded with Pudgee®
foam. (See Appendix
4 for sources.)

posterior stop to limit plantarflexion. I recommend taking this approach to management of knee hyperextension and consider the knee splint to be a training aid that helps build quadriceps control.

If the knee hyperextension splint fails or is poorly used or tolerated—or if the supinatory forces generating hyperextension at the knee are too great—manage it with an AFS. Rang et al. (1986) suggest that a little knee flexion is better than recurvatum. Begin by setting the hindfoot in slight (2 degree) pronation. The talar plantarflexion will facilitate knee flexion through the closed chain. Once the primary condition of functional alignment of the foot structures has been satisfied, and still more control is needed, the ankle-foot splint (either SAFS or HAFS) is molded in 5 degrees of dorsiflexion. If the child requires added knee control, a low wedge can be added to the heel of the shoe.

If lateral deviation persists in the stance knee, the device is posted at the lateral-plantar aspect of the heel and forefoot. This action prohibits the foot from rolling outward, taking the shaft section with it. A 1/4-inch lateral buttress, attached to the outer surface of the shoe and sole, can also help to reduce the problem of rolling outward. Evaluate the foot to determine evidence of either forefoot valgus deformity or plantarflexed first ray as contributing factors. If either of these problems exists, posting within the plantigrade shell at the forefoot can help reduce the lateral roll.

Knee Flexion Contracture

As noted previously, the clinician must alleviate limitation of knee extension mobility in conjunction with management measures to reduce functional equinus deformity (Cary et al. 1975; Westin et al. 1983; Bleck 1987; Harrington et al. 1983-84). (See Chapter 6 for more information regarding long-leg serial casting.) Otherwise, the results of intervening below the knee will be disappointing. This is because the contracture at the knee joint—into flexion and/or internal (medial) genicular position—will force the child who is wearing the SAFS or HAFS either to resume toe-stepping or to buckle into a crouched posture (Rang et al. 1986).

Forefoot Varus Deviation

Forefoot varus deviation is a common finding in equinovalgus deformity. Consideration should be given to posting as needed, to molding to produce a plantigrade foot portion in the splint, and then perhaps to partially support the varus forefoot in weight-bearing.

Forefoot Valgus Deviation

This deformity is acquired. Typically it accompanies supination and equinovarus deformities in the more proximal foot and ankle structures.

Distinguishing true forefoot valgus (which includes all metatarsal heads) from a rigid plantarflexed first ray is a necessary component of therapeutic intervention, because the methods of management differ (Tiberio 1988). The purpose of intervening with orthoses is to prohibit the lateral aspect of the forefoot from lowering to the ground at the expense of hindfoot neutrality and stability.

The complete valgus forefoot is supported merely on a wedge-shaped post along the plantar surface of all the metatarsal heads. This is to accommodate the valgus angle relative to the varus posting under the lateral four metatarsal heads while leaving a depression for the first metatarsal head. The result is a functionally level forefoot in weight-bearing. Here, too, refrain from posting the forefoot at all in young children.

Leg Length Discrepancy

Children with neuromotor impairment already face serious biomechanical difficulties related to sensorimotor control of posture and function. Even the smallest consistently detectable anatomic leg length discrepancy demands a significant effort to compensate for the imbalance. Postural adjustment does not occur with subtlety in these children. Therefore, it is a good practice to intervene to align the feet if necessary and to lift the shoe on the shorter leg when a true shortening appears. Do this when the shortening has not been caused by hip subluxation.

The idea that "it is better for the child with hemiplegia to have a shorter leg because it helps to clear the foot in swing" is frequently encountered, but it is an unacceptable rationalization. The shortened leg imposes the need for numerous biomechanical and functional compensations in both the more affected and less affected limbs. Equinus is promoted by the need to reach the floor while maintaining the pelvis aligned on the transverse plane. Pronation frequently develops in the opposite foot. In addition, Staheli et al. (1968) came to the following conclusions concerning children with hemiplegia:

- Femoral "anteversion" (that is, antetorsion) averages 40 degrees on the more affected side, which is an average of 11 degrees greater than on the less affected side.
- Longitudinal growth inhibition is greatest in the tibia, leaving the femur unaffected.
- Limb muscle atrophy and shortening increase with age.

These conclusions suggest a lack of adequate magnitude of the externally applied forces of compression and torque that model bones and hypertrophy muscle and connective tissue. Full weight-bearing on the extremity during movement generates greater magnitude of both of these forces than partial weight-bearing.

It may be preferable to relieve foot drop in swing with a hinged ankle-foot device, allowing 5-10 degrees of plantarflexion as needed for optimum toe clearance and progression in stance. After this a lift can be added that equals the functional leg length and levels the pelvis. Certain children with hemiplegia go through the phenomenon of compression-induced, accelerated bone growth after having a lift applied to the shoe on the shorter side. After these children wear the lift for a few months (together with a hinged ankle-foot splint if needed), it can be determined—by means of the same evaluative criteria that brought about the application of the lift—whether the lift is needed any longer. Even months later it can be reapplied if shortening occurs again. This approach is appropriate because periodic adjustments are made to suit the current biomechanical requirements for optimum function

Managing Crouch Deformity with Splints

Chapter 4 discussed the multiple problems of alignment and function that have been identified in crouch deformity. As the chapter pointed out, the primary contributing factor to crouch deformity is weakness in the triceps surae group. This weakness results in failure to stabilize the tibia from falling forward over the plantigrade foot in stance. Energy consumption and muscle fatigue eventually can lead to the child's refusal to use ambulation as a primary means of locomoting. This often occurs by adolescence (Figure 5.32).

History and Rationale

In normal gait, an ankle plantarflexion/knee extension force couple occurs at midstance, when the body's center of mass passes in front of the extended knee. Knee extension is thereafter controlled and maintained by the eccentric, reverse action of the plantarflexors, which contract briefly and explosively as the foot enters push-off (Rodgers 1988; Harrington et al. 1983-84; Sutherland et al. 1978; Sutherland et al. 1980). The plantarflexors stabilize the tibia against the calcaneus. As they anchor the tibia above the heel, the heel lifts at the end of stance. The movement of the body over the forefoot and the hyperextending toes increases step length as the swing leg advances. In this manner, the length of the foot increases step length.

When the ankle falls into dorsiflexion during stance phase, the knee extension force of the soleus muscle is compromised. When this happens, the knee also sinks into flexion. The center of mass remains behind the knee joint throughout the stance phase, and the knee remains anterior to the vertical force vector (Figure 5.33) (Harrington et al. 1983-84; Sutherland et al. 1978). There is no moment of heel-off at the end of stance; the foot leaves the floor as a unit, and step length—maximized primarily by hyperdorsiflexion in the stance ankle—is reduced (Schafer 1987).

Most traditional orthotic interventions for crouch deformity have met with little success in either prohibiting the deviations in alignment at the leg and foot, or in significantly reducing the work load of walking (Frost 1971; Lehmann 1986). Hip-knee-ankle-foot-orthoses (HKAFOs) that are locked at the knee joint cause too much interference with ambulation, although their effect on postural alignment of the legs can be dramatic.

If the ankle joint is rigidly supported against dorsiflexing, the brace that supports it functions as a first-class lever, with the fulcrum at the distal end under the metatarsal heads. Floor reaction forces are transferred to the proximal end of the brace—in most cases, the proximal tibia (Harrington et al. 1983-84). (Figure 5.34—compare with Figure 5.32.) The rigid support provided in turn reduces energy costs (Lehneis 1976).

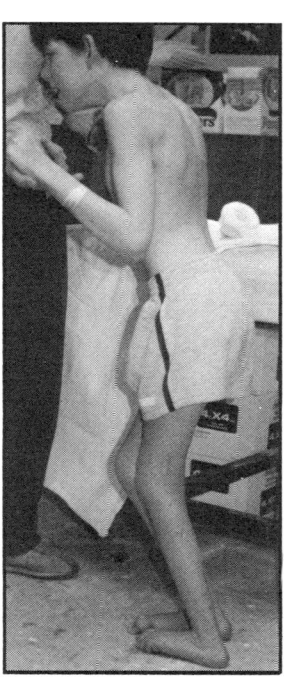

Figure 5.32
Crouch deformity—
preadolescence.
Note full foot contact;
calcaneus deformity
(excess dorsiflexion).

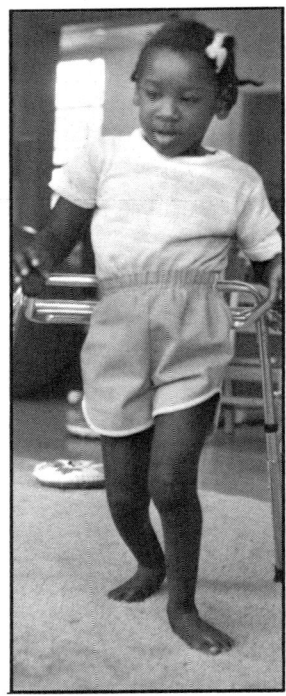

Figure 5.33
Crouch gait: The center of mass remains posterior to the knee joint. Stabilizing action of the plantarflexors on the tibia is lacking. Note pronation at the feet.

Saltiel (1969) described this principle in relation to the patella-tendon-bearing, laminated knee-locking ankle-foot orthosis. He developed this original version of the floor reaction ankle-foot orthosis for the management of polio-induced paralysis in the lower extremity. The design consists of one continuous piece of laminate with a molded foot support, a plantarflexed ankle position, and an extension of the laminate plastic material over the most proximal aspect of the tibia. The design provides a distal fulcrum at the metatarsal heads for extension at the knee; it does this by using floor reaction forces in weight-bearing.

The Anterior Floor Reaction Orthosis (AFRO)

At Newington Children's Hospital in Newington, Connecticut, Harrington et al. (1983-84) applied the concept developed by Saltiel to the problems of the cerebral palsied child who crouches. Harrington's group modified the design into the anterior floor reaction orthosis (AFRO). They eliminated the feature of weight-bearing on the patella tendon by trimming down the proximal border. They then observed that forward progression in gait was impeded while a child was wearing bilateral AFROs. They modified the angle at the ankle, setting it as needed for optimum ambulatory function—at up to 5 degrees of dorsiflexion relative to the frontal plane (Harrington et al. 1983-84).

Prerequisites for use—The Newington group outlined prerequisites upon which favorable results of the use of the AFRO are contingent. These criteria include the following:

- The presence of some trunk balance and/or ability to use auxiliary walking aids.
- The presence of a minimum of Grade 3 (fair) quadriceps strength.
- The absence of hip and knee flexion contractures exceeding 10 degrees, presumably measured in standing. (The authors do not specify their measurement methods.) Of 11 children studied at Newington, all required elongation of hamstrings either surgically or by serial casting before they could use the AFRO (Harrington et al. 1983-84; Waters et al. 1985).
- Careful determination in setting the angle of ankle dorsiflexion, allowing forward progression in walking without compromising the goal of achieving knee extension support. This concern is especially important if intervention is bilateral.

Reported outcome—For the 11 children studied, intervention with AFROs resulted in a significant reduction in crouch gait. Three of the children were assessed using computerized gait analysis. The following parameters of gait function showed improvement in those who underwent computerized analysis:

- Single limb support time and stability.
- Stride length.
- Walking velocity.
- Endurance. Although energy consumption remained unchanged in this study, stride length and velocity gains rendered overall gait more efficient.

Crouch-Control Ankle-Foot Splints

History and Rationale

In 1982, while preliminary studies of Newington's AFRO were awaiting publication, the staff at Children's Rehabilitation Center (CRC) was engaged in the design of a similar device. With the assistance of Mike Smith, the orthopedic technician, I designed the solid crouch-control ankle-foot splint (SCAFS) (Figures 5.34 to 5.37). The SCAFS operates on principles that are similar to those applied to the Newington AFRO, and our experiences with the SCAFS somewhat paralleled those of the Newington group. Four years later, I added a hinge to the SCAFS (Figures 5.38 to 5.41).

The solid CAFS, which was made of Aquaplast®, was first designed to prohibit three postural problems: pronation of the STJ complex; knee hyperflexion; and ankle hyperdorsiflexion. This splint encompasses the foot and lower leg and is applied by inserting the foot and leg through an opening on the posterior aspect (Figure 5.36). Effective transfer of floor reaction forces to the knee depends upon the structural features of a rigid plantar surface at the forefoot and toes (Figure 5.37) and an ankle section that resists dorsiflexion forces (Lehmann 1986; Harrington et al. 1983-84; Lehneis 1976).

This device is built with functional calcaneal midposition as a key biomechanical feature. The plaster contoured footboard (discussed previously) is used to mold a thin footplate of 1/16-inch Aquaplast-T®. The footboard is designed to provide the minimum degree of forefoot varus post needed to maintain the calcaneus between vertical and 2 degrees varus alignment. The resulting footplate is then posted extrinsically (to maintain the forefoot/hindfoot alignment) before incorporating it into the floor of the splint. The footplate, combined

Figure 5.34
Solid crouch-control ankle-foot splint (SCAFS) applied. (Compare with Figure 5.32.) Limitations of the solid ankle on forward progression in gait has led to development of the hinged CAFS (HCAFS).

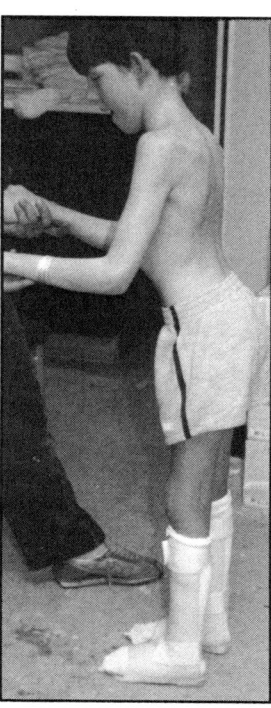

Figure 5.35
SCAFS addresses multiple alignment problems related to crouch deformity. (Compare with Figure 5.33.)

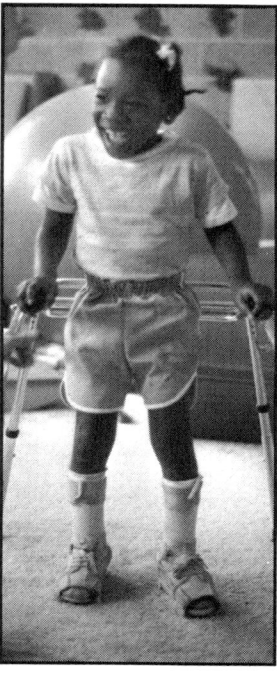

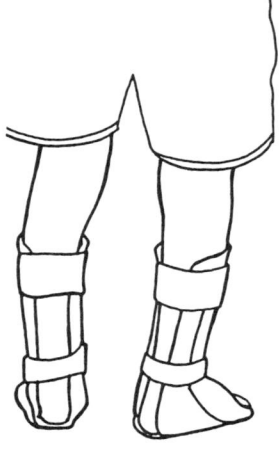

Figure 5.36
The CAFS (solid
or hinged) is applied
through the posterior
opening.

with the shell, employs the closed kinetic chain to restore the leg structures to functional position. Thus the lower leg, via the talar alignment, gains improved alignment relative to the sagittal and frontal planes (Figure 5.38).

The child for whom this device was originated was a preadolescent boy with asymmetric diplegia (or double hemiplegia, considering his upper extremity involvement), hydrocephalus (status post ten shunt revisions), and crouch posture. He had recently undergone hamstring lengthening. As a child, multiple operations on his feet and ankles (including calcaneal osteotomy) had left him with severe calcaneus deformity on one side (hyperdorsiflexion of the talocrural joint) and weakness on the other. Both feet were curling into cavus as he relied on long toe flexors, intrinsics, and ankle dorsiflexors for compensatory stabilization.

For more than a year, he had used bivalved plaster "inhibitory" cast boots with contoured footboards as Yates (1977) suggested. He was able to walk with a rolling walker in his casts. The length of his feet increased that year, indicating a reduction in the trend toward cavus deformity. As he grew, the casts became unwieldy and cosmetically unacceptable and were discontinued.

The child then entered a growth spurt, and his crouch deformity became a threat to his independence in walking. He was issued a pair of standard leather and metal knee-ankle-foot orthoses (KAFOs), which promptly became useful only as sleeping splints. Otherwise, they were too impractical because he was unable to don them independently or to operate the knee locks on both sides.

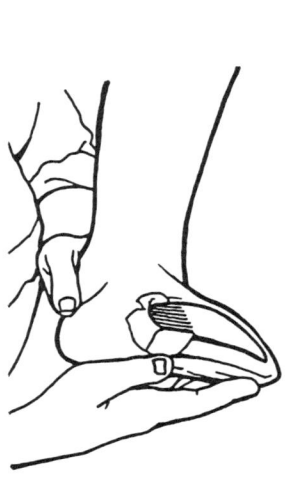

Figure 5.37
The CAFS (solid or
hinged): The rigid toe
support acts as a
fulcrum for directing
floor reaction forces
to promote knee
extension.

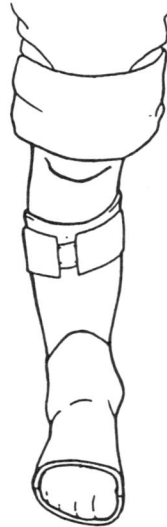

Figure 5.38 Functional alignment of the subtalar and midtarsal joints is a significant feature of the CAFS, because restoration of optimum biomechanical alignment of the foot structures aids in restoring alignment to the proximal joints. A posted, contoured footplate provides support via the floor of the device. The dorsal shell controls major deviations.

Because it was evident that ankle weakness was the source of the boy's postural problems, Smith and I wrapped some splinting material over the dorsum of his ankle, foot, and tibia while maintaining his foot and ankle in midposition. These rudimentary SCAFSs, despite their bulk and lumpiness, effectively reduced his crouch posture and improved his ambulatory status. He resumed walking in school and at home.

Over the next two years, CRC produced 40 SCAFS devices for 15 children. The staff encountered the same difficulties as did the Newington group: limitations on efficient forward progression, primarily imposed by the 90-degree angle at the ankle. This was particularly true when these splints were applied bilaterally. In response, the device was adjusted by adding heel posts to tip the shaft forward a few degrees and thereafter set the angle of the ankle at 5 degrees of dorsiflexion in order to reduce this limitation.

The HCAFS—In June 1986, during a seminar in St. Louis, I turned my attention to the inability of the SCAFS to address adequately two problems:

- Weakness in the triceps surae muscle group (the fixed ankle does not permit plantarflexion).
- Limitation of forward progression.

A participant posed the provocative question, "Why don't you put a joint in it?" The hinged crouch-control ankle-foot splint (HCAFS) was promptly created with the following features:

- Support for the STJ complex in functional calcaneal midposition.
- A strong block against sinking into abnormal ankle and knee flexion though single-limb stance (Figure 5.39).
- Articulation that allows the normal 20 degrees of plantarflexion after heel-off. This provides the opportunity to strengthen the plantarflexors in their normal role as tibial stabilizers at the appropriate moment of gait (Figure 5.39).
- Availability of the normal 15-20 degrees of plantarflexion that occur after initial contact. This plantarflexion separates the ankle motion from the knee at the onset of the stance phase, unlike a fixed-ankle device (Figure 5.41).
- Adjustment capability to determine the optimum functional angle of ankle dorsiflexion.

This development was a significant improvement over the solid CAFS. However, at that time it was felt that the forefoot might model out of varus deformity, so it was typically left unposted. I have altered the design recently to provide a contoured forefoot varus posted inner footplate, if needed, to help reduce compensatory pronation and stress at the hindfoot. Crouch deformity that calls for this level of external stabilization usually occurs in children older than age 8-10 years, when the issue of forefoot remodeling has waned.

The HCAFS approaches the foot and ankle from the dorsum because of the nature of the stress tolerance of this splinting material. Any attempt to replicate the design of the AFRO using Aquaplast® fails because the flexibility of the material permits the ankle area of the

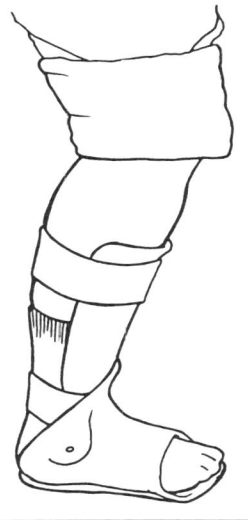

Figure 5.39
Hinged crouch-control AFS (HCAFS) offers the same block against excess dorsiflexion as CAFS; allows 5 degrees dorsiflexion.

Figure 5.40
HCAFS allows normal motion into 20 degrees of plantarflexion after midstance . . .

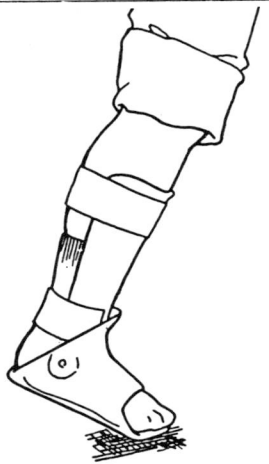

Figure 5.41
. . . and allows plantarflexion after initial contact as an isolated motion, separate from the knee.

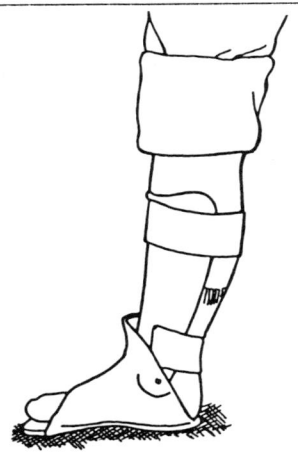

splint to bend into dorsiflexion under the stress of the type of loading that occurs in crouch deformity. Furthermore, the AFRO does not provide for ankle plantarflexion.

The feature of ankle angle for forward progression can be more easily controlled in the HCAFS by setting the splint at 5-7 degrees of dorsiflexion while molding. Then there can be an evaluation of the functional effect of reducing the available excursion between the shaft and foot sections by inserting closed-cell PPT® padding, which compresses very little, until the ideal angle is achieved. (See Appendix 4 for sources.) That ideal angle is then maintained permanently by replacing the trial padding with an equal thickness of splint material and then trimming away the residual dorsal tongue.

Research is needed, however, to ascertain the effectiveness of the HCAFS in facilitating strengthening and timely activity of the ankle plantarflexors in gait. The sole of the device, which extends to support the toes, seems to combine with the stabilization at the ankle in a way that resembles the knee-ankle force couple discussed previously. Normal individuals who wear the device report that as the knee moves in front of the ankle after midstance, a lever force (perceived proprioceptively) facilitates active plantarflexion needed to propel past the toe at the end of terminal stance phase. They consistently report sensing activity in the triceps surae group after midstance. The staff of the departments of physical therapy and orthotics at the Shriners Hospital in Tampa, Florida, have used the HCAFS in variable designs since 1986. They report a notable increase in girth of the calf musculature in children who use them (Lundy 1989).

More research is also needed to revise the design to minimize bulky excess where possible. Modifications have already begun at the suggestion of the pediatric therapists in Austin, Texas. These changes might eliminate the separate sole piece by molding the foot section like a supramalleolar splint, doubling the softened splint material over the dorsum of the dorsiflexed ankle. (I have found this technique troublesome so far, because the material wrinkles on the anterior ankle.) Furthermore, with a stronger material—such as polypropylene or copolymer—the flap-like extension of the foot piece over the distal shaft piece might be trimmed considerably to two small peaks or a band that lies anterior to the malleoli. If toe drop occurs in swing, the two components of the HCAFS can be connected with an elastic strap of suitable strength to gain toe clearance.

The modified supramalleolar device—A modification of the supramalleolar orthosis has been used for the child with mild inclination to crouch posture. The malleolar extensions are extended proximally and anteriorly to the dorsum of the ankle and distal lower leg. An anterior strap is attached. The posterior opening proximal to the calcaneus allows the ankle to plantarflex (Hylton et al. 1988). This design could be replicated with splint material to determine its effectiveness and used either alone or in combination with a shaft piece.

Advantages of the HCAFS

As an alternative to the SAFS with an anterior shell (bivalved SAFS) or to the AFRO, the HCAFS offers the following advantages for controlling crouch posture:

- The potential to build plantarflexion strength with mobility.
- Broader distribution of the heavy anterior-medial displacement of weight over the surface of the lower leg.

Indications for Hinged and Supramalleolar Crouch-Control Splints

Crouch-control splints are indicated under the following conditions:

- Weakness in the triceps surae muscle group and hyperextensibility of the Achilles tendon, resulting in exaggerated ankle dorsiflexion in stance and gait.
- Knee flexion contracture of less than 10 degrees with the hip extended; less than 30 degrees with the hip flexed 90 degrees (popliteal angle).
- Hip flexion contracture less than 10 degrees.
- A foot supple enough to be manipulated into correct alignment at the STJ.

Contraindications for Crouch-Control Splints

- Contracture of hip flexors and/or hamstrings exceeding 10 degrees with the legs extended.
- Popliteal angle exceeding 30 degrees.
- Strong equinus that is evident in combination with knee flexion in stance and swing. In such cases, the HCAFS would only decorate the existing deformity.
- Genu recurvatum.
- Poor trunk control, with the child unable to adapt to the ankle and knee support without fear of falling backward and responding by flexing forward. In this case the splint might be introduced gradually as an aid to improving standing balance, rather than as an ambulatory device.

Management of Problems Associated with Crouch Deformity

Hamstrings extensibility and knee control—Waters et al. (1985) urge the correction of knee flexion contractures of 30 degrees before definitive orthotic fitting is undertaken in order to permit normal limb alignment. (They do not indicate their method of measurement.) Chapter 6 contains more information regarding progressive casting to reduce hamstrings contracture.

If genu recurvatum is a postoperative sequela of hamstrings lengthening, a knee hyperextension splint is the first choice of intervention, combined with a splint of appropriate design to support the foot structures and allow optimum sagittal-plane ankle motion. These devices are used as training aids until the quadriceps strength improves and recurvatum resolves. Strengthening of the plantarflexors continues, preferably with the pronated foot supported by a splint of appropriate design.

If the knee hyperextension splint, combined with a distal splint, falls short of reducing genu recurvatum, a copolymer knee-ankle-foot orthosis with an adjustable knee flexion strap stop can be implemented. The knee joint is prohibited from extending past 3-5 degrees of flexion by adjusting the tension in a posterior strap that connects the plastic thigh cuff with the shaft piece of the AFO section. The ankle joint is allowed to plantarflex if possible. The clinician should use this device temporarily as a training aid, releasing the knee joint in small increments as the child gains control. Fabricating this device with splinting material is difficult, if not impossible. This device should be closely monitored and discontinued as soon as severe genu recurvatum has resolved. Prolonged intervention with this control system can result in crouch deformity. Triceps surae strengthening is a major feature of implementation of the KAFO for recurvatum, because the triceps surae group is also needed to control knee joint alignment on the sagittal plane in gait. (See below.)

Triceps surae strengthening—The triceps surae group is difficult to strengthen in a child with neuromotor impairment, particularly in a functional activity. The biomechanical ankle platform system (BAPS) is an elliptical board that is mounted on a half-ball of variable diameter. It is designed to accept weights that, by their location on the platform, offer resistance to ankle and foot motions while the patient either sits or stands. This unit offers a combination of strengthening and functional integration. It can be used as a supplemental strengthening activity for managing crouch posture and muscle weakness following tendo-Achilles lengthening. (See Appendix 4 for sources.)

A similar strengthening device can be fabricated for children by using one or two thicknesses of Tri-Wall® corrugated board or plywood. (See Appendix 4 for sources.) The half-sphere on the undersurface can be made of a rubber ball, sliced in half and glued to the underside of the board. For more control of foot motions, a groove can be carved in the undersurface. In this groove, dowels of varying diameter can be placed. These dowels allow graduated increments of motion of the board within a single plane. Weights placed on the posterior section of the board offer resistance to plantarflexion. The child can begin to use the strengthening board in standing position by holding onto stall bars or poles or an adult's hands. Two small boards, one for each foot, might be desirable for disassociated functional training and strengthening.

Foot support for such strengthening activities can be provided either by the HCAFS, a modified SFS, an HAFS that allows full plantarflexion, or a contoured plaster footboard. Strengthening in pronation would defeat the purpose of achieving optimum activation of the triceps surae group across its appropriate axis.

By reducing the influence of hyperdorsiflexion at the ankle, the HCAFS can also be used as an evaluative tool. The HCAFS aids in making surgical decisions regarding the influence on gait of the hamstrings and hip flexors vs. the distal musculature.

The solid-ankle floor reaction orthosis (AFRO) has been used successfully in patients with myelomeningocele, muscle disease, and polio. This indicates that the problem of weakness in the distal musculature, rather than a specific diagnosis, is the primary consideration, along with the prerequisite criteria listed above (Harrington et al. 1983-84; Yang et al. 1986). The crouch-control splints can be used in similar applications.

Summary

An element of common sense unifies all of this talk of closed-chain biomechanics, optimum alignment of foot structures, and the functional influences of hinged, solid, ankle-foot, and foot support devices. Clinicians should keep the foot structures aligned in their optimal weight-bearing arrangement, whatever the deformity, without unnecessarily blocking motion. When the bones are arranged appropriately, the muscles can operate at their optimum advantage. If a deformity is caused by weakness (as is often the case with crouch posture), strengthening of the weakened muscles is an essential feature of intervention. In this case a splint or orthosis should participate in, rather than oppose, that effort. If the child is young enough to have modeling potential within the foot structures, the clinician should try not to interfere with that process.

These principles and interventions are an important aspect of the habilitation of children with neuromotor disabilities. But they are only that—an aspect of management; they cannot be expected to change the future for children who struggle for control of their bodies. This realm of management—like neurodevelopmental treatment, joint mobilization, manual therapy, movement training, adaptive equipment, and sensory integration—is a boost up another rung of the developmental ladder. Casting and splinting offer a mechanical advantage to proceed to develop antigravity strength and control within the limits of each child's motor system's capacity to do so.

Sound understanding of biomechanical principles provides a fund from which to draw for continued creative thinking and development. Methods will inevitably change with advances in technology and improved materials, but all clinicians who wish to can participate in the developmental process.

References

Agnew, P., DPM. December 8, 1988. Personal communication.

Baker, L. D., and L. M. Hill. 1964. Foot alignment in the cerebral palsy patient. *Journal of Bone and Joint Surgery* 46-A(1):1-15.

Baumann, J. U., and M. Zumstein. 1985. Experience with a plastic ankle-foot orthosis for prevention of muscle contracture. *Developmental Medicine and Child Neurology* 27:83. (Abstract)

Bleck, E. E. 1982. Developmental orthopedics III: Toddlers. *Developmental Medicine and Child Neurology* 24(4):533-555.

Bleck, E. E. 1987. Orthopaedic management in cerebral palsy. *Clinics in Developmental Medicine No. 99/100.* Philadelphia, PA: J. B. Lippincott.

Bleck, E. E., and U. J. Berzins. 1977. Conservative management of pes valgus with plantar flexed talus, flexible. *Clinical Orthopaedics and Related Research* 122:85-92.

Browning, Timothy, Certified Orthotist. June 23, 1985. Personal communication, Daytona, Florida.

Bunch, W. H., and V. M. Dvonch. 1985. Cerebral palsy. In *Atlas of orthotics,* 2d ed., edited by W. H. Bunch and members of the American Academy of Orthopedic Surgeons, 259-269. St. Louis, MO: C. V. Mosby.

Cailliet, R. 1983. *Foot and ankle pain, 2d ed.* Philadelphia, PA: F. A. Davis.

Carlson, J. M. 1985-86. Double flexure designs for orthotic ankle joints. *Scientific abstracts section—Orthotics and Prosthetics* 39(4):60.

Carlson, J. M. November 25, 1987. Personal communication.

Carlson (incorrectly cited in the article as Colson), J. M., and G. Berglund. 1979. An effective orthotic design for controlling the unstable subtalar joint. *Orthotics and Prosthetics* 33(1):39-49.

Cary, J. M., R. Lusskin, and R. G. Thompson. 1975. Prescription principles. In *Atlas of orthotics, 2d ed.,* edited by W. H. Bunch and others of the American Academy of Orthopedic Surgeons, 235-244. St. Louis, MO: C. V. Mosby.

Child Prosthetic and Orthotic Studies. 1981. Ankle-foot orthosis with flange: Fabrication and fitting instructions. *Inter-clinic Information Bulletin, Prosthetics and Orthotics,* 17(12):5-12. NYU Postgraduate Medical School, 317 East 34th Street, New York, NY 10016.

Coram, S. January 15, 1989. Personal communication. Springfield, OH.

D'Amico, J. C. 1984. Developmental flatfoot. In *Symposium on podopediatrics—Clinics in podiatry,* edited by J. V. Ganley, 535-546. Philadelphia, PA: W. B. Saunders Co.

Deusinger, R. H. 1984. Biomechanics in clinical practice. *Physical Therapy* 64(12):1860-1868.

Dolan, C. M. E., C. Mereday, and G. Hartman. 1969. *Evaluation of NYU insert brace.* New York: New York University Postgraduate Medical School, Department of Prosthetics and Orthotics.

Fasano, V. A., G. Broggi, G. Barolat-Romana, and A. Scuazzi. 1978. Surgical treatment of spasticity in cerebral palsy. *Child's Brain* 4:289-305.

Fishman, S., N. Berger, J. E. Edelstein, and W. P. Springer. 1985. Lower limb orthoses. In *Atlas of orthotics, 2d ed.,* edited by W. H. Bunch and members of the American Academy of Orthopedic Surgeons, 201-212. St. Louis, MO: C. V. Mosby.

Fixsen, J. A. 1982. The foot in childhood. In *The foot and its disorders, 2d ed.,* edited by L. Klenerman, 55-81. Boston, MA: Blackwell Scientific Publications.

Ford, C., R. C. Grotz, and J. K. Shamp. 1986. The neurophysiological ankle-foot orthosis. *Clinical Prosthetics and Orthotics* 10(1):15-23.

Franco, A. H. 1987. Pes cavus and pes planus: Analysis and treatment. *Physical Therapy* 67(5):688-694.

Frost, H. M. 1971. Cerebral palsy: The spastic crouch. *Clinical Orthopaedics and Related Research* 80:2-8.

Goldner, J. L. 1982. Foot and ankle deformities in cerebral palsy (static encephalopathy). In *Disorders of the foot, vol. 1,* edited by M. H. Jahss, 282-334. Philadelphia, PA: W. B. Saunders.

Gray, G. W. 1986. *Enhancing our clinical abilities through biomechanics.* Presentation—SCAPTA, Charleston, WV. May 17.

Gritzka, T. L., and C. Gerlach. 1986. Serial short-leg casts for the treatment of equinus deformity in cerebral palsy. *Developmental Medicine and Child Neurology* (Abstract) 27:83.

Harrington, E. D., R. S. Lin, and J. R. Gage. 1983-84. Use of the anterior floor reaction orthosis in patients with cerebral palsy. *Orthotics and Prosthetics* (Spring):34-42.

Harris, S. R., and K. Riffle, 1986. Effects of inhibitive ankle-foot orthoses on standing balance in a child with cerebral palsy: A single-subject design. *Physical Therapy* 66(5):663-666.

Helfet, A. J. 1956. A new way of treating flat feet in children. *Lancet* 1:262.

Henderson, W. H., and J. W. Campbell. 1967. UCBL shoe insert: Casting and fabrication. *Technical report 53.* Berkeley and San Francisco: University of California Biomechanics Laboratory.

Hoffer, M. M., R. T. Knoebel, and R. Roberts. 1987. Contractures in cerebral palsy. *Clinical Orthopaedics and Related Research* 219:70-77.

Huber, S. R. 1985. Therapeutic application of orthotics. In *Neurologic rehabilitation, vol. 3,* edited by D. Umphred, 616-631. St. Louis, MO: C. V. Mosby.

Hylton, N., B. Cusick, and R. P. Jordan. 1988. *Dynamic casting and orthotics.* Presentation—unpublished lecture notes and instructional materials. Neurodevelopmental Treatment Association annual meeting. Kansas City, MO, May 23.

Irwin-Carruthers, S. H., L. M. Davids, C. K. van Rensburg, and D. S. Magasiner. 1985. Early physiotherapy in selective posterior rhizotomy. *Fisioterapie* 41(2):45-49.

Jordan, R. P. 1984. Therapeutic considerations of the feet and lower extremities in the cerebral palsied child. In *Symposium on podopediatrics—Clinics in podiatry,* edited by J. V. Ganley, 547-561. Philadelphia, PA: W. B. Saunders Co.

Jordan, R. P. November, 12, 1987. Personal communication.

Jordan, R. P., J. Cusack, and B. Resseque. 1983. *Foot function and its relationship to posture in the pediatric patient with cerebral palsy and other neuromuscular disorders.* Symposium, sponsored by the Neurodevelopmental Treatment Association, New York: May 20-22.

King, H. A., and L. T. Staheli. 1984. Torsional problems in cerebral palsy. *Foot & Ankle* 4(4):180-184.

Lehmann, J. F. 1986. Lower limb orthotics. In *Orthotics, etcetera, 3d ed.,* edited by J. B. Redford, 278-351. Baltimore, MD: Williams and Wilkins.

Lehneis, H. R. 1976. The use of modern materials in new design concepts in lower extremity orthotics. In *The advance in orthotics,* edited by G. Murdoch, 157-165. Baltimore, MD: Williams and Wilkins.

LeLievre, J. 1970. Current concepts and correction in the valgus foot. *Clinical Orthopaedics and Related Research* 70:44-55.

LeVeau, B. F., and D. B. Bernhardt. 1984. Developmental biomechanics: Effect of forces on the growth, development, and maintenance of the human body. *Physical Therapy* 64(12):1874-1881.

Levitt, S. 1982. *Treatment of cerebral palsy and motor delay, 2d ed.* Boston, MA: Blackwell Scientific Publications.

Lockard, M. A., 1988. Foot orthoses. *Physical Therapy* 68(12):1866-1873.

Lundy, M. 1989. Personal communication. April 25.

McCollough, N. C. 1974. Rationale for orthotic prescription in the lower extremity. *Clinical Orthopaedics and Related Research* 102:32-45.

McCollough, N. C. 1985. Biomechanical analysis systems for orthotic prescription. In *Atlas of orthotics, 2d ed.,* edited by W. H. Bunch and others of the American Academy of Orthopedic Surgeons, 34-75. St. Louis, MO: C. V. Mosby.

McCrea, J. D. 1985. *Pediatric orthopedics of the lower extremity: An instructional handbook.* Mount Kisco, NY: Futura.

Meyer, P. R. 1974. Lower limb orthotics. *Clinical Orthopaedics and Related Research* 102:58-71.

Molnar, G. E. 1985. Cerebral palsy. In *Pediatric rehabilitation,* edited by G. E. Molnar, 420-468. Baltimore, MD: Williams and Wilkins.

Molnar, G. E. 1986. Orthotic management of children. In *Orthotics, etcetera, 3d ed.,* edited by J. B. Redford, 352-387. Baltimore, MD: Williams and Wilkins.

Peacock, W. J., and L. J. Arens. 1982. Selective posterior rhizotomy for the relief of spasticity in cerebral palsy. *South Africa Mediese Tydskrif* 62:119-124.

Peacock, W. J., and R. W. Eastman. 1981. The neurosurgical management of spasticity. *South African Medical Journal* 28:849-850.

Perry, J. 1974. Kinesiology of lower extremity bracing. *Clinical Orthopaedics and Related Research* 102:18-31.

Perry, J. 1975. Cerebral palsy gait. In *Orthopaedic aspects of cerebral palsy: Clinics in developmental medicine. Nos. 52/53,* edited by R. L. Samilson, 71-89. Philadelphia, PA: J. B. Lippincott.

Ploeger, D. N., and R. C. Rockman. 1987. Improving function in the spastic child. *Physical Therapy Forum* VI(7):1 and 3.

Rang, M., R. Silver, and J. de la Garza. 1986. Cerebral palsy. In *Pediatric orthopaedics,* 2d ed., edited by W. W. Lowell and R. B. Winter, 345-396. Philadelphia, PA: J. B. Lippincott.

Redford, J. B. 1986. Principles of orthotic devices. In *Orthotics, etcetera, 3d ed.,* edited by J. B. Redford, 1-20. Baltimore, MD: Williams and Wilkins.

Regnauld, B. 1986. *The foot: Pathology, aetiology, semiology, clinical investigation and therapy.* New York, NY: Springer-Verlag.

Riley, P. O., W. A. Hodge, and R. W. Mann. 1987. Posture and balance with cerebral-palsied children. *Developmental Medicine and Child Neurology* (Abstract) 29(5):3.

Rodgers, M. M. 1988. Dynamic biomechanics of the normal foot and ankle during walking and running. *Physical Therapy* 68(12): 1822-1830

Root, M. L., W. P. Orien, and J. H. Weed. 1977. *Normal and abnormal function of the foot.* Los Angeles, CA: Clinical Biomechanics Corp.

Root, M. L., W. P. Orien, J. H. Weed, and R. J. Hughes. 1971. *Biomechanical examination of the foot, vol. 1.* Los Angeles, CA: Clinical Biomechanics Corp.

Rose, G. K. 1962. Correction of the pronated foot. *Journal of Bone and Joint Surgery* 44-B(3):642-648.

Rose, G. K., E. A. Welton, and T. Marshall. 1985. The diagnosis of flat foot in the child. *Journal of Bone and Joint Surgery* 67-B(1):71-78.

Rosenthal, R. K. 1984. The use of orthotics in foot and ankle problems in cerebral palsy. *Foot & Ankle* 4(4):195-200.

Rosenthal, R. K., S. D. Deutch, W. Miller, W. Schumann, and J. E. Hall. 1975. A fixed-ankle, below-knee orthosis for the management of genu recurvatum in spastic cerebral palsy. *Journal of Bone and Joint Surgery* 57-A(4):545-547.

Salek, B. 1981. *Corrective footwear in young children with neuromuscular disorders.* Presentation for the Fall meeting of the Neurodevelopmental Treatment Association, Philadelphia. November 8.

Saltiel, J. 1969. A one-piece laminated knee-locking short leg brace. *Orthotics and Prosthetics* 23:68-75.

Schafer, R. C. 1987. *Clinical biomechanics: Musculoskeletal actions and reactions, 2d ed.* Baltimore, MD: Williams and Wilkins.

Selby, L. 1988. Remediation of toe-walking behavior with neutral-position, serial-inhibitory casts: A case report. *Physical Therapy* 68(12):1921-1923.

Sellers, J. S. 1988. Relationship between antigravity control and postural control in young children. *Physical Therapy* 68(4):486-490.

Smith, E. M., and R. C. Juvinall. 1986. Mechanics of orthotics. In *Orthotics, etcetera, 3d ed.*, edited by J. B. Redford, 21-50. Baltimore, MD: Williams and Wilkins.

Spencer, A. M., and V. A. Person. 1984. Casting and orthotics for children. In *Symposium on podopediatrics—Clinics in podiatry,* edited by J. V. Ganley, 621-629. Philadelphia, PA: W. B. Saunders Co.

Staheli, L. T., W. R. Duncan, and E. Schaefer. 1968. Growth alterations in the hemiplegic child. *Clinical Orthopaedics and Related Research* 40:205-212.

Staheli, L. T., and L. Giffin. 1980. Corrective shoes for children: A survey of current practice. *Pediatrics* 65(1):13-17.

Staros, A., and M. LeBlanc. 1975. Orthotic components and systems. In *Atlas of orthotics,* edited by members of the American Academy of Orthopedic Surgeons, 184-215. St. Louis, MO: C. V. Mosby.

Sutherland, D. H., and L. Cooper. 1978. The pathomechanics of progressive crouch gait in spastic diplegia. *Orthopedic Clinics of North America* 9(1):143-154.

Sutherland, D. H., L. Cooper, and D. Daniel. 1980. The role of the ankle plantar flexors in normal walking. *Journal of Bone and Joint Surgery* 62-A(3):354-363.

Tachdjian, M. 1985. *The child's foot.* Philadelphia, PA: W. B. Saunders.

Tardieu, C., A. Lespargot, C. Tabary, and M. D. Bret. 1988. For how long must the soleus muscle be stretched each day to prevent contracture? *Developmental Medicine and Child Neurology* 30:3-10.

Tardieu, G., and C. Tardieu. 1987. Cerebral palsy: Mechanical evaluation and conservative correction of limb joint contractures. *Clinical Orthopaedics and Related Research* 219:63-70.

Tardieu, G., C. Tardieu, P. Cobeau-Justin, and A. Lespargot. 1982. Muscle hypoextensibility in children with cerebral palsy: II. Therapeutic implications. *Archives of Physical Medicine and Rehabilitation* 63:103-107.

Tiberio, D. 1988. Pathomechanics of structural foot deformities. *Physical Therapy* 68(12):1840-1849.

Valmassy, R. L. 1984. Biomechanical evaluation of the child. *Symposium on podopediatrics—Clinics in podiatry,* edited by J. V. Ganley, 563-579. Philadelphia, PA: W. B. Saunders.

Waters, R. L., and B. R. Lunsford. 1985. Energy expenditure of normal and pathologic gait. In *Atlas of orthotics,* 2d ed., edited by W. H. Bunch and members of the American Academy of Orthopedic Surgeons, 151-159. St. Louis, MO: C. V. Mosby.

Westin, G. W., and S. Dye. 1983. Conservative management of cerebral palsy in the growing child. *Foot & Ankle* 4(3):160-163.

Wilson, J. M. 1987. Developing ambulation skills. In *Therapeutic exercise in developmental disabilities,* edited by B. H. Connolly and P. C. Montgomery, 83-94. Chattanooga, TN: Chattanooga Corporation—Education Division.

Wilson, J., T. S. Park, and M. B. Wiley. 1988. *Selective posterior rhizotomies for cerebral palsy patients.* Seminar, sponsored by KAPTA. Unpublished lecture notes and instructional materials. September 10-11.

Yang, G. W., D. S. Chu, J. H. Ahn, H. R. Lehneis, and R. M. Conceicao. 1986. Floor reaction orthosis: Clinical experience. *Orthotics and Prosthetics* 40(1):33-37.

Yates, H. L., and D. H. Mott. 1977. Inhibitive casting. In *Proceedings: First William C. Duncan Seminar on Cerebral Palsy.* Seattle, WA: University of Washington.

Zachazewski, J. E., E. D. Eberle, and M. Jefferies. 1982. Effect of tone-inhibiting casts and orthoses on gait. *Physical Therapy* 62(4):453-455.

CHAPTER **6**

Serial Casts—an Approach to Management of Static Soft Tissue Contracture

Objectives for the Reader

- To be able to discuss the development of the use of plaster casts in management of children with cerebral palsy.

- To differentiate between "inhibitive" and corrective serial cast procedures.

- To recall the indications for casting rather than splinting the foot and ankle.

- To recall the contraindications for undertaking a serial cast procedure.

- To recall the principles of molding the cast for optimum alignment of foot structures and elongation of contracted muscle and connective tissue.

- To describe various posting modifications designed to influence the angle of gait in the below-knee cast.

- To describe the precautions needed for positioning and treatment in below-knee casts, relative to the fixed ankle and stresses on the knee joint ligaments.

- To discuss indications and precautions pertaining to long-leg serial casting to gain knee extension mobility.

- To be able to discuss alternative nonsurgical measures for increasing muscle and tendon extensibility.

History and Rationale

For more than 30 years, plaster casts (also known as weight-bearing plasters, standing position plasters, plaster splints, and inhibitory casts) have been used successfully as a conservative intervention for children with cerebral palsy (Figures 6.1 and 6.2). Reports of their use have come from England, South Africa, Australia, Germany, France, and the United States (Wilson et al. 1962; Domisse 1963; Groen et al. 1964; Bobath et al. 1966; Hayes et al. 1970; Hausermann 1972; Kahn et al. 1973; Yates et al. 1977; Cusick 1980; Westin 1980; Sussman 1980; Sussman et al. 1981; Tardieu et al., 1982; Cusick et al. 1982; Levitt 1982; Goldner 1982; Westin et al. 1983; Sussman 1983; Duncan et al. 1983; Wilson 1984; Otis et al. 1985; Molnar 1985; McCrea 1985; Baumann et al. 1985; Bertoti 1986; Gritzka et al. 1986; Hoffer et al. 1987; Hinderer et al. 1988; Tardieu et al. 1987; Tardieu et al. 1988). Probably many other authors and countries belong on this list. These authors propose the following aims of casting the lower extremities in children with hypertonic neuromotor impairment:

- To provide a more normal proprioceptive awareness of stance posture and weight distribution.
- To prohibit the expression of abnormal postural and tonic foot reflex patterns.
- To gain distal positional stability to facilitate gains in proximal antigravity postural control and strength.
- To regain extensibility in the soft tissues under stretch—if not in the first application, then by repeating the procedure in a progressive series.

Westin et al. (1983) began using plasters in the 1950s as a first line of intervention to reduce muscle contracture related to hypertonus. They advocate using long-leg casts. This is because the common occurrence of hamstrings contracture in children with cerebral palsy is an important functional deterrent. In a 27-year follow-up study, they report that of 194 subjects with cerebral palsy, casts were used in the management of 84 percent. Of the total study group, 61 percent

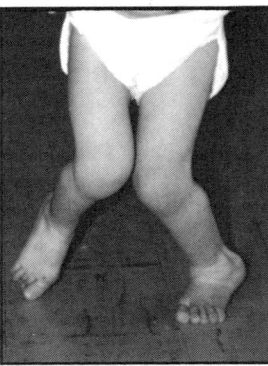

Figure 6.1
Pre-cast stance posture in a 4-year-old child with spastic diplegia.

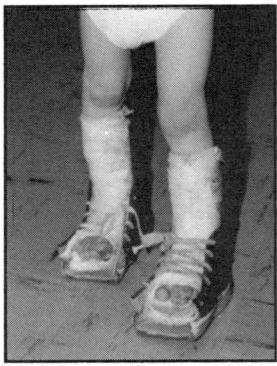

Figure 6.2
Casts are applied and used as a therapeutic modality for movement training.

never needed surgical lengthening, 23 percent underwent surgery in addition to casting, and 16 percent had neither procedure.

Hayes et al. (1970) present a comprehensive review of four years of clinical experience using long-leg weight-bearing plasters in the management of 57 children, 23 with hemiplegia and 34 with bilateral involvement. Most of the children were between 5 and 9½ years of age at the time of casting. The authors suggest that it is within this age range that rapid growth occurs, weight is gained, emotional tension increases (apparently related to peer interaction and schooling), and a change occurs in environmental circumstances (particularly the classroom situation).

Following the cast-use episode, Hayes et al. (1970) note improvements in gait pattern, joint mobility, postural alignment, and (in some cases) hand and speech function and emotional state. They report that even though some children sustained significant improvement in gait pattern for only three to six months, many of them retained minor gains that were then increased by replastering 12 to 18 months later. Among those who held their gains for one year, some continued to maintain for four years, while others needed "resplinting." They propose that at minimum, casts can help halt regression in mobility or function during a stressful growth period in the child's life, without adding the pain and fear of surgery.

Ten years before Hayes and Burns published their findings and recommendations, Duncan (1960) reported on the identification of the newborn's tonic foot reflexes—sustained responses to localized proprioceptive stimuli. For example, the tonic toe grasp reflex is elicited with the application of pressure and/or vibration to the center three metatarsal heads on the plantar surface of the foot. The eversion/abduction reflex is a response to stimulus applied to the lateral surface of the fifth metatarsal head. The inversion/adduction reflex is a response to stimulus applied to the medial aspect of the first metatarsal head. The dorsiflexion response occurs after stimulus is applied to the plantar aspect of the calcaneus.

Duncan then discovered that in many children with spasticity, these reflexes persist and strengthen and their "reflexogenous" or sensitive areas expand (Duncan 1960). Yates et al. (1977) then applied this knowledge to the design of a "footboard." (Figure 6.3 depicts a modified version.) The contoured footboard, which Yates makes with plywood and plaster, has since been used as an adaptation of the solid and bivalved below-knee, standing position cast for children with functional contracture of the ankle plantarflexors. The footboard is routed out on the uppermost surface to reduce sensory input to the reflexogenous areas of the foot. In that way it reduces the tonic foot reflex responses. In addition, a depression is routed into the contact area for the calcaneus. The depression allows the calcaneus to remain in the center or to tip medially or laterally as needed; it is a mechanical aid to help in aligning the hindfoot. Plaster is added to the uppermost surface to provide support for the toes in extension, the cuboid notch, the medial longitudinal arch, and around the calcaneus. Additional plaster added under the first metatarsal head is intended to inhibit the eversion reflex. Or, plaster is added under the

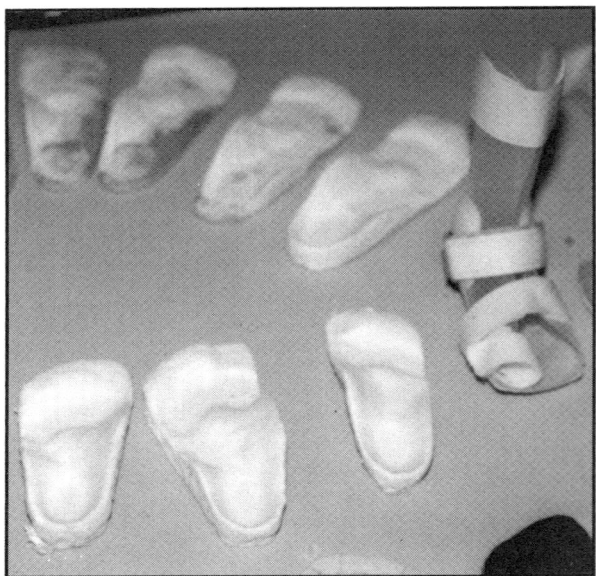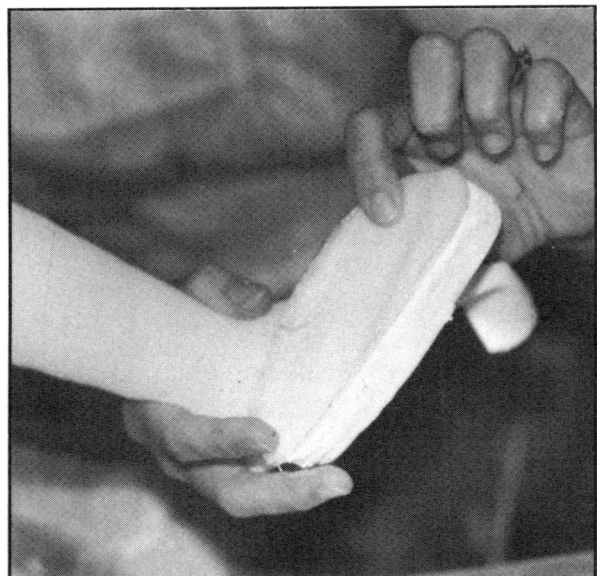

Figure 6.3 Contoured plaster footboard can be applied to the plantar surface of the foot during cast application. When used for casting equinovalgus deformity, the footboard is molded to maintain the hindfoot structures in true neutral alignment. The clinician can apply the below-knee cast with the child supported in sitting position when using the footboard.

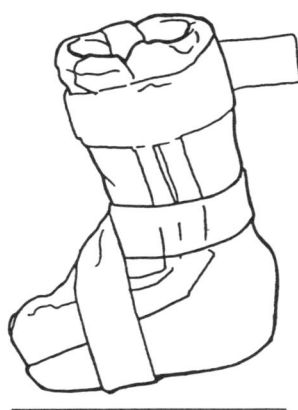

Figure 6.4
Bivalved plaster and fiber glass cast boot.

fifth metatarsal head and fifth toe, presumably to inhibit the inversion reflex. The contact surface of the footboard is padded with thin bubble wrap—or a reasonable substitute—and built into the cast as a contoured support for the foot (Yates 1979). The combined footboard and plaster cast were described by Mott and Yates as the "inhibitive cast," known also as "the Seattle cast" (Yates et al. 1977; Duncan et al. 1983; Molnar 1985). The footboard is made the same way and incorporated into casts made by Hylton (1988) and Hinderer et al. (1988).

In 1977, the staff at Children's Rehabilitation Center in Charlottesville, Virginia, learned that solid plaster, below-knee "inhibitory casts" were used as distal support for the plantigrade foot and ankle. These casts were a way to introduce the child to appropriate sensations of weight distribution under the foot. They also helped facilitate the achievement of postural control. They were not used in the presence of fixed contracture of the ankle plantar flexors. Rather, full range of passive dorsiflexion was defined as an indication for cast use (Mohr 1977). CRC used these casts quite routinely in nonoperative management and following soft-tissue surgery at the hips and knees. They served as a stabilization influence on the foot and ankle during rehabilitation (Sussman et al. 1981; Sirna et al. 1986).

Two years later, with the help of Linda Yates, the staff introduced bivalved casts with footboards (described in detail above) to CRC (Yates 1979). For reasons related to available manpower and time, Polyflex® splint material replaced plywood bases and plaster for footboard construction. Between 1977 and 1981, CRC made 224 sets of casts for 145 children with cerebral palsy (Cusick et al. 1982) (Figure 6.4). The clinicians at CRC continued to observe that upright stability skills improved significantly in the casts, although any attempts to quantify these observations fell short of achieving an objective measure of performance related specifically to cast use.

In 1981, CRC began to make foot splints with Aquaplast-T® for use following cast removal and as an interim measure between using bivalved casts and the delivery of prescribed orthoses. The staff soon realized that the splints, which had been molded specifically to align properly the structures of the foot and ankle, generally sufficed instead of the bivalved casts as a distal support system, particularly for young children. Before long, they replaced casts with splints when a distal support system was needed in general management, following soft tissue surgery, in the management of head trauma, and as an evaluative tool. The staff rapidly revised their indications for using casts in management, drawing them in as a secondary intervention when plastic support systems proved inadequate to withstand the stress of strong hypertonus. They also used them when the weight of the cast was considered an advantage in providing stability and proprioceptive information.

Watt et al. (1986) studied the short- and long-term effects of a three-week period of "inhibitory cast" wear. Their study involved 28 children with cerebral palsy, ages 18-60 months (average age 31 months), all of whom demonstrated functional hypertonus of typical bilateral and unilateral distribution, with at least 5 degrees of passive ankle dorsiflexion available with the knee extended. During the three weeks of cast wear, a program of therapeutic exercises was carried out at least twice weekly. At the same time, the child's parents were instructed in a program to be carried out on a daily basis at home. Following cast removal, therapeutic exercise was continued for six months, either on a regular treatment schedule or through a home program.

The clinicians assessed five features of function and physical status prior to cast application, and also at two weeks and five months after cast removal:

- Muscle tone, using conventional (that is, unquantifiable) neurological assessment techniques.
- Motor skills and equilibrium reactions.
- Passive range of ankle dorsiflexion.
- Gait pattern.
- Standing posture.

The only feature in which the researchers noted a statistically significant difference was passive joint mobility into ankle dorsiflexion. This gain in extensibility was retained in full for the two-week post-cast period but was generally lost at five months. The average gain in range of motion retained at the five-month evaluation was three degrees.

In regard to gait pattern, 30-40 percent of the children showed improvement of foot contact on the floor at the five-month follow-up, with fewer showing improvement on the left foot than the right.

Following cast removal, solid ankle-foot orthoses were used as a follow-up and maintenance measure. Night splinting was not discussed, and hinged ankle-foot devices were evidently not available to the study population, as they were not mentioned in the report.

The study by Watt et al. ascertains that a single three-week episode of cast wear for preschoolers with hypertonus and no static contracture probably has limited effect on long-term mobility gain at the ankle. It has a positive impact on gait pattern for some.

The researchers do not discuss the influence of age on bone growth rate as a factor in the recurrence of functional contracture. Rang et al. (1986) and Tardieu et al. (1982) address this issue with regard to the physiologic capacity within the spastic muscle to adapt adequately to bone growth. In younger children, the rate of bone growth is at its highest. Therefore, the potential for recurrence of contracture is also greatest. For this reason, Rang et al. (1986) advise refraining from undertaking tendo-Achilles lengthenings on children under the age of 4 years.

Watt et al. (1986) have also provided clinicians with suggestions for methods of obtaining quantifiable data about such interventions. These suggestions are a valuable contribution to the field.

The indications for casting—particularly the requirement that passive dorsiflexion mobility to five degrees be available—have changed, as has the cast application technique used in Watt's study. These changes reflect several factors: the relative novelty of this form of intervention, at least in this country; the knowledge that has accumulated in the field over time; the development of alternative methods of management; and the inevitable adjustments in thinking about criteria that ride on the heels of new information. Because the literature was sparse on this modality in the late 1970s, those in the field who were open to exploring new procedures did, in fact, "reinvent the wheel" before moving forward. Times have indeed changed.

Is Casting "Inhibitive" or "Facilitative"?

On the subject of inhibition, several authors have recently described their experiences using below-knee "inhibitive" and "tone-reducing" casts and splints (Jordan et al. 1983; Harris et al. 1986; Jordan 1984; Yates et al. 1977; Duncan et al. 1983; Otis et al. 1985; Bertoti 1986; Zachazewski et al. 1982; Hinderer et al. 1988) and "neurophysiological" and "tone-reducing" ankle-foot orthoses (Ford et al. 1986; Zachazewski et al. 1982). These devices incorporate design features that are intended to inhibit hypertonus that has resulted from any or all of four problems:

- Persistent tonic reflexes in the foot.
- The positive support reflex.
- Abnormal toe grasp.
- Abnormal alignment of foot structures.

The TRAFO®, which was developed by Paul Jordan and sold by the Langer Biomedical Group, Inc., is a bivalved rendition of the plaster bivalved cast. It is made with a combination of resin-based and fiber glass casting materials. It is often made with a severe bevel under the toe portion of the sole. The TRAFO® is designed to maintain neutral subtalar joint alignment of the foot and ankle structures as a means of facilitating improved function (Jordan 1984).

Research findings have yet to quantify or substantiate tone- reducing effects of any of these devices (Watt et al. 1986; Carlson 1984; Mills 1984). This is despite an abundance of clinical evidence of improved function—and, in the use of solid casts, empirical evidence of increased mobility in the casted joints—provided by numerous clinicians since 1962.

Hinderer et al. (1988) undertook a study to compare the influence on gait of bivalved casts made *with* the inhibitory footboard described above, and of a cast made *without* the footboard by a "trained" orthopedic technician. Both casts were finished so as to mask any evidence of their fabrication technique. No mention was made of the technician's training in the anatomy, kinesiology, or biomechanics of the foot, or of the technician's attention to alignment of the subtalar and midtarsal joints during molding. Only the tone-reducing cast fabrication technique was described in enough detail that it could be replicated. The ankle joint in both casts was set at 90 degrees. Both casts were trimmed to mid-calf height. Each child underwent a baseline period of no cast use, followed by use of one type of cast. This was followed by a return to no cast use, followed by use of the other type of cast. The schedule of wearing the cast was different for each child. One of the children wore casts approximately nine hours per day. The other child averaged between six and seven hours of wear per day. Both children continued with their NDT-based physical therapy programs throughout the study.

The full battery of data was collected successfully on only one child of the two who were evaluated. The patient was 5 years 9 months of age, with a diagnosis of mild asymmetric diplegia, truncal hypotonia, moderate ataxia, and normal intelligence. She was independent in ambulation for short community distances. The other child exhibited mild spastic diplegia and mild mental retardation. Evidently, problems with compliance interfered with obtaining standard performance on the latter child's videotaped activities, and that component of the data was discarded.

Analysis of gait included footprint data, which featured stride length, step symmetry, base of support, and angle of progression; videotape analysis of functional activities such as walking on variable surfaces, squat-to-stand, and standing balance; and reports of observations of attending therapists and parents.

The comparative results showed significant improvement in stride length in both children while they were using the "tone-reducing" casts rather than the standard casts or no casts at all. Improvements were also noted in the female patient in several functional activities in which performance seemed to have worsened in standard casts. The authors attribute the difference in performance to the features of the footboard, "which positions the toes and feet in neutral position by supporting the toes and the longitudinal, peroneal, and metatarsal arches" (p. 374).

These authors do not define "neutral position" in biomechanical terms relative to true congruity of foot structures. This author presumes that they mean that the calcaneus is aligned in vertical position and the forefoot is plantigrade within the cast, which is not the current biomechanical description of neutrality of foot position. The angle of 90 degrees at the ankle was described but not discussed as a potential feature of interference to forward progression past midstance in gait. The authors did not evaluate range of motion or "tone" before and after cast use. These casts—like the bivalved casts used for several years at CRC—were used in the context of a removable orthosis featuring immense positional stability.

The study by Hinderer et al. (1988) is a valuable addition to the physical therapy literature because it offers ideas that can be used by others in single-subject research of the effectiveness of orthotic, casting, and splinting interventions for the child with cerebral palsy.

Carlson (1984) undertook a similar single-subject study of a young child with diplegia who used bilateral bivalved below-knee "inhibitive" casts (not described) for approximately six hours per day. Features of gait were recorded during a baseline period of four weeks. This was followed by six weeks of using the casts followed by four weeks of not using the casts. The author recorded positive gait changes, including a decrease in maximum anterior pelvic tilt, a decrease in genu recurvatum in stance, and increased control of plantarflexion after heel strike. The author attributes these changes to improved execution of therapeutic activities and to adjustments in postural alignment while the casts were worn. The researchers did note a negative effect: a delay in heel-off in stance with the casts removed. Carlson suggests that perhaps this occurred secondary to a dysfunction of the plantar flexors that was unmasked by a decrease in positive support reaction. Or the negative effect may have been caused by the decreased capability of the same muscle group to generate torque force.

With the development of improved splinting materials and orthotic techniques, the previous role that casts played (as stabilizers of the foot and ankle to enhance proximal adjustments) has been usurped in many cases by well-built ankle-foot splints and orthoses.

The Changing Role of Casts

Serial, or progressive, corrective casting is a process by which casts are applied and removed in succession. The purpose of this process is to regain or increase extensibility in the soft tissues surrounding the casted joint. Casting is undertaken gradually enough to allow the cellular physiologic changes, which are a feature of growth, to occur. The role of casts has been redefined for use in cerebral palsy because of evidence that in solid, serial applications, casts are effective in managing soft tissue contracture related to persistent hypertonus of mild or moderate degree (Cary et al. 1975; Westin 1980; Goldner 1982; Tardieu et al. 1982; Westin et al. 1983; Booth et al. 1983; Griffith 1983; Harrington 1983-84; McCrea 1985; Baumann et al. 1985; Gritzka et al. 1986; Hoffer et al. 1987; Tardieu et al. 1988; Cusick 1988).

Tardieu et al. (1982) and Tardieu et al. (1987) state that there are two types of contracture in cerebral palsy. The more common is hypoextensibility related to imbalance of hyperactivity between the agonist and the antagonist muscles. In this type of hypoextensibility, growth regulation capability within the tissue is normal. The muscle can respond to a stretch stimulus applied in a relaxed state, which is required for muscle and connective tissue to grow in length (Rang et al. 1986; Tardieu et al. 1987). Such growth occurs by the addition of sarcomeres—which occurs more slowly than does concurrent lengthening of connective tissue—and responds favorably to gradual progressive casting (Tardieu et al. 1987). The results of surgical lengthening in this group are unpredictable (Truscelli et al. 1979; Tardieu et al. 1987). Tardieu et al. (1987) attribute failures in surgical correction for this group to inadequate postoperative provision for day and night braces opposing muscle imbalance. They do not define the criteria by which they determine a successful surgical outcome, however, except in terms of the imbalance—which might remain, reverse, or improve—and of recurrence, overcorrection, or success.

The other, less common, type of hypoextensibility is more passive in nature, revealing a dysfunction in trophic, or growth, regulation. Evidence of persistent contractions is lacking. Muscle growth does not keep pace with bone growth, so contracture worsens steadily with growth. Casting for this group has no lasting effect, and surgery is effective only until the bone grows again. There is no effect at all from bracing or physiotherapy. The long-term recurrence rate of equinus deformity is high (Truscelli et al. 1979).

In 1982, Tardieu et al. advised using an average of three casts in a three-week period to gain extensibility in the triceps surae group. They reported an average gain of 20 degrees in the maximum angle of dorsiflexion in 17 children with hypoextensibility in the triceps surae. This hypoextensibility was accompanied by sustained plantarflexion hyperactivity, including actual muscle shortening. These children underwent progressive casting. Their casts extended from the foot to either below or above the knee. The above-the-knee casts addressed involvement of the gastrocnemius muscle. An additional 17 children outside the study group showed an average gain of 15 degrees of dorsiflexion range with progressive casting.

Tardieu et al. claim a 90 percent success rate for their progressive casting technique. They use it as their "treatment of choice for children with unbalanced triceps surae activity" (p. 107). In 10 children who revealed triceps surae hypoextensibility (contracture) and no persistent hyperactivity in the muscle, casting was unsuccessful. Two of the same authors, Guy and Catherine Tardieu (1987), state the following: "When the soleus muscle is immobilized by plaster cast in a shortened position, the muscle fibers lose 40 percent of their sarcomeres. The immobilization of this muscle at its maximum length results in production of 19 percent more sarcomeres. These changes take place within four weeks. They result in a change of the shape of the active tension-extension curve, which depends only on sarcomere number. All these changes are quite reversible" (p. 65).

Baumann et al. (1985) report that during a period of 8 years, successful management of equinus deformity was observed through the use of "reflex inhibiting casts" and a double-shell, plastic sleeping orthosis. The orthosis is designed to sustain the influences of the casts. The authors provided 1200 such orthoses for children on their caseload, beginning at age 3 years. These children continued the night bracing throughout their skeletal growth. The authors state: "While the effects of so-called reflex inhibiting casts is limited to a few weeks or months, the results show that their combination with the subsequent use of these special plastic splints at night permits long-term prevention of calf muscle contractures. As a result, operations for equinus deformity have become a rare exception in this group of patients" (p. 83).

Rang et al. (1986) suggest that progressive casting is a feasible intervention for the milder degrees of equinus in younger children, provided that the clinician is strictly attentive to the prevention of heel sores.

These observations regarding the effectiveness of serial casts in reducing soft tissue contracture have been substantiated in clinical application by this author. In 1985, serial casting procedures were instituted at the Division of Developmental Disabilities, Medical University of South Carolina, with the support of local attending orthopedists in Charleston, South Carolina. An informal review of the caseload (from noncomputerized records) reveals that from January 1985 through December 1987, I made 176 casts for 35 children who ranged in age from 2 to 26 years. In 1987, I made 13 full-length casts (including the ankle and knee joints) for three children who were 4 and 6 years of age. (See the case study at the end of this chapter for a discussion of long-leg casting.) Two of the older patients had sustained head injury more than four years prior to casting and were poor surgical candidates, and one was a preschooler with clubfoot deformity and mild neuromotor dysfunction. For these three patients, 23 below-knee casts were made. (The child with clubfoot went on to a second surgery after two rapid recurrences of her deformity following cast removal.) The remaining 140 casts were applied to 32 children with hypertonic cerebral palsy, between 2 and 10 years of age. Among this group, one child with hemiplegia went on to have surgical lengthening of the Achilles tendon.

From May 1988 to March 1989, as a full-time graduate student and consultant to Cardinal Hill Hospital and Lexington Physical Therapy, Inc., in Lexington, Kentucky, I made 103 casts for 24 patients with congenital or traumatic neuromotor impairment whose ages were between 4 and 23 years. Ten of these patients carry the diagnosis of spastic cerebral palsy. Five were within seven months post head injury. Three have rare syndromes with neurologic impairment leading to knee flexion and/or equinus contracture.

Eight of these patients wore long-leg casts as a component of the cast series, thus generating a total of 34 long-leg casts. Two patients used cylinder long casts exclusively. Six used full-length casts, beginning with below-knee casts for the first one or two casts in the series. Sixty-nine casts were applied below the knee on 16 patients. Most cast-wear durations for inpatients between changes totalled three days; for outpatients, one week. One patient, who lived 90 miles away, wore each solid cast for nine days between changes.

In all cases, range of motion increased significantly (that is, at least 7 and as much as 50 degrees) in the casted joints, including contracted subtalar and midtarsal joints. One of these patients has been scheduled for tendo-Achilles lengthening, nine months post-casting. The overall duration of solid cast use averaged 19.95 days for this group of 24 patients. These results are similar to those reported by Tardieu et al. (1982), Westin et al. (1983), and Gritzka et al. (1986).

There are disadvantages as well as advantages to selecting this intervention measure, however, and the clinician must clearly communicate them to the child's caregivers. These considerations are outlined below:

Disadvantages of Serial Casting

- Muscle atrophy might occur with progressive casting, though this usually resolves within three months (Westin et al. 1983; Booth 1987). Atrophy has been observed in the gastrocnemius muscle following stretch casting of the triceps surae group, but the soleus muscle hypertrophied at the same time (Booth 1987).

- Plaster is inconvenient for caregivers. It must not get wet, and it is heavy.

Lighter-weight casts can be made with fiber glass cast tape, or with a combination of plaster and fiber glass materials (Snavely et al. 1986). I prefer the combination, incorporating a thin inner layer of plaster to achieve the desired contours and angles in the foot and ankle, and a thick outer layer of fiber glass cast tape for strength and durability (Cusick 1988). Gluing a crepe sole to the fiber-glass-covered bottom eliminates the need for adding extra plaster for durability under the sole. Extra plaster is undesirable because it adds more weight.

However, any hardened fiber glass cast must be removed with a cast saw. Plaster casts made with Gypsona® plaster can be soaked off in 20 to 30 minutes. Precautions must be taken to protect plumbing, however, when Gypsona® is removed.

- The family routine is disrupted because the traditional bath time or other activities are eliminated for the duration of the casting episode. (Some parents retain the daily bath by wrapping the casts in plastic and taping them tightly to prevent seepage of water, then using the kitchen sink with the child's lower legs resting on the counter.) The bath often becomes the child's longed-for ultimate reward for enduring the cast series.

- Making casts is time consuming if the clinician is meticulous about technique. I can usually remove and apply two below-knee casts within 90 minutes, including preparing the work space, pre-cutting and laying out materials, positioning the child and caregiver, and cleanup. Making plantar footboards adds 40 minutes to the initial procedure. The same footboards are modified as needed and reused with each cast change. The same procedures for two full-length casts usually require up to 2½ hours of time per cast change, without preparation and cleanup assistance.

- Cast removal, particularly if the cast is reinforced with fiber glass, requires the use of a noisy, scary cast saw. Most children (though not all) become upset by it, with good reason, regardless of whether or not they were maimed by a careless cast remover in the past.

The first step toward minimizing fear is to name the machine a "vibrator," a "tickler," a "buzzer," or something other than a "saw" or a "cutter." Another very effective way to reduce the patient's fear is to diminish the noise. Cotton ear plugs or dense foam earmuffs are distributed to everyone in the room before turning on the "buzzer." Beyond these measures, all the junk food, portable tape players, and photo albums in the world will not distract a frightened child from the clinician's mission. Precautions taken to protect the skin during the padding phase of cast application, expedience, a firm grip, and cognizance of the nature of the materials that must be cut are the best combination of qualities and skills.

The child's skin can be protected from the cast saw by incorporating strips of cast foam or a thin layer of adhesive-backed felt (3 cm wide) under the plaster along the anticipated cut line on both the medial and lateral sides of the leg. The padding strips eliminate the use of layers of protective cotton roll padding that can bottom out and create unwanted space inside the cast.

The combined materials of plaster and fiber glass offer an unusual amount of resistance to the oscillating saw blade. Friction develops, which generates heat. The person who is removing the cast *must stop at frequent intervals to check and cool the blade* before proceeding, to prevent the appearance of heat blisters on the skin under the cut line. The risk of raising heat blisters is greater when protective foam strips are omitted during cast application than when such protective strips are used.

If the person removing the cast is using a saw with a sharp blade, knows the proper procedures for cutting into—rather than along—a cutline, and takes precautions against burns induced by friction, then a surprise kick offers the only risk of cutting the child with the saw.

Casts made of Gypsona® plaster bandage soak off easily, offering the clinician and family an alternative to using the cast "vibrator" at all. (See Appendix 4 for sources.) Casts made with most other types of plaster begin to unravel only after more than two hours of soaking in water. When fiber glass is used as an outer layer, the vibrator is again necessary for removal.

- Pressure sores still happen, even with the most fastidious fabrication technique. The dorsum of the ankle and the malleoli can be protected fairly certainly with padding, but the posterolateral surface of the calcaneus remains at risk, apparently because of a combination of abrasion and the rigidity of the cast (Rang et al. 1986). The best defense against heel sores is prompt cast removal for the child who can communicate discomfort, and frequent cast changes (that is, every three days) for those who cannot.

The caregiver can participate in heel sore prevention by learning all the trouble signs, by closely monitoring the child's behavior for adverse changes, by promptly contacting the attending clinician with relevant concerns, and by proceeding to soak off the cast made with Gypsona® or a comparable plaster material at the smallest risk that a pressure sore is developing.

Casts made with other types of materials require a cast saw for removal. The attending clinician must therefore maintain 24-hour responsibility for the prevention of heel sores by prompt removal of the cast, after having clearly communicated the warning signs to all caregivers. Unless the clinician owns a saw and is practicing privately, access to the cast saw should be arranged during off hours, if necessary, for the duration of the casting series.

Protective padding is another preventative measure. Orthopedic felt has been used to prevent heel sores, but the results are inconsistent enough for the clinician to consider using other materials. Products that I have discovered to offer greater success than standard orthopedic felt include 1/2-inch T-Stick® and 3/8-inch Pudgee® foam padding, combined with a thin (1/8-inch) layer of cotton padding (Figure 6.5). The best results with either type of foam used alone seem to occur if the nonweight-bearing surface of the calcaneus is well padded with subcutaneous tissue, or when the foam is used for casting small children between 3 and 4 years of age. The plaster must be drawn snugly around the padded calcaneus during cast fabrication in order to prevent the heel from pistoning within the cast.

- Night spasms might occur. Tardieu et al. (1982) recommend applying the cast to stretch the soleus muscle only slightly, which avoids traumatizing the existing sarcomeres. Progressive casting

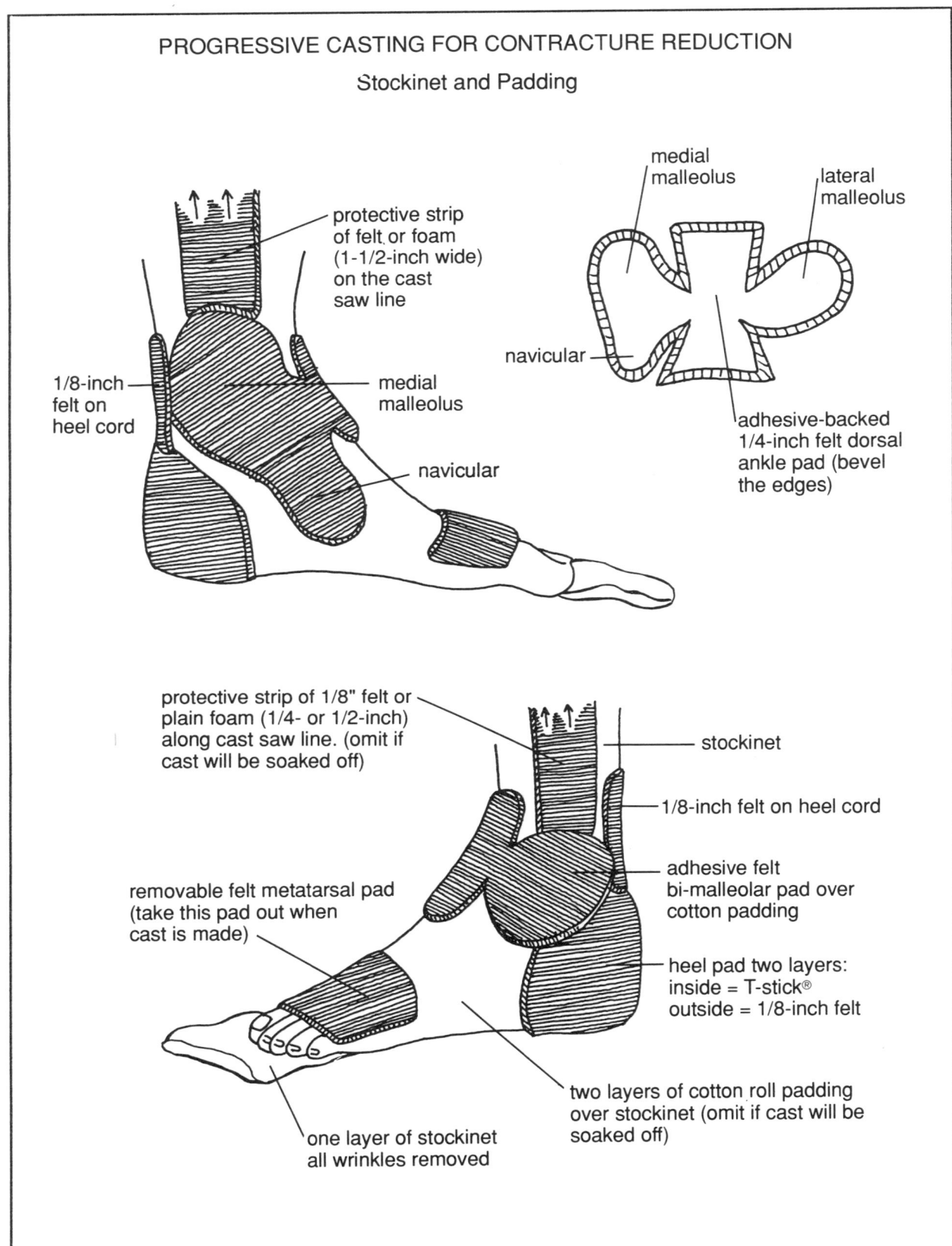

PROGRESSIVE CASTING FOR CONTRACTURE REDUCTION

Stockinet and Padding

protective strip of felt or foam (1-1/2-inch wide) on the cast saw line

medial malleolus

lateral malleolus

navicular

adhesive-backed 1/4-inch felt dorsal ankle pad (bevel the edges)

1/8-inch felt on heel cord

medial malleolus

navicular

protective strip of 1/8" felt or plain foam (1/4- or 1/2-inch) along cast saw line. (omit if cast will be soaked off)

stockinet

1/8-inch felt on heel cord

adhesive felt bi-malleolar pad over cotton padding

removable felt metatarsal pad (take this pad out when cast is made)

heel pad two layers:
inside = T-stick®
outside = 1/8-inch felt

one layer of stockinet all wrinkles removed

two layers of cotton roll padding over stockinet (omit if cast will be soaked off)

Figure 6.5

is a gradual process. Connective tissue regains extensibility more quickly than muscle fibers. Spasms in the calf muscles occur occasionally during sleep in a cast, evidently in response to overstretching of the muscle belly. This is a miserable event for the child and the family because the spasm is impossible to relieve with common household remedies such as aspirin, and a hot bath and massage are both prohibited by the nonsoakable plaster or fiber glass cast. Prompt cast removal is the optimum solution, easily undertaken at home if the cast is made of a soakable type of plaster material. If not, all caregivers should have a prescription for an appropriate dose of muscle relaxant, to be filled as needed, from the child's physician. This medication can relieve the child's discomfort due to spasm, and the cast can be removed professionally the following day.

- There is a risk of peroneal nerve damage.
- There may be stiffness at the knees. The integrity of ligaments supporting casted joints, and of their attachment sites to bone, is diminished for several months following any prolonged period of immobilization. Disuse signals osteoclasts to resorb bone at the insertion sites. The ligaments fail to turn over fibrils in response to strain signals that dictate their optimum configuration. The lack of stimulation normally provided by movement results in formation of a random, rather than parallel, matrix of extracellular fibers. The parallel arrangement of ligament fibrils is necessary for maximum strength against tensile forces and produces optimum stiffness. The random matrix of fibrils therefore depletes the stiffness of the ligament (Akeson et al. 1987).

Evans et al. (1960) studied the effects of immobilization, combined with weight-bearing, of the knee joint in rats. They discovered that fibrofatty connective tissue begins to proliferate into the intercondylar space and is well established within 30 days. They observed a marked development of invasive adhesions between this fibrofatty connective tissue and the underlying cartilage between 30 and 60 days. After 60 days, thinning and ulceration of articular cartilage were found in areas of compression. All of the knees were stiff following prolonged immobilization, but full mobility was regained after a period that nearly doubled that of the immobilization. The weight-bearing activity did not affect the reactive connective tissue proliferation and the formation of adhesions.

The same infiltration of fibrofatty connective tissue into immobilized joint spaces, and eventual fibrous ankylosis, was also observed in human amputation and autopsy studies following immobilization totalling 12 months or more (Enneking et al. 1972). Furthermore, the increased joint stiffness "probably results from random insertion of new fibers into the nylon hose-like meshwork of the normally extensible capsular and/or synovial fabric in the posterior part of the knee" (Akeson et al. 1987, p. 33).

These studies of the effects of immobilization on joints offer a biochemical rationale for keeping immobilization periods to a minimum, whether or not weight-bearing is allowed, and for protecting immobilized joints from abnormal strains in the early period following cast removal (Akeson et al. 1987).

I usually change long casts for inpatients every three days, taking time at cast changes to regain full range of movement in the knee joint with repetition of knee flexion and extension activities. I have also recently begun to open a hole for mobilization of the patella within the cast. This is at the suggestion of a workshop participant who reported learning to do so from the staff at Newington Children's Hospital in Newington, Connecticut. Such access to and tracking of the patella has apparently led to freedom from post-cast stiffness observed in the casted knee joints. Aside from exposing and mobilizing the patella, all other features of cast application remained the same as those that were used previously. The incidence of knee stiffness following long-leg cast series was higher when the patella was enclosed in the cast, although the duration of stiffness following cast removal was less than the stiffness after the casting series.

- Following a long-leg cast course of four to five weeks' duration, even when full mobilization and weight-bearing activities are undertaken at cast changes, pain on weight-bearing on the casted leg is a common finding for several weeks. I surmise that the new and unusual approximation of joint surfaces within the knee joint, having gained full range of motion, requires a period of adjustment and modeling. Perhaps fibiofatty tissues infiltrate the joint space as well, and the weakened ligaments and attachment sites might be painful.

This weight-bearing discomfort passes, typically within six to eight weeks. In the interim, I recommend seeking a physician's authorization for the child to use mild pain relievers. I also recommend applying elastic knee supports, such as an Ace® bandage or inflatable splints, to help make the transition period more comfortable. Caregivers must be trained and competent in proper use of such interventions, to avoid constricting the blood supply. Such problems might be avoided by using long casts in stages of two to three weeks each, with night-splinting in the interim, and by allowing the child time to regain functional level before resuming another short casting course. Such casting episodes might be separated by four- to six-week intervals until adequate extensibility is restored.

- The range of motion gained by casting might diminish in six to twelve months, depending upon any of the following factors: effectiveness of follow-up management, growth rate, changes in activity level (either increased or decreased), illnesses, the physiology of the muscle tissue, and family stresses. If, in fact, the muscle hypoextensibility type is appropriate for management with casts, repetition of the progressive casting series might be required every year or two to maintain or regain extensibility.

Rang et al. (1986) state that muscle growth is a response to stretch, which is usually induced by bone growth and normal movement while the muscle is in a relaxed state. Tardieu et al. (1988) suggest that to prevent contracture from developing in the soleus muscle, a minimum of six hours of stretch above the minimum threshold is needed per 24-hour period. When the stretching time was as short as two hours per day, they observed progressive contracture in the soleus muscle of a child with cerebral palsy. They further suggest that if night splints fail to maintain extensibility, one probable cause is that the splints fail to position the ankle above its minimal threshold of stretch (Tardieu et al. 1988).

The same authors propose in other writings that the pathophysiology of the muscle tissue is a factor. If the trophic regulation capability of the contracted tissue is disordered, contracture will recur with bone growth regardless of splinting, casting, or bracing. Such disorder is evident in soft tissues that exhibit little difference between initial and final resistances to passive elongation (Tardieu et al. 1982; Tardieu et al. 1987).

- The attending clinician must remain on 24-hour call for the duration of the casting series. That person bears the primary responsibility for securing prompt and safe cast removal if the cast is made of materials that require use of a cast saw.

Advantages of Serial Casting

- When criteria for using casts are met, serial casting usually achieves the goal of improving soft tissue extensibility (Westin et al. 1983; Tardieu et al. 1982; Tardieu et al. 1988). If the clinician takes the necessary precautions for the prompt removal of casts in the event of any associated problem, the potential for gaining mobility with this method is worth exploring.

- A serial cast course followed by consistent night splinting may serve to prevent the need for surgical lengthening of muscle tendon (Westin et al. 1983; Gritzka et al. 1986; Baumann et al. 1985; Hoffer et al. 1987). The recurrence rate for tendo-Achilles lengthenings is highest among those children who undergo the operation early in life. The rapid rate of growth in the early years seems to account for this problem of recurrence. Casting can at least delay the inevitable procedure until the risk of recurrence is less (Rang et al. 1986). By undertaking serial casting, it is clear to the caregivers that the team is making every effort to prevent surgery, if possible.

- Casting does not produce the risks of surgery—anesthesia, infection, over-lengthening of muscles, adhesions, and myositis ossificans.

- Hospitalization is unnecessary for most casting episodes (unless the associated social circumstances are complicated); thus separation from family and home does not become an issue.

- Compared to surgery, the cost of casting is significantly less.

- Unlike surgical lengthening, serial cast applications do not result in permanently weakened or atrophied muscle (Westin et al. 1983).

- If the deformity recurs, the process can be repeated. It is recommended, however, that such repetition be limited to twice per year. If recurrence happens very rapidly, such as within 6 weeks, the clinician should obtain a surgeon's opinion of the value of undertaking a third casting episode. The pathophysiology of the muscle contracture might render casting ineffective (Truscelli et al. 1979; Tardieu et al. 1982; Tardieu et al. 1987).

- The availability of Gypsona® and comparable plaster bandages that soak off easily greatly reduces stress on the child and family caused by dependence upon medical professionals and cast saws for prompt cast removal. The risk of skin breakdown drops markedly with such ease of removal. Caregivers are given permission to remove these casts if they are concerned at all about skin conditions or spasm, and attending clinicians are advised to remove promptly casts that are made of other types of casting material in response to the same concerns.

If a casting course of six weeks' duration fails to correct fixed soft-tissue deformity in the triceps surae, posterior tibialis, peroneal muscles, or hamstrings, or if contracture recurs rapidly, then orthopedic surgery is usually considered and often undertaken, and a splint or orthosis is used afterward as needed (McCrea 1985; Cary et al. 1975; Westin et al. 1983; Goldner 1982; Rang et al. 1986; Hoffer et al. 1987). Postoperative results are often disappointing, however, particularly if the muscle hypoextensibility is related to a dysfunction of trophic regulation (Truscelli et al. 1979; Tardieu et al. 1987). Furthermore, even following surgical procedures, those patients must be followed until maturity and often require repeat cast immobilization (Westin et al. 1983).

Post-Casting Follow-Up and Support

Further research will help clinicians determine the comparative effectiveness of various styles of splints and orthoses—both night splints and daytime support systems—in maintaining mobility and functional gains after serial casting. As discussed previously in this chapter, Baumann et al. (1985) use a double-shell solid ankle-foot orthosis for night splinting following cast use. Gritzka et al. (1986) use either fixed or free dorsiflexion AFOs to maintain functional gains following serial cast applications. Of Gritzka's study group of 70 patients with mild to moderate hypertonus, a one-year follow-up evaluation revealed that 70 percent had a heel-strike or foot-flat gait in AFOs and had maintained a functional range of ankle dorsiflexion. They suggest that correction can be maintained in free dorsiflexion AFOs.

Some children who undergo a casting series use follow-up systems including hinged ankle-foot or supramalleolar splints combined with night splinting in an SAFS. If they lose mobility at the ankle joint within a year and return for a second series of casts, this recurrence should be regarded not as a failure but as a signal to intervene promptly and appropriately. One to two casting episodes per year, particularly during periods of rapid growth, should be considered within the realm of appropriate management.

Indications for Serial Casting

The following indications for serial casting have been derived from the literature and from the author's recent clinical experience in the areas of head injury rehabilitation and cerebral palsy management:

- Persistent hypertonus in a child with mild to moderate involvement. The hypertonus results in static, soft tissue contracture, which features a significant difference between the point of initial resistance and the maximum endpoint. Initial resistance indicates existing tendon and connective tissue length. The maximum endpoint indicates maximum excursion of the muscle belly. The finding pertaining to the initial endpoint of resistance is more significant to functional ability than the final endpoint (Tardieu et al. 1982; Tardieu et al. 1988).

- Passive ankle dorsiflexion, with STJ in neutral position, is less than 5 degrees past neutral (or less than 95 degrees).

- Strong resistance to passive ankle dorsiflexion through the full range, regardless of the child's activity level or leg position. This resistance indicates shortening of connective tissue and tendon (Tardieu et al. 1982; Tardieu et al. 1988).

- Knee flexion contracture (hamstrings and/or gastrocnemius). The opposite hip is held in extension. On the leg to be tested, the clinician should maintain the ankle at its endpoint of dorsiflexion, flex the hip 90 degrees, and extend the knee. A popliteal angle of 30 degrees or more from vertical (or from full knee extension) is indication for intervention to reduce knee flexion contracture.

- Following hamstrings lengthening for severe flexion contracture, nerves and blood vessels may be shortened so that full surgical correction is prohibited. In that case, serial casts can be used to complete the lengthening procedure gradually.

Adequate equipment and therapy services must be available to provide the child in casts with alternative positioning (particularly frequent standing) and intensive therapeutic exercise for the cast wear duration. The child who wears casts—particularly long casts—without maintaining activities and exercise might effectively "turn to stone" and take several months to return to pre-casting activity levels.

A capable caregiver should be available and instructed to monitor for toe grasping on the cast itself as a compensatory balancing mechanism. This person should also inspect the child's feet and the casts at regular intervals for fit and evidence of discomfort and for skin irritation, swelling, or circulatory impairment, as well as for cracks or dents in the cast itself.

Contraindications for Serial Casting

- Long-standing static contracture that remains evident for more than three years following head trauma. If surgery is not a viable option, the clinician might try a cast series, but it will be a slow process, with potentially few, if any, gains.
- Static hypoextensibility in cerebral palsy. If the shortened muscle group is not activated, as in persistent hypertonus, a disorder of trophic (growth) regulation is likely to exist (Tardieu et al. 1982).
- Open sores or wounds (Booth et al. 1983).
- Swelling. The clinician should wait until any swelling has subsided before applying or reapplying a cast.
- Severe decerebrate/decorticate extensor spasticity (Booth et al. 1983).
- Severe full plantarflexion contracture (Booth et al. 1983).
- Presence of bony obstruction or abnormality.
- Acute heterotopic ossification (as often occurs after head injury). Application of stretch to the inflamed tissues can aggravate the condition (Evans 1981).

The clinician should not undertake casting in the absence of adequate therapy services, either at a clinic or at home. Furthermore, there must be no lack of attention to or equipment for carry-over positioning and handling. If the child's caregivers cannot be trusted to keep return appointments or to remain living in the area, or simply to act in the child's best interests during the casting episode, the clinician should take one of two courses: Arrange for the child to be admitted to a children's center for the duration of the casting series, or do not use solid casts.

Guidelines for Using Casts to Reduce Deformity

Most serial cast procedures require a total commitment of three to six weeks from start to finish, because the final cast should be applied for five to ten days to maintain the desired range of motion once it is achieved. It appears that this much time is needed to achieve the physiologic changes in soft tissue structure that are needed for lasting results (Tardieu et al. 1982; Booth et al. 1983; Otis et al. 1985; Tardieu et al. 1987). (Some clinicians limit cast wear to two weeks.)

Below-Knee Casts

- In managing equinovalgus deformity, attempt to find the neutral (congruent) alignment of the STJ complex, and assess the relationship of the foot and leg structures in neutrality. The pronation component of equinovalgus or pronation deformity may have resulted in enough shortening of the lateral ligaments and connective tissues and of the peroneal muscles to prohibit the achievement of full STJ congruity at the time the cast series is initiated. If this is the case, take extra precaution to protect the medial bony prominences with padding. Replicate the optimum congruent alignment of both the hindfoot and forefoot when applying the cast for equinovalgus or pronation deformity. For example, if the calcaneal bisection is aligned in 6 degrees of varus in STJ neutral position, set it that way in the cast. Similarly, gently plantarflex the medial rays and accommodate any remaining forefoot varus deviation in the cast. By eliminating dorsiflexion components of triplanar motion at the subtalar and midtarsal joints by locking them in congruity, excursion into dorsiflexion occurs entirely at the talocrural joint.

Equinovarus and cavus deformities, on the other hand, would only be enhanced by setting the foot structures in neutral (congruent) position, because neutral position in children typically results in a varus deviation. Reduce supination deviations in this foot: gently dorsiflex and abduct the forefoot around the oblique axis of the midtarsal joint (MTJ); evert the calcaneus; mold into the lateral longitudinal arch; and elongate the medial plantar fascia.

An alternative approach to molding the foot structures is to make a contoured plaster footboard prior to cast application. Such a footboard can be designed to align the foot structures either in neutral position for equinovalgus deformity or in slight pronation for equinovarus deformity. The footboard is then padded and inserted under the plantar aspect of the otherwise padded foot, outside the stockinet, during cast fabrication (Figure 6.3). As the foot structures gain extensibility and their alignment can be improved, the footboard may need revising. Check the mobility and alignment of the foot structure with each cast change and adjust the contours of the footboard accordingly before using it in the next cast.

- Use only one layer of stockinet and specifically pad the bony prominences, the dorsum of the ankle, the dorsum of the metatarsal heads, the non-plantar surface of the calcaneus (with foam plus thin felt combined), and—if a saw will be used for removal—the future cast cut line. Add a thin (1/8-inch) adhesive felt pad over the Achilles tendon (Figure 6.5). Do not wrap cotton roll padding around the entire foot and leg. Close contact between the plaster and the limb is desirable. Extra roll padding usually packs down and creates more room for movement within the cast. Movement brings about skin sores.

In choosing casting materials, consider their advantages and disadvantages. Less plaster and more fiber glass will reduce weight and setting time, increase cost, and prohibit soaking the (Gypsona® plaster) cast off. Consider your management priorities and level of skill in choosing a casting medium and its proportions. Fiber glass is never necessary for a resting cast. The child's activity level is likely to decrease in a resting cast because the angle of ankle plantarflexion is greater than the angle of the casts that will follow. Elastic plaster bandages afford improved conformity, but there is an increased risk of circulatory constriction.

- If you did not make a plaster footboard, the plaster slipper inner cast offers another method of securing the foot structures in the optimum alignment allowed by existing extensibility in the muscle and connective tissue (Figure 6.6). After padding for protection of bony prominences, gently mold the foot structures toward the desired alignment as the slipper sets.

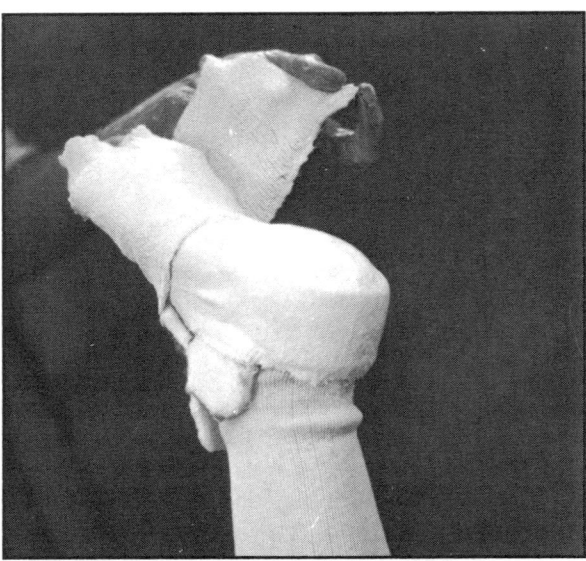

Figure 6.6 During cast application in prone position, a slipper cast insert is sometimes used to align the foot structures in optimal position before molding the ankle. Align the pronated hindfoot in neutral (congruent) position and gently plantarflex and adduct the MTJ. Evert the calcaneus and dorsiflex and adduct the MTJ around its oblique axis when casting the supinated foot. Applying the cast in two stages allows attention to molding into the contours under the foot. The prone position permits the clinician full visual access to the contours and structure of the foot and ankle during molding.

- Set the initial "resting" cast at a comfortable angle of dorsiflexion without compromising the foot position. This angle might be 25 degrees of plantarflexion or more in the resting cast. Do not use force to dorsiflex the ankle (Figure 6.7). Gentle pressure at the threshold of contracture elongates the muscle belly and connective tissues. Increasing the pressure (and thus the angle of ankle dorsiflexion) adds length to the connective tissues but overstretches the muscle fibers.
- Mold closely around the entire available surface of the calcaneus, including its inclination into the medial and lateral longitudinal arches (Figures 6.7 and 6.8). Mold beside the Achilles tendon and behind the malleoli.
- Post to create a supporting base for the foot and the toes. The surface that will contact the floor must be absolutely flat under the tarsus and metatarsals to permit stable and efficient alignment in standing without causing the child to topple in any

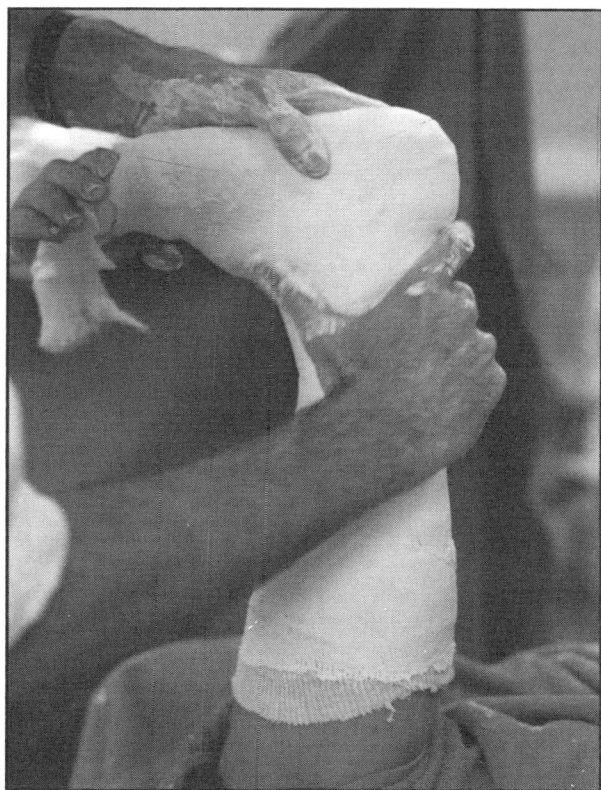

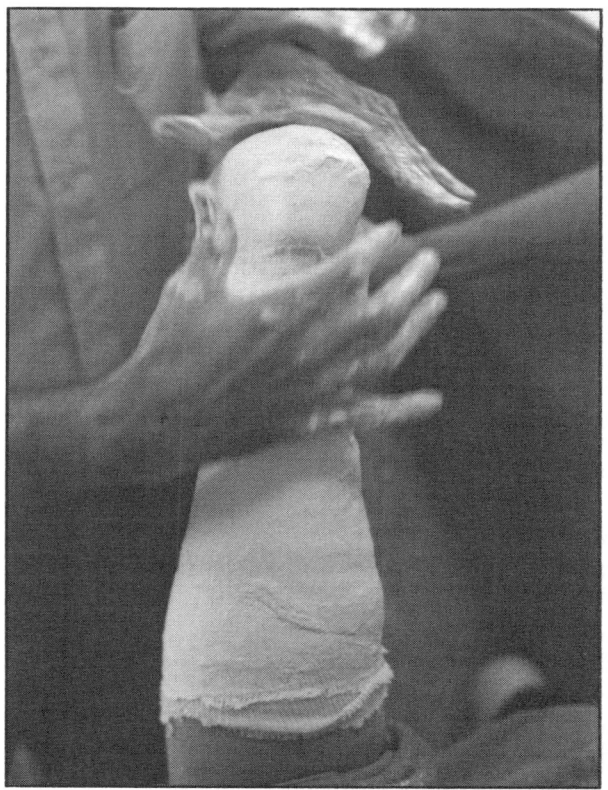

Figure 6.7 Apply the initial (resting) cast at the comfortable endpoint of dorsiflexion (miniumum point of passive resistance) with the knee flexed. Maintain optimal STJ/MTJ position.

Figure 6.8 Mold closely around the entire calcaneus, including the medial and lateral longitudinal arches, Achilles tendon insertion, and the area beside the Achilles tendon.

direction. Set the sole and shaft sections at 5 degrees of dorsiflexion (Figure 6.9). The plantar surface should be parallel with the transverse plane when the lower leg is aligned on the sagittal plane, except in the case of significant distal varum (Figure 6.9-A).

- Use a flat sheet of Plexiglas® or rigid plastic to bevel the plaster at the anterior and posterior edges of the plantar surface of the cast. Align the beveled edges in support of a smooth angle of progression (Figure 6.10).

- The concept of gait extension modifications to adjust the angle of gait can be applied to casts (Jordan 1984). For example, to encourage reduction of in-toeing, bevel the plaster at the lateral heel and the medial toe portions of the plantar surface of the cast to reduce any obstruction to a weight-bearing progression from the lateral heel at foot contact to the medial forefoot at toe-off (Figure 6.10).

- Use fiber glass tape to add strength for the active child (Figure 6.11).

- If the cast is not removable by soaking, mark the location of the cut line padding strips for safe removal either by yourself or, if the child lives far away, by another qualified clinician (Figure 6.12).

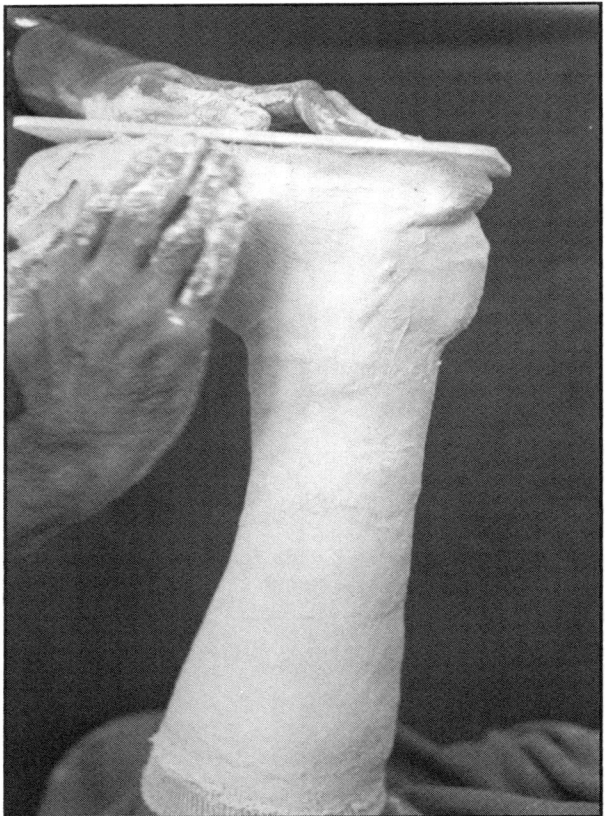

Figure 6.9 Post to stabilize the distal limb segments in optimum alignment for weight-bearing. Build an angle of 5 degrees of anterior pitch between the floor and the shaft section.

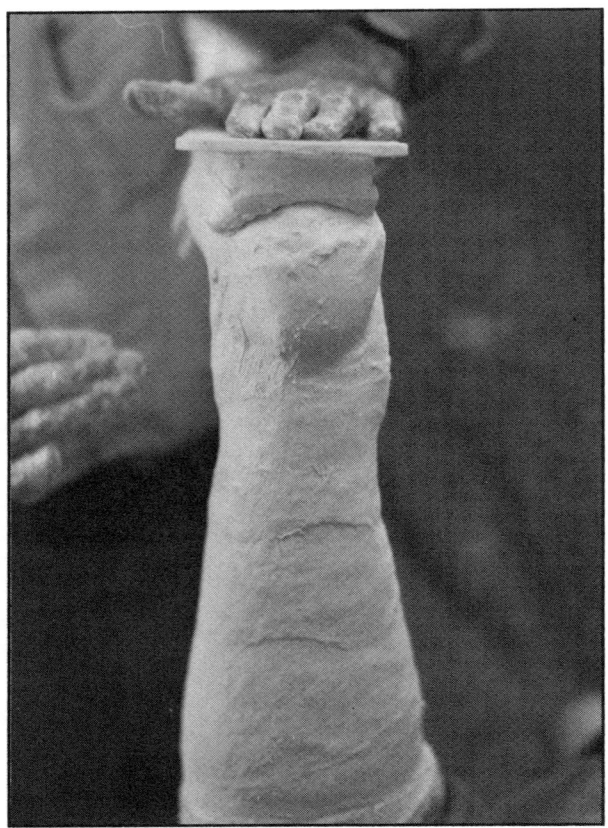

Figure 6.9-A Post for frontal plane stability.

- Add a crepe sole or a terry cloth slipper with a rubber sole to protect the fiber glass from wearing thin on tar and cement and to reduce any skidding that might occur on tile floors.

Prohibit any walking and strenuous activity for at least 24 hours, to allow the inner layers of a standard plaster cast to dry completely. When using plaster and fiber glass combinations, this waiting period can be reduced in proportion to the amount of plaster used. Fiber glass casts set fully within a few hours.

With most plaster casts, this precaution is essential, because children who overuse their feet, particularly the long toe flexors, for stabilizing themselves can deform the inner contour of the wet cast and create space in which pistoning of the foot can occur. The likelihood of rubbing a heel sore increases with movement inside the cast, and the structural support for the foot structures can be compromised. (Extend the waiting period to two days if it is raining or intensely humid—decrease it if you live in a very dry area.)

Many clinicians advocate using fiber glass cast tape for casting (Snavely et al. 1986). I prefer plaster for solid, serial casts mainly because I am more familiar with its properties. Since soakable plaster has become available, I am inclined to use it rather than fiber glass, because it is easier to remove.

Figure 6.10
Bevel under the heel and toe to facilitate smoothness of progression in a walking cast.

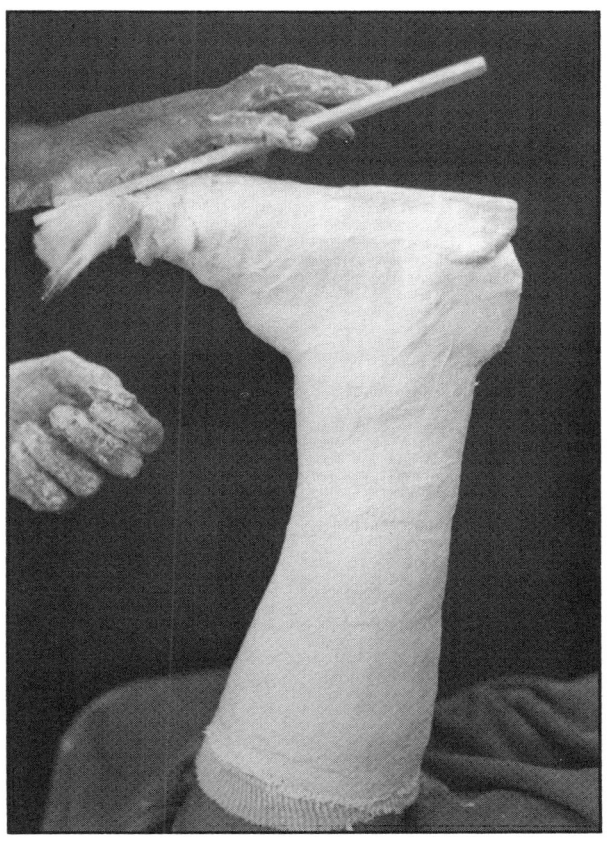

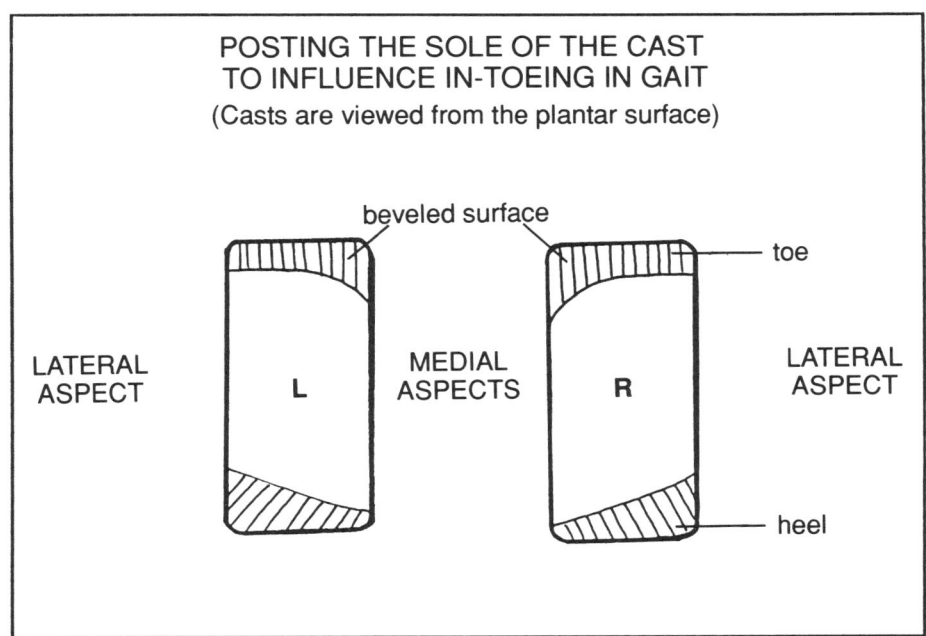

POSTING THE SOLE OF THE CAST
TO INFLUENCE IN-TOEING IN GAIT
(Casts are viewed from the plantar surface)

beveled surface

toe

LATERAL
ASPECT

L

MEDIAL
ASPECTS

R

LATERAL
ASPECT

heel

Figure 6.11 Add a fiber glass outer layer for durability.
Increasing fiber glass and decreasing plaster reduces its weight.
Mark the cast along the padding lines for possible removal by another.

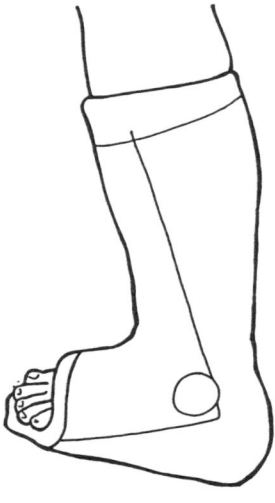

Figure 6.12
Mark trim lines on the finished cast.

Care and Management Following Each Cast Application

During the first 24 hours, prohibit weight-bearing and alert the nursing staff (including the night shift if the child is in the hospital) and other caregivers and family to check the following signs every one to two hours:

- Pulse at the child's toes
- Circulatory status, via capillary refill
- Color of nail beds
- Veins, for duskiness
- Swelling
- Complaints of "tingling"

For relief of the above symptoms, try flaring the edge of the cast at proximal and distal ends to relieve constriction. (Such an adjustment is very difficult when the cast is made using fiber glass cast tape.) If the toes feel cool in plaster casts, consider the interior dampness of the cast. Do not remove the cast unless other signs of constriction accompany the coolness. If flaring the ends does not relieve these symptoms, elevate the foot until cast removal (as promptly as possible) can be arranged.

Other signs may require *immediate* action:

- Evidence of pain
- Evidence of muscle spasm

Have caregivers contact you immediately regarding these concerns. Be prepared to remove the cast promptly.

After the complete setting period, continue to check for:

- Night spasms. If night spasms occur, remove the casts and reapply them at a reduced angle of stretch.
- Refusal to bear weight on (either) casted foot.
- Changes for the worse in sleeping patterns or general affect (particularly if the patient is nonverbal or comatose). If an ordinarily playful and active child demonstrates a significant withdrawal or a dimming of spirits, suspect a pressure sore is developing and remove the cast(s).
- Wetness that could cause softening of the cast.
- Objects, such as coins, dropped into the cast.
- Unusual odors coming from the cast.
- Cracks or dents in the plaster.

Review cast care procedures with all attending staff and family. Explain the properties of plaster under varying environmental conditions and stress the importance of detecting evidence of impairment of circulation, skin breakdown, or spasm. Instruct the caregivers to call you at work or at home immediately if they observe any of the trouble signs, and provide them with your telephone numbers.

At the time of cast application, if you have used standard types of plaster, fiber glass, or combinations of those materials in cast construction, make arrangements for the immediate removal of a cast. Prepare the caregivers to recognize and respond appropriately to any circumstances that suggest that skin breakdown or circulatory constriction is occurring. If the patient lives far away from your facility, provide the caregiver with a letter of authorization for a qualified clinician to remove the cast(s) at the caregiver's request and without delay. Explain the purpose of the casts in your letter, and provide your telephone numbers at work and at home for verification. Mark each cast to indicate the location of protective padding strips and instruct the caregivers about the purpose of the markings.

If you have used soakable plaster, the caregivers should voice their concerns to the attending clinician and may then proceed to remove the cast, if necessary.

When it is time to continue the series:

- Change the cast as often as every three days if you have the time and energy. Frequent cast changes reduce the chance of skin sores developing, but they are time-consuming, so many clinicians change the casts every 7 to 14 days (Booth et al. 1983; Hayes et al. 1970). If you change casts frequently, do not be tempted to try to gain extensibility too quickly. Consider the time needed for sarcomere production in the muscle fibers and the relatively greater speed with which the connective tissues lengthen compared with the muscle tissue. Keep the lengthening process a gradual one (Tardieu et al. 1987).

- Take some time at cast changes to gently mobilize the foot and ankle joints. Keep in mind the possibility that weakening is occurring in the ligaments, so avoid vigorous mobilizations. Allow some activation of the immobilized muscles, both to promote some guarded weight-bearing and to evaluate muscle activation and control. If isolated muscle action is evident at the ankle joint, do some strengthening activities before applying the next cast. Keep the joints lubricated and free of adhesions.

- A minimum total of three to four weeks for a progressive casting series is recommended because of the time needed for physiologic cellular adaptation to occur in the soft tissues (Hayes et al. 1970; Tardieu et al. 1982; Otis et al. 1985; Tardieu et al. 1987). Whether solid casts, bivalved casts, or splints are required throughout the immobilization period is not yet established by researchers and would be determined by clinical evaluation.

- When adequate range of dorsiflexion has been achieved without compromising the alignment of the foot structures, Booth et al. (1983) suggest applying a holding cast to maintain the ankle in dorsiflexion (5-10 degrees past neutral) for an additional five to ten days. The time spent in the holding cast allows more time for physiologic cellular adaptation and might prolong the duration of the resulting improved extensibility. Consistent night splinting might suffice as an alternative, with daytime stabilization of foot structures for function.

Treatment in Below-Knee Casts

The below-knee cast imposes some mechanical limitations on movement that can be overcome only with the facilitator's assistance. Because many children who have undergone tendo-Achilles lengthenings or subtalar arthrodeses wear casts for up to six weeks, they too need every advantage for biomechanical efficiency.

A schedule of three sessions per week of therapeutic exercise is recommended as a minimum for children in below-knee casts (Mohr 1977). The casts do not interfere with processes such as mobilization and functional strengthening of the trunk and proximal limb musculature, activation and strengthening of the knee extensors and flexors, or activation of equilibrium responses in all positions (Cusick 1980; Sussman 1980; Sussman et al. 1981; Sirna et al. 1986). Attending therapists should provide close monitoring of the status of the child's skin, circulatory reflux, and functional influences of the casts for the duration of wear, while promoting optimum antigravity function. Many children seek compensatory stability by gripping the surface of the cast with their toes. Problems related to malalignment or destruction from wear can hinder the habilitation effort. Casts are not a convenient substitute for therapy. They are an adjunct.

The following suggestions are derived from years of experience in coping with these problems, with the guidance of Lois Bly (1980) and Joan Mohr (1977).

Managing Casts in Various Positions

Prone and supine—The feet are heavy in casts, and lateral rotation occurs at the knee joint. The rotation at the knee joint stresses the collateral knee ligaments. The weight of the boots can leave the knee joint unstable. Nurses and parents are the most likely caregivers to check on the sleeping child. They should have photos at the bedside with instructions for proper positioning.

Encourage the child to sleep in side-lying positions. Use extra pillows or blanket rolls to support the trunk and upper leg comfortably, and to minimize rotary and frontal plane stresses to the knee joint. Adjust prone and supine sleeping positions to realign the feet closer to the sagittal plane; the feet should be off the end of the mattress in prone, and propped with pillows in supine.

Quadruped and kneeling—Rotation of the lower legs can contribute to a "windblown" appearance of the lower legs, even in casts. Windblown legs roll or twist in the same direction (Figure 6.12). When the twist occurs below the knee, the weight of the casts in quadruped and kneeling positions can disrupt a symmetrical weight distribution at the trunk and hips. As the lower legs roll to the right side, for example, the hips and pelvis tend to shift to the left. Here are three ways to address these concerns:

- Square the anterior edge of the toe support (Figure 6.11).
- Work on a mat table or a firm double- or triple-thickness mat. Lower the foot off the edge of the mat.
- Use a towel roll under the dorsal surface of the cast for motor training in these positions (Figure 6.14).

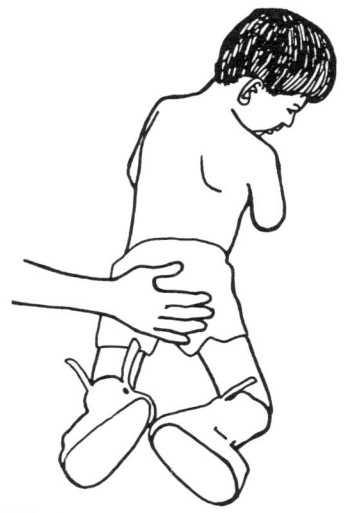

Figure 6.13 Lateral rotation of the lower leg in fixed-ankle devices can block normal weight shifts of the center of gravity.

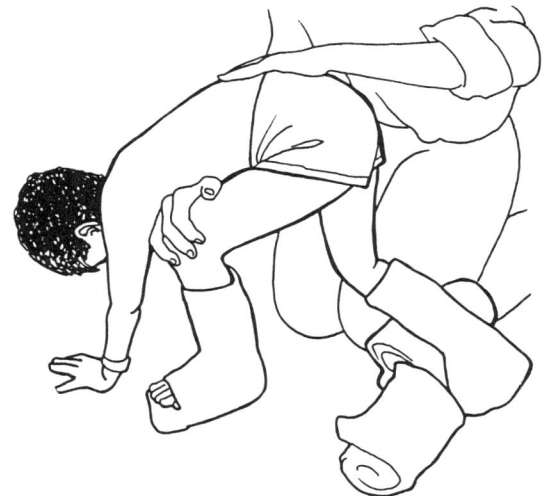

Figure 6.14 A towel roll, large dowel, or small bolster can be used to align the foot during movement training.

Half-kneeling and standing—The angle that the shaft of the cast forms with the floor, relative to the frontal plane, will determine the facility of executing weight transfers forward over the casted foot. Within the limit of normal function, the greater the degree of dorsiflexion, the easier the transition forward. In half-kneel-to-stand transitions, the therapist might need to assist the child to tip the lower leg forward during the transition. When the child must repeat such transitions for strengthening, insert a portable rubber wedge, such as a door stop, under the cast to raise and stabilize the heel.

For standing, set the angle of the ankle at 5 degrees of dorsiflexion in the holding casts, as long as the appropriate or desirable position of the foot is not compromised. If ankle joint mobility is limited, as is typical early in the series, you may achieve the functional effect of adequate dorsiflexion by one of the following methods:

- Post the sole of the cast accordingly with plaster.
- Wedge the heel of the cast with splint material. If the cast is covered in fiber glass, the thermoplastics can adhere.
- Use a temporary heel wedge of crepe sole or firm foam, either placed under the heel at the time of the transition, or taped to the sole of the casts with moleskin or fiber-filled strapping tape.

Standing and walking—The angle that the shaft forms with the floor, relative to the frontal and sagittal planes, will significantly affect the child's capacity to progress forward in walking and will change the distribution of weight across the plantar surface of the foot. The potential problems of standing alignment and ambulatory function related to cast construction are discussed below.

Problems of Malalignment

- Unequal thickness that can be observed while comparing the soles of the left and right cast boots. This oversight can impose a leg-length discrepancy and pelvic obliquity on a child who might not otherwise have these problems.

- Uneven thickness of the sole under the foot that can result in deviation of the shaft on the frontal plane (mediolaterally). In this case:

  — Valgus or varus forces are evident at the knee.

  — Lateral or medial excursions of the trunk increase.

- The angle between the shaft and the floor is 90 degrees or less (that is, plantarflexed). This configuration can result in any one or more of the following functional problems:

  — Knee hyperextension, because full foot contact is achieved by lowering the heel to the ground.

  — Backward stepping is easier then forward stepping, as a result of floor reaction forces that prohibit forward progression past midstance.

  — Increased knee flexion, to avoid pressure from the proximal cast on the anterior tibia.

  — Increased abduction or adduction of the foot, apparently executed to achieve forward progression by removing the casted foot from the line of progression. This maneuver effectively shortens the foot, and thus the distal lever arm. It is a compensation for inadequate excursion into dorsiflexion, and it might signal or produce laxity in the soft tissue structures of the knee joint.

  — "Running" in preference to walking, usually on the beveled toes of the cast.

Problems of Rotary Deviations

Excessive lateral rotation—An angle of gait exceeding 15-20 degrees to the sagittal plane distributes loading forces of extraordinary magnitude over the medial aspect of the stance foot and knee. Check the sagittal plane angle between the shaft and sole of the cast. If the child is younger than 8 years, and the sagittal plane angle at the ankle is adequate to allow smooth forward progression (that is, 5 degrees), consider beveling the lateral corner of the toe-break area of the sole. The beveled corner originates from the most distal point on the medial plantar surface of the cast and ends on the lateral edge of the same surface, at a point proximal to the fifth metatarsal head

(Figure 6.10). Creating this angled toe-break results in a flat plantar surface of the cast longer on the medial edge than on the lateral edge. You can expect this angled toe-break to encourage a reduction in out-toeing by creating a path of least resistance that favors forward progression over the outer aspect of the forefoot (Spencer et al. 1984; Jordan 1984).

Medial rotation—Medial rotation in gait is often caused by medial genicular position, medial tibiofibular torsion and/or residual femoral antetorsion. This problem might also offer evidence of functional contracture of the hip flexors and adductors. A combination of all of these factors is possible in the ambulatory child with neuromotor impairment (McCrea 1985). Presumably, thousands of repetitions of active hip lateral rotation with extension, executed over several years, are needed to resolve femoral antetorsion and to achieve adequate lateral tibiofibular torsion in a child's growing bones.

Because it involves soft tissue, however, medial genicular knee malalignment can be managed more rapidly by one or more of the following methods:

Passive derotation in infancy—McDonough (1984) and Ganley (1984) advocate long-leg serial casting in infancy, to gain enough extensibility gradually in the knee joint ligaments to allow the lower leg to be rotated laterally beyond the sagittal plane. The casts are applied with the knee flexed at least 30 degrees.

Passive derotation in childhood—McCrea (1985) suggests long-leg serial casting for children (no specified age range), maintaining the knee in 30 degrees of flexion and the foot encased in plaster. He divides the cast circumferentially distal to the knee joint at weekly intervals, rotates the lower leg laterally to the next tolerable endpoint, and repairs the cut with plaster to secure the new position. He suggests that the rotary deviation should reduce within four weeks, including one full cast change at two weeks. McCrea does not discuss this procedure in the context of the child with hypertonic neuromotor deficit, however. The process of using progressive casting to reduce medial genicular knee deformity might require more time in the presence of spasticity.

Using casts to reduce the contractures that maintain genicular knee position might provide the soft tissue extensibility needed to facilitate the active, gait-induced correction of in-toeing. The influence of the gait extension modification to the plantar surface of the cast (described below) might thus be enhanced by a preparatory progressive casting series. Research is needed to ascertain this possibility.

Active derotation of medial genicular position through application of torque and floor reaction forces—The same concept about the in-toeing gait extension modification of the SFS that was discussed in Chapter 5 applies to the cast boot. By your beveling the anterior medial corner of the sole of the cast more deeply than, and at an angle to, the lateral anterior section, the child between ages 2 and 12 years might respond by increasing the angle of gait (Spencer et al. 1984; Jordan 1984). The resulting length of the flat surface of the sole is greater on the lateral than the medial aspect (Figure 6.10).

The beveled sole might encourage the child to progress forward most efficiently by maneuvering the foot to complete the stance phase by rolling off of the medial forefoot (Jordan et al. 1983; Spencer et al. 1984; McCrea 1985).

Unless the child is able to walk without relying on the upper extremities for support, the lateral rotary forces applied in the stance phase of gait do not seem to be adequate to bring about the desired increase in the angle of gait. Independent ambulation, without assistive devices, appears to be a key ingredient for effecting this correction of in-toeing secondary to soft tissue contracture.

Serial Long-Leg Casts

The knee joint is included in a progressive cast course in order to address limitation of motion at the knee imposed by shortening of the hamstrings and/or the gastrocnemius muscle, and as a means of reducing medial genicular position (described above) (Tardieu et al. 1982; Westin et al. 1983, Valmassy 1984; McDonough 1984; Ganley 1984; McCrea 1985). I have no knowledge of using serial casting to gain knee flexion mobility.

Management of Knee Flexion Contracture

When it is evident that the gastrocnemius is shortened, alone or in combination with the hamstrings, the below-knee cast can be extended over the knee joint to the proximal thigh. I suggest beginning a long-leg cast series by casting the foot and ankle first, through one or two changes, before adding the knee joint. Prevention of spasm is the rationale for this procedure, because fewer two-joint muscles are elongated simultaneously.

To determine the angle at which to set the knee joint in the cast, place the child in sitting position with the posterior walls of the pelvis vertical. Then extend the knee. When the pelvis tips posteriorly, the end point of knee extension in sitting has been reached. Set the knee at that angle (Figure 6.15).

If for some reason the child cannot sit for the test, set the knee joint at the popliteal angle determined in supine, with the ankle dorsiflexed to its comfortable endpoint (that is, with the foot and ankle casted). By limiting the stretch on the muscle fibers within the knee flexors, the risk of night spasm is likely to be reduced.

The illustrated case study on T. S. (which is discussed at the end of this chapter) is fairly typical of my experience with long-leg casts, although I might recommend using Gypsona® for ease of removal by the caregiver, or reducing the amount of plaster and applying fiber glass to reduce the weight and bulk of the casts. Also, I now cut out a hole to expose the patella for mobilization during casting and suggest casting in stages of two weeks each, allowing four weeks between stages to regain full function at each new level of extensibility.

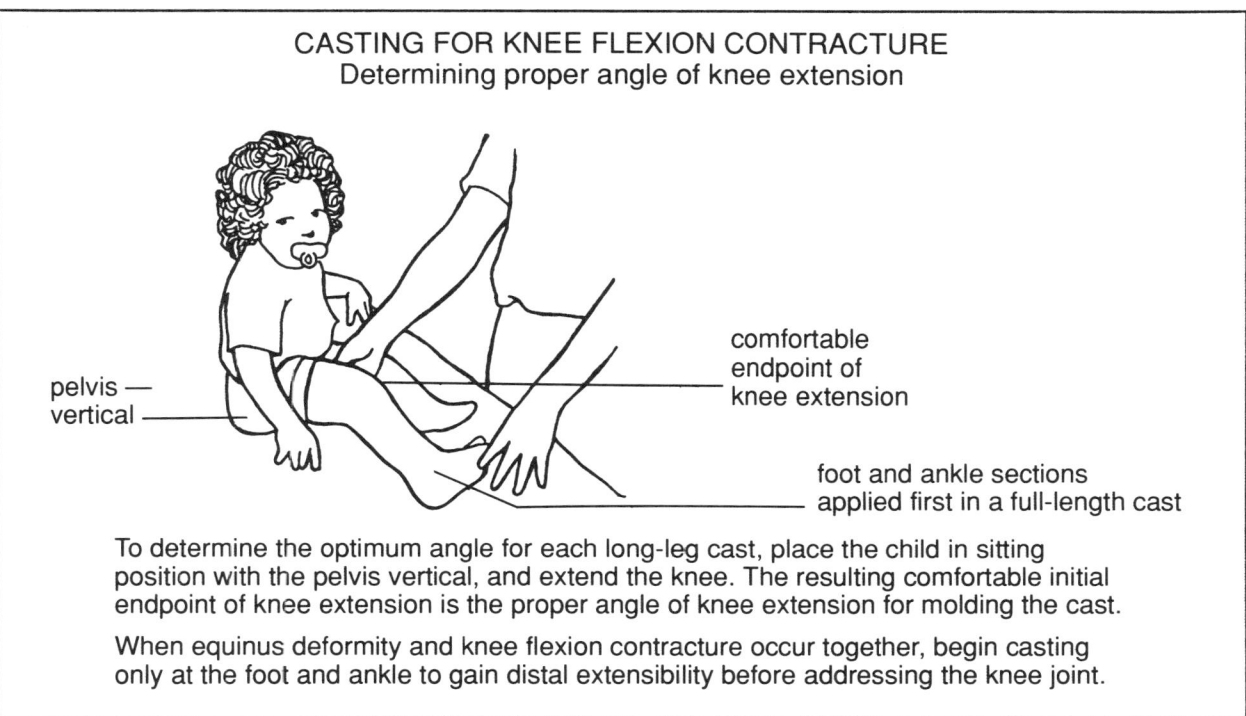

CASTING FOR KNEE FLEXION CONTRACTURE
Determining proper angle of knee extension

pelvis — vertical

comfortable endpoint of knee extension

foot and ankle sections applied first in a full-length cast

To determine the optimum angle for each long-leg cast, place the child in sitting position with the pelvis vertical, and extend the knee. The resulting comfortable initial endpoint of knee extension is the proper angle of knee extension for molding the cast.

When equinus deformity and knee flexion contracture occur together, begin casting only at the foot and ankle to gain distal extensibility before addressing the knee joint.

Figure 6.15

Hamstrings contracture—The hamstrings might be contracted (for example, in crouch deformity) while the ankles allow full or excessive mobility. In this instance, a cylinder cast is indicated, with stabilizing foot splints as needed to align the foot structures. Determine the knee joint angle for immobilization by extending the knee with the child in sitting. Stop when the pelvis tilts posteriorly.

By cutting a small window in the cast around the patella, the patella can be mobilized and its proper tracking facilitated during treatment (Figures 6.16, 6.17, and 6.18). Such an adaptation requires careful padding around the patella to allow safe removal of plaster in that area. As discussed previously, the exposed and mobilized patella seems to grant a measure of freedom from knee joint stiffness following cast removal. Take some time during cast changes to mobilize the knee joint and to strengthen the musculature before applying the next cast.

For casts made of standard plaster and fiber glass materials, I use foam or adhesive-backed felt strips along the saw line on the medial and lateral aspects of the leg to protect the skin during cast removal (Figure 6.16). A thick Pudgee® or T-Stick® foam pad around the proximal ankle area also helps to prevent skin irritation and breakdown from pressure. Molded heel support cups with medial and lateral uprights would be useful for this purpose. The uprights are toothed and designed to be incorporated into the distal cast; they prevent the cast from slipping down with gravity.

I consider fiber glass cast tape a feasible casting medium for cylindrical long casts because of the generally smooth contours of the leg compared with the foot and ankle. The light weight of the fiber glass

LONG-LEG CAST PADDING

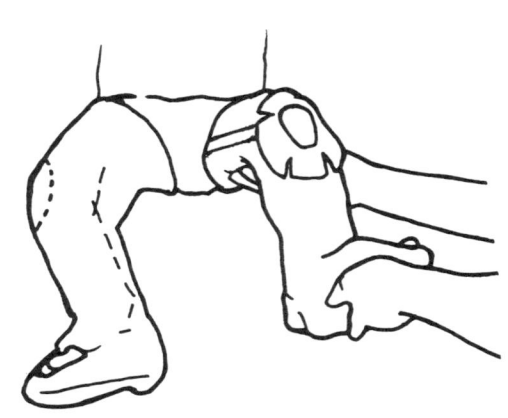

- Apply one layer of stockinet to the proximal thigh.

- Apply T-Stick® or Pudgee® to the proximal popliteal space (not shown).

- Apply 1/4-inch thickness adhesive felt (see padding schematic, Figure 6.17) to anterior knee joint.

- Add protective felt (1/8-inch) or foam strips to medial and lateral aspects of knee and thigh if the cast is to be removed with a saw.

- Apply four layers of cotton padding (Webril®) to the proximal thigh.

Figure 6.16

THE PATELLAR PAD

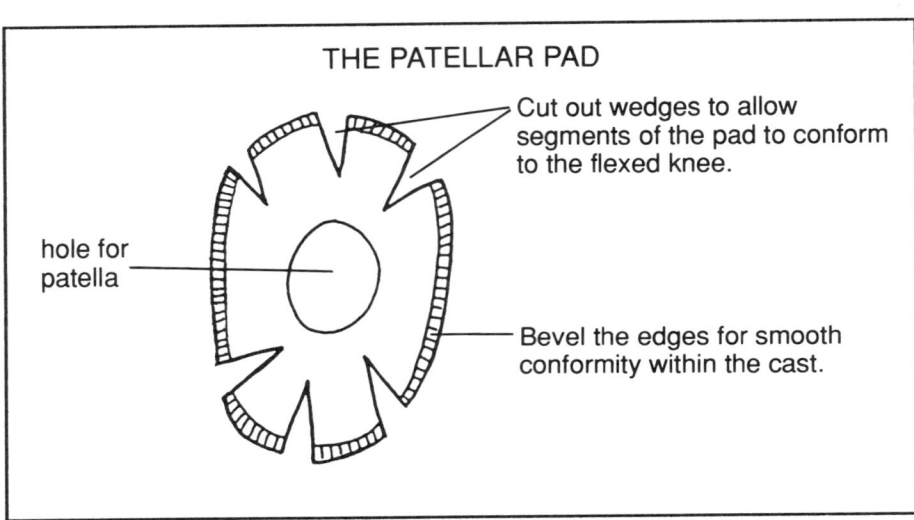

Cut out wedges to allow segments of the pad to conform to the flexed knee.

hole for patella

Bevel the edges for smooth conformity within the cast.

Figure 6.17

FULL-LENGTH CASTS
(Holes expose patellae)

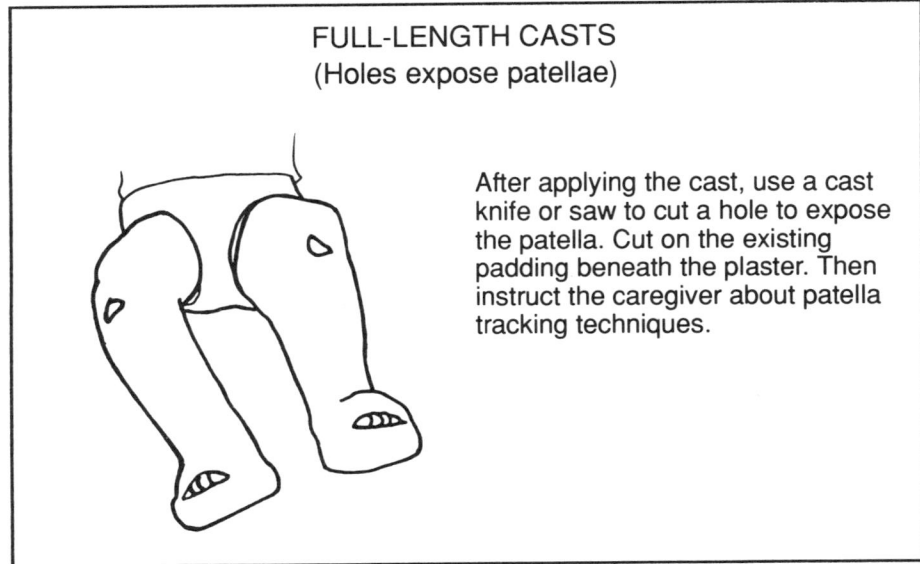

After applying the cast, use a cast knife or saw to cut a hole to expose the patella. Cut on the existing padding beneath the plaster. Then instruct the caregiver about patella tracking techniques.

Figure 6.18

material compared with plaster can be a significant advantage to the family and therapist, particularly during therapeutic exercise in casts. Fiber glass casts cannot be soaked off, however, and are several times more expensive than plaster.

Treatment in Long-Leg Casts

Hayes et al. (1970) suggest that the effects of casting are dependent more upon time spent bearing weight in them than upon the duration of cast wear alone. They note that casting episodes in which weight-bearing is not offered commonly result in a considerable increase in knee flexor spasm upon cast removal. I find that unless the patella is exposed and tracked, weight-bearing in casts does not prevent post-cast knee joint stiffness in extension. As was discussed previously under the disadvantages of serial casts, researchers have shown that fibrofatty connective tissue proliferates into the joint space and forms adhesions in the knee joint when weight-bearing is allowed in the cast.

Hayes et al. (1970) commonly used long-leg casts in management. The total time spent in plasters was usually between 20 and 35 days, prolonged by approximately one week after observation of "generalized reduction of spasm" (p. 109). With careful attention to initial positioning and regular position changes, they used the time spent in plasters to establish new patterns of weight-bearing and to effect such treatment goals as the following:

- Strengthening and mobilizing the trunk.
- Improvement of weight-bearing postural alignment through the trunk, pelvis, and hips.
- Facilitation of balancing reactions.
- Activation of the muscles of hip extension, abduction, and lateral rotation.
- Independent walking without aids.
- Prevention of "spasm shunting from the plastered limb to other parts of the body" (the means was not specified) (p.109).

I concur with Hayes and Burns that each serial cast course must be accompanied by a vigorous therapeutic exercise program that emphasizes ample weight-bearing of two to three hours per day. I would add the following to their protocol:

- Joint mobilization as needed for the anterior and inferior aspects of the hip joint capsule.
- Strengthening for the shoulder girdle, trunk, and neck musculature.
- Patellar mobilization and stabilization, using the window cut in the cast, during activities that require activation of the quadriceps muscles.

There is a risk of inducing a preference for a sedentary lifestyle in a child who wears casts but does not actively move in them.

Alternative Interventions to Reduce Contracture

In recent years, clinicians have been exploring the effectiveness of various techniques in reducing existing contracture in the triceps surae group. These techniques are in their preliminary stages and offer some encouraging alternatives to cast immobilization and surgical lengthening procedures. Among them:

The "Bioboot"

Coram (1989) is using a removable cast boot. It is made using a resin-based casting material that resembles fiber glass casting tape but retains flexibility after setting. The insole of the boot consists of a contoured plaster footboard made on an inverted piece of vinyl flooring. The footboard is constructed to maintain the pronated foot structures in true STJ neutral position and the toes in neutral extension. The ankle joint is set at the existing tolerable endpoint for dorsiflexion (which might be 10-15 degrees of plantarflexion in the first boot). The boot is trimmed to the height of a high-top basketball sneaker, and the dorsum wraps entirely around the midfoot. The distal lower leg is allowed to come forward over the stabilized foot.

The "bioboot" is used in daily therapy sessions for one hour, during which the child is guided into weight-bearing activities involving varying increments of squatting over the plantigrade foot. Each boot in the series is constructed in relatively less plantarflexion as the triceps surae group gains extensibility, and therapeutic exercise continues. Clinical evidence indicates that the intense therapy program combined with the boots can result in dramatic increases in extensibility and thus reduction of contracture within two weeks. However, it is not yet known whether the gains in extensibility are occurring in the connective tissue or within the muscle fibers. Connective tissue lengthens more rapidly than muscle tissue. If the muscle belly is not lengthening as well, the affected muscles retain a limited excursion and thus a limited capacity for strength (Rang et al. 1986; Tardieu et al. 1987). Muscle lengthening might, however, be occurring during the maintenance period, when the use of the boots is reduced to twice weekly and night splinting is provided.

The Hinged Ankle-Foot Stretch Splint

Carpenter (1989) designed a hinged ankle-foot splint (HAFS) stretch splint. The hindfoot is molded into optimal position and secured in the splint by running a wide Velcro® strap over the dorsum of the instep and through slots in the splint on both sides of the calcaneus. The strap then attaches on the outside surfaces of the heel area of the splint. The foot piece and shaft section are connected to each other with 1/2-inch surgical tubing or with the strongest grade of Thera-Band® elastic strap. The elastic connecting band is attached to brackets that are made of splinting material and fastened to both the lateral and medial aspects of the proximal shaft and the distal foot pieces. The tension generated in the tubing or elastic strap applies a constant pull on the foot piece into dorsiflexion. (In the presence of clonus, the elastic straps are replaced by nonstretch straps and a toothed buckle.)

The hinged stretch splint is used on a gradually increasing program, beginning with 15 to 20 minutes three times per day, with the tension in the elastic bands set at a perceivable but tolerable level. If discomfort in the triceps surae group persists for more than 30 minutes following removal of the splint, the tension is reduced. If no discomfort occurs, the tension is increased slightly. After several days of using the splint for 15 to 20 minutes per session, the time is increased by 15-minute increments to two hours. When the patient can tolerate two hours of splint wear, three times per day, the splint is used at night, and the daytime program is discontinued. As long as the splint is applying a gentle dorsiflexion stretch, the tension is adequate.

Clinical evidence is encouraging for the use of this splint for adults with head trauma and cerebral vascular accident. It is a long-term intervention, and its effects require investigation on all levels to determine optimum protocols for various types and severity of contracture. It offers a favorable alternative to plaster casting in the acute phases of recovery following head trauma, because of its removability for medical purposes. At this writing, I am not aware that its use for children with cerebral palsy has been evaluated.

Peripheral Alcohol Nerve Blocks

Diamond (1988) blocked the sciatic branches to the medial hamstring and the tibial and obturator nerves as an adjunct to the treatment programs underway for 120 children during a period of 18 months. The patients ranged in age from 18 months to 21 years. In this study, 106 patients were diagnosed as having cerebral palsy. The researchers noted that sciatic blocks were performed most frequently (for crouch posture), but the longest duration of effect occurred with tibial nerve blocks for equinus deformity. They supplemented tibial nerve blocks with serial casting for five patients, all of whom showed full reduction of contracture after one course of casting. The authors concluded that "the peripheral nerve block is a safe, easily performed procedure of benefit to CP patients in whom gross motor function has plateaued" (p. 13).

Neuromuscular Stimulation

Bowser et al. (1985) studied the effectiveness of this modality for treating children ages 2½ to 9 years with various distributions of spastic cerebral palsy. Twelve of these children revealed plantarflexion contractures. The children used a portable electrical stimulator for 15 to 30 minutes twice daily. Intermittent stimulation was applied to the peroneal nerve or the anterior tibialis muscle. The authors observed gains in active range of dorsiflexion totalling 5 to 10 degrees or more in all except one child. They saw 11 children progress to using the stimulator in gait to improve dorsiflexion in the swing phase. The authors have not reported the amount of time it takes to effect the changes they have observed. They suggest that "neuromuscular stimulation is a non-invasive physiological approach that results in a significant decrease in contractures and improved range of motion at the ankle" (p. 94). The increasing availability of such portable stimulation units should offer ever greater numbers of clinicians access to this modality as a contracture-reducing intervention. Nevertheless, it appears that by activating the body's reciprocal innervation mechanism, an appropriate contracture reduction process is effected. It is hoped that other researchers will verify these suppositions.

Summary

Casts have been used effectively for decades as a contracture management procedure. They present the patient and family with considerably fewer risks than surgical muscle lengthening. Casts represent a conservative approach that can be supplemented by surgery if necessary. Yet many facilities do not offer serial casting as a management option. If inconvenience is a factor, I suggest that therapists and orthopedic technicians assume the burden of time and effort imposed by the procedure. No standard therapeutic exercise program offers a patient a potential 45-degree gain in knee extension mobility in four to six weeks of treatment. The hours spent in therapy trying to elongate tight muscles and joint capsules could be devoted to activating and strengthening the lengthened muscles and their antagonists in improved functional patterns. Movement training could proceed without the impedance of contracture. True muscle growth can occur with a casting course, so the potential for gaining strength through casting increases. Surgery, which lengthens tendons and fascia, usually leaves a shortened muscle belly, and its potential excursion (strength) limited.

No inexperienced clinician should undertake to apply or remove a cast without training and direct supervision by another clinician who is more qualified and experienced in the technique being used. Every cast application and removal carries abundant risks of skin abrasion or laceration. Each procedure must be approached with a reverence and regard for all precautions, and a readiness to remove the cast promptly in response to any measure of concern.

The success of splints and orthoses often depends upon the availability of adequate extensibility in the muscle and connective tissues. The following chapter presumes that such extensibility exists. Chapter 7 addresses the principles of therapeutic splinting, including molding for correction, handling the elastic thermoplastic materials, and evaluating the finished products.

Case Study: Long-Leg Serial Casting

This case describes the treatment of only the third patient on my caseload to undergo long-leg casting. I will, therefore, occasionally interject newer approaches and ideas of which I was unaware at the time of treatment.

T. S. demonstrates severe spastic diplegia with a mild athetoid component. She was 6 years and 10 months at the initiation of the casting series and was unable to stand or walk without full assistance because of problems of scissoring, bilateral hip flexion and adduction contractures, knee flexion contractures, and profound bilateral equinovalgus deformity. Her orthopedist suggested that her athetoid component, though evident only in her fingers and oral motor control, rendered surgery somewhat unpredictable. The orthopedist ordered bilateral "clamshell" braces with thick rocker-bottom soles, and a "saddle-type" walker. Because T. S.'s orthotist and attending physical therapist both expressed the opinion that more joint mobility was required before measuring for braces, she was referred to me for casting.

Her range of motion at the outset of casting was as follows, with little difference comparing left to right sides:

- Hip extension—lacks 25 degrees from neutral position.
- Hip abduction—30 degrees with the hip extended.
- Knee extension (popliteal angle)—lacks 60-64 degrees of full knee extension (Figure 6.19).
- Knee extension with hip extended—lacks 20 degrees left side, 10 degrees right.
- Ankle dorsiflexion—full with neutrally aligned STJ, after overcoming strong resistance to passive motion throughout the available range. Initial resistance to passive dorsiflexion was encountered at 0 degrees plantarflexion on the right, 4 degrees plantarflexion on the left.

T. S.'s casting course is outlined next. Table 1 presents the changes that were observed in her knee flexion contractures.

October 23—Bilateral below-knee casts were applied, with the ankles set at 2-3 degrees of dorsiflexion on the right, 0 degrees on the left, because these angles presented a slight stretch past minimum threshold (Figure 6.20). Orthopedic felt padding was used to protect the malleoli, the dorsum of each ankle, and the heel. (I would now use T-Stick® and 1/8-inch felt to protect the heel area.) The plantar surface under each heel was wedged with plaster to allow some weight-bearing in standing, in consideration of her knee flexion contractures and the ankle joint position within each cast.

She used canvas knee extension splints at night and, when possible, during the day during the first week. This was an effort to prepare her for the long casts that were planned. Joint mobilization and

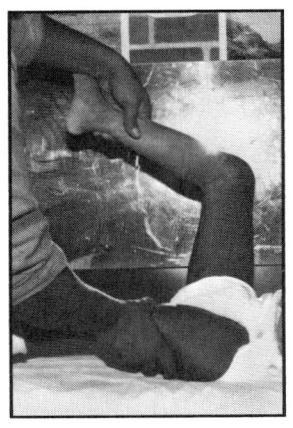

Figure 6.19
October 23: Pre-cast status of knee flexion contracture (popliteal angles):
R = -64 degrees
L = -60 degrees

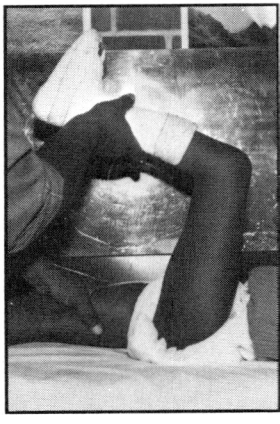

Figure 6.20
October 23: Applied below-knee casts with canvas-covered knee extension splints.

strengthening for the trunk, hip, and knee extensors was recommended to her attending therapist as a complement to casting. Her mother was instructed in cast care and precautions.

October 30—During this week, a school nurse became concerned over her impression that there was swelling in the right foot and referred T. S. to her doctor, who determined that all was well. However, to be safe, the right cast was removed and the skin inspected. Excellent skin condition, and no resistance to dorsiflexion was observed. The right below-knee cast was replaced, with the ankle joint set at 5 degrees dorsiflexion.

Then, both casts were extended above the knee. A felt pad was inserted under the anterior proximal area of each below-knee cast, to protect the tibia from pressure, and stockinet and cotton roll padding were applied above the tibias to the proximal thighs. (I now use one layer of stockinet to the groin, thin felt strips on medial and lateral thigh and knee joints, and four layers of cotton roll padding at proximal thigh.)

A large felt pad was then applied over the anterior aspect of each knee joint. (I now cut a hole in this pad to expose the patella for tracking.) Plaster bandage was wrapped, beginning by overlapping the below-knee cast by 2-3 cm, and terminating at the upper thigh. (I now use Pudgee® foam or T-Stick® on the popliteal surface also, particularly over the hamstrings tendons of insertion.)

The knees were extended only to an angle of approximately 40 degrees of flexion so T. S. would be able to continue to tolerate the sitting position. The plaster was molded close to the posterior aspect of the knee joint to support the proximal tibia against posterior displacement. (Now, I would increase the initial knee angle to 50-55 degrees, or the available range in sitting with the pelvis vertical.)

T. S. began standing in therapy after the casts were dried, using an adapted prone stander (modified to accommodate her flexed knees) both at school and at home. The angle of knee flexion prohibited functional weight-bearing.

November 9—Both knee portions were removed, along with the left below-knee cast. Hamstrings contractures had reduced from over 60 degrees to 41 on the left and 34 degrees on the right (Figure 6.21). Knee extension with the hips extended, however, was still incomplete in both knees.

The left heel had developed a small closed pressure area. Extra padding was applied to the area with cast reapplication. (Since this series, I have learned that a U-shaped pad of adhesive-backed felt, 1/4-inch thick, applied over a layer of Pudgee® foam or T-Stick® around the perimeter of a sore can lift overlying plaster from the site. This pad often can also help promote the healing of a closed sore. At the time I was treating T. S., I was using only standard felt and cotton roll padding material, and I was careful to cover the calcaneus.)

The knees were set at 20 and 25 degrees of flexion in the next pair of casts. The soles were posted by wedging the heels so as to allow optimum weight distribution in standing (Figure 6.22).

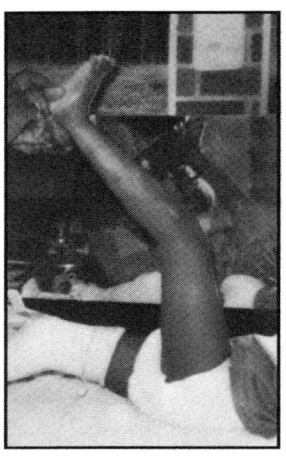

Figure 6.21
November 9, cast change;
popliteal angles:
R = -41 degrees
L = -34 degrees

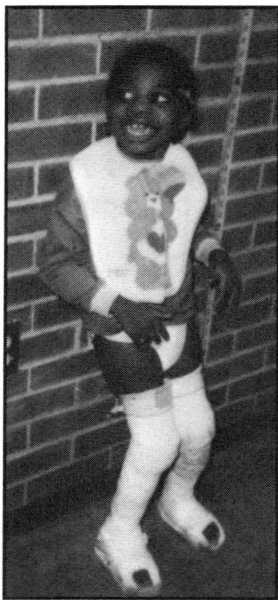

Figure 6.22
Set knees in 20 and 25 degrees of flexion. Posted soles to allow standing with optimum stability.

A standing program was instituted in school and at home. T. S. could stand for 30 to 40 minutes with minimal support and appeared to enjoy doing so. Hip flexion contracture persisted, however.

November 17—No complaints or difficulties since November 9. Removal of the knee portions revealed a popliteal angle of 25 degrees on the right and 22 degrees on the left, with the hip flexed 90 degrees. With hips extended, however, passive extension of the right knee was full, and the left knee lacked 15 degrees. Right ankle mobility was full, with the foot structures aligned in neutral. The status of her left heel was unchanged.

The right knee was set in a functional 5 degrees of flexion. The left was set at 15 degrees, or the maximum comfortable range.

November 30—The mother reported that T. S. was "lazy" about standing in the days preceding this visit. On cast removal small closed pressure sores were noted, one on each heel.

Popliteal angle measured 8 degrees on the right and 16 degrees on the left, with the hip flexed 90 degrees (Figures 6.23 and 6.24).

For evaluative purposes, a crouch-control ankle-foot splint (CAFS) was made for each leg. These splints enabled T. S.'s team to assess the feasibility of a below-knee support system before prescribing an alternative device such as a knee-ankle-foot orthosis (KAFO) that covers and locks the knee joint. The crouch-control ankle-foot splints also provided some distal stabilization at the ankle, which aided T. S. in maintaining the upright position so she could build strength in the quadriceps and triceps surae group. The design of the splints helped heal her heel sores as well, as there is no contact between the posterior heel and the splint (Figure 6.25).

A hinge was added to the right ankle to promote the use of the ankle plantarflexors as stabilizers of the tibia. A cylindrical cast was applied to the left leg, setting the knee at 5 degrees with the foot excluded. This last cast was applied in an effort to gain a few more degrees of extension mobility in the left knee and to offer her some mechanical assistance as she gained strength in the right (uncasted) knee. Cast removal by her physician was scheduled to occur at her next clinic visit on December 17.

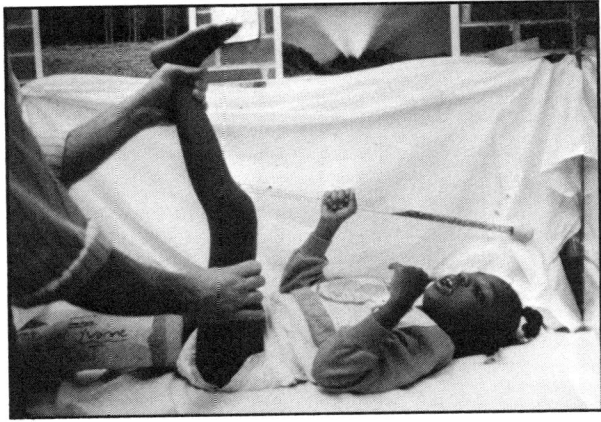

Figure 6.23 November 30:
left popliteal angle: -16 degrees

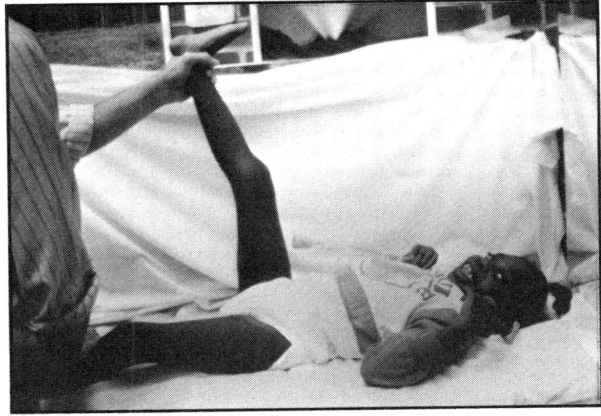

Figure 6.24 November 30:
right popliteal angle: -8 degrees

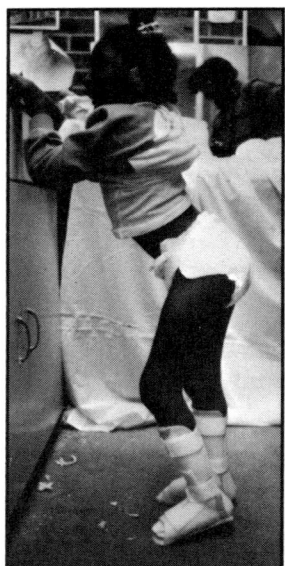

Figure 6.25
Provided evaluative bilateral crouch-control ankle-foot splints: L = solid / R = hinged. Applied long-leg cylindrical holding cast to left leg in 5 degrees of knee flexion. (Hip flexion contracture persists.)

December 17, Follow-up—During the week following the right cast removal, T. S. complained of right knee pain, refusing to take weight on the right (uncasted) leg. It was recommended that she use the canvas knee splint for security against buckling and that her mother contact the doctor for clearance to use children's aspirin to reduce pain or inflammation during this adjustment period.

February 15, Follow-up—Telephone contact with the mother: T. S. is doing well. A pair of bivalved polypropylene ankle-foot orthoses (AFOs) had been ordered for her at the clinic visit in December. Her heels had healed well. She was beginning to gain strength in her extensors. Her mother reported that she was pleased with T. S.'s progress, and that her physician was impressed with the results of casting.

Long-term goal—T. S. will be able to assist actively in transfers and ambulate with contact support over short distances by taking full weight on her feet and supporting herself reliably with help. Surgical lengthening of the iliopsoas is needed to reduce anterior pelvic tilt.

	10/23	10/30	11/9	11/17	11/30	12/17
Maximum Popliteal Angle						
Right	64	64	41	25	8	*
Left	60	60	34	22	16	*
Casted Knee Flexion Angle						
Right	N/A	40	20	5	N/A	*
Left	N/A	40	20	15	5	*
*Cast removed, no data						

Table 1. T. S. Serial Casting Course—total of 45 days—3 cast changes on the right leg, 4 cast changes on the left. October 30: Added plaster above the knee—set the knees at 40 degrees of flexion (not shown).

References

Akeson, W. H., D. Amiel, M. F. Abel, S. R. Gartin, and S. L-Y. Woo. 1987. Effects of immobilization on joints. *Clinical Orthopaedics and Related Research* 219:28-36.

Baumann, J. U., and M. Zumstein. 1985. Experience with a plastic ankle-foot orthosis for prevention of muscle contracture. *Developmental Medicine and Child Neurology* 27:83. (Abstract)

Bertoti, D. B. 1986. Effect of short leg casting on ambulation in children with cerebral palsy. *Physical Therapy* 66(10):1522-1529.

Bly, L. 1980. Personal communication. Charlottesville, VA. May 16.

Bobath, K., and B. Bobath. 1966. *Neurodevelopmental and orthopedic treatments of cerebral palsy.* Western Cerebral Palsy Centre, London, England. (Unpublished paper—instructional materials.)

Booth, B. J., M. Doyle, and J. Montgomery. 1983. Serial casting for the management of spasticity in the head-injured adult. *Physical Therapy* 63(12):1960-1965.

Booth, F. W. 1987. Physiologic and biochemical effects of immobilization on muscle. *Clinical Orthopaedics and Related Research* 219:15-20.

Bowser, B. L., and M. M. Dimitrijevic. 1985. Effects of neuromuscular stimulation on passive ankle dorsiflexion in children with cerebral palsy: A preliminary report. *Developmental Medicine and Child Neurology* 27(5):116-117. (Abstract)

Bunch, W. H., and V. M. Dvonch. 1985. Cerebral palsy. In *Atlas of orthotics,* edited by W. H. Bunch and members of the American Academy of Orthopedic Surgeons. St. Louis, MO: C. V. Mosby.

Carlson, S. J. 1984. A neurophysiological analysis of inhibitive casting. *Physical & Occupational Therapy in Pediatrics* 4(4):31-42.

Carlson, S. J. 1988. Gait changes in a child with cerebral palsy during an inhibitive casting program. *Physical & Occupational Therapy in Pediatrics* 8(1):93. (Thesis abstract)

Carpenter, D. 1989. Personal communication. Scranton, PA. February 4.

Cary, J. M., R. Lusskin, and R. G. Thompson. 1975. Prescription principles. In *Atlas of orthotics,* compiled by the American Academy of Orthopedic Surgeons. St. Louis, MO: C. V. Mosby.

Coram, S. 1989. Personal communication. Cincinnati, OH. March 9.

Cusick, B. D. 1980. Developmental programs for children in below-knee casts. In *Proceedings: Orthopedic aspects of developmental disabilities, 2d ed.,* edited by J. M. Wilson and L. A. Davis. Division of Physical Therapy, Department of Medical Allied Health Professions, School of Medicine, Wing C 221 H, University of North Carolina, Chapel Hill, NC.

Cusick, B. D. 1988. *Serial casts: Their use in the management of spasticity-induced foot deformity, 2d ed.* Words at Work; distributed by Therapy Skill Builders, Tucson, AZ.

Cusick, B. D., and M. D. Sussman. 1982. Short-leg casts: Their role in the management of cerebral palsy. *Physical & Occupational Therapy in Pediatrics* 2(2/3):93-110.

Diamond, M. 1988. Peripheral alcohol nerve blocks as an adjunct to the management of spasticity. *Developmental Medicine and Child Neurology* 30(5):13. (Abstract.)

Domisse, G. 1963. The role of surgery in cerebral palsy. *South African Medical Journal* 16(2):188-190.

Duncan, W. 1960. Tonic reflexes of the foot: Their orthopedic significance in normal children and in children with cerebral palsy. *Journal of Bone and Joint Surgery* 42-A(5):859-868.

Duncan, W. R., and D. H. Mott. 1983. Foot reflexes and the use of the "inhibitive cast." *Foot & Ankle* 4(2):145-148.

Enneking, W. F., and M. Horowitz. 1972. The intra-articular effects of immobilization on the human knee. *Journal of Bone and Joint Surgery* 54-A:973-976.

Evans, C. D. 1981. *Rehabilitation after severe head injury*. New York, NY: Churchill Livingstone.

Evans, E.B., G. W. N. Eggars, J. K. Butler, and J. Blumel. 1960. Experimental immobilization and remobilization of rat knee joints. *Journal of Bone and Joint Surgery* 42-A:737-740.

Ford, C., R. C. Grotz, and J. K. Shamp. 1986. The neurophysiological ankle-foot orthosis. *Clinical Prosthetics and Orthotics* 10(1):15-23.

Ganley, J. V. 1984. Corrective casting in infants. In *Symposium on podopediatrics—Clinics in podiatry*, edited by J. V. Ganley, 501-516. Philadelphia, PA: W. B. Saunders Co.

Goldner, J. L. 1982. Foot and ankle deformities in cerebral palsy (static encephalopathy). In *Disorders of the foot, vol. 1*, edited by M. H. Jahss, 282-334. Philadelphia, PA: W. B. Saunders.

Griffith, E. R. 1983. Spasticity. In *Rehabilitation of the head injured adult*, edited by M. Rosenthal, E. R. Griffith, M. R. Bond, and J. D. Miller, 125-140. Philadelphia, PA: F. A. Davis.

Gritzka, T. L., and C. Gerlach. 1986. Serial short leg casts for the treatment of equinus deformity in cerebral palsy. *Developmental Medicine and Child Neurology* 28(5):6-7. (Abstract)

Groen, T. E., and G. Domisse. 1964. Plaster casts in the conservative treatment of cerebral palsy. *South African Medical Journal* 38:502-505.

Harrington, E. D., R. S. Lin, and J. R. Gage. 1983-84. Use of the anterior floor reaction orthosis in patients with cerebral palsy. *Orthotics and Prosthetics* (Spring):34-42.

Harris, S. R., and K. Riffle. 1986. Effects of inhibitive ankle-foot orthoses on standing balance in a child with cerebral palsy: A single-subject design. *Physical Therapy* 66(5):663-666.

Hausermann, U. 1972. Application of standing-position plaster in cerebral palsy (indications, reasons and technique). *Rehabilitation* (©Georg Thieme Verlag, Stuttgart) 11:9-19.

Hayes, N. K., and Y. R. Burns. 1970. Discussion on the use of weight-bearing plasters in the reduction of hypertonicity. *Australian Journal of Physiotherapy* 16(3):108-117.

Hinderer, K. A., S. R. Harris, A. H. Purdy, D. E. Chew, L. T. Staheli, J. F. McLaughlin, and K. M. Jaffe. 1988. Effects of "tone-reducing" vs. standard plaster casts on gait improvement of children with cerebral palsy. *Developmental Medicine and Child Neurology* 30(3):370-377.

Hoffer, M. M., R. T. Knoebel, and R. Roberts. 1987. Contractures in cerebral palsy. *Clinical Orthopaedics and Related Research* 219:70-77.

Howell, D. W. 1988. Therapeutic exercise and mobilization. In *Physical Therapy of the Foot and Ankle*, edited by G. C. Hunt, 257-284. New York: Churchill Livingstone.

Hylton, N. 1988. Personal communication and course hand-out. Kansas City, MO. May 23.

Jaffe, M. B., J. P. Mastrilli, C. B. Molitor, and A. S. Valko. 1985. Intervention for motor disorders. In *Head injury rehabilitation: Children and adolescents*, edited by M. Ylvisaker, 175-194. San Diego, CA: College-Hill Press.

Jordan, R. P. 1984. Therapeutic considerations of the feet and lower extremities in the cerebral palsied child. In *Symposium on podopediatrics—Clinics in podiatry*, edited by J. V. Ganley, 547-561. Philadelphia, PA: W. B. Saunders Co.

Jordan, R. P., J. Cusack, and B. Resseque. 1983. *Foot function and its relationship to posture in the pediatric patient with cerebral palsy and other neuromuscular disorders.* Symposium—sponsored by the Neurodevelopmental Treatment Association, New York: May 20-22.

Kahn, N., and J. Hylton. 1973. Casting used as an adjunct to neurodevelopmental treatment. *NDT Newsletter* (Newsletter of the Curative Workshop of Milwaukee—United Cerebral Palsy of Wisconsin, Inc.) 5(2):1-3.

Levitt, S. 1982. *Treatment of cerebral palsy and motor delay, 2d ed.* Boston, MA: Blackwell Scientific Publications.

McCrea, J. D. 1985. *Pediatric orthopedics of the lower extremity: An instructional handbook.* Mount Kisco, NY: Futura.

McDonough, M. W. 1984. Angular and axial deformities of the legs of children. In *Symposium on podopediatrics—Clinics in podiatry*, edited by J. V. Ganley, 601-620. Philadelphia, PA: W. B. Saunders Co.

Mills, V. M. 1984. Electromyographic results of inhibitory splinting. *Physical Therapy* 64(2):190-193.

Mohr, J. D. 1977. Personal communication, Charlottesville, Virginia. March 8-10.

Molnar, G. E. 1985. Cerebral palsy. In *Pediatric rehabilitation*, edited by G. E. Molnar. Baltimore, MD: Williams and Wilkins.

Otis, J. C., L. Root, and M. A. Kroll. 1985. Measurement of plantar flexor spasticity during treatment with tone-reducing casts. *Journal of Pediatric Orthopaedics* 5:682-686.

Rang, M., R. Silver, and J. de la Garza. 1986. Cerebral palsy. In *Pediatric orthopaedics, 2d ed.*, edited by W. W. Lovell and R. B. Winter, 345-396. Philadelphia, PA: J. B. Lippincott.

Sirna, E., and M. D. Sussman. 1986. Immediate mobilization of patients after tendo-Achilles lengthening. *Developmental Medicine and Child Neurology* 28(5):17. (Abstract)

Snavely, K. M., M. L. Brown, and R. T. Hellman. 1986. New directions in fiber glass casting. *Developmental Medicine and Child Neurology* 28(5):54. (Abstract)

Spencer, A. M., and V. A. Person. 1984. Casting and orthotics for children. *Symposium on podopediatrics—Clinics in podiatry*, edited by J. V. Ganley, 621-629. Philadelphia, PA: W. B. Saunders Co.

Sussman, M. D. 1980. Use of casts as an adjunct to physical therapy management of cerebral palsy patients. In *Proceedings: Orthopedic aspects of developmental disabilities, 2d ed.*, edited by J. M. Wilson and L. A. Davis, 47-59. Division of Physical Therapy, Department of Medical Allied Health Professions, School of Medicine, Wing C 221 H, University of North Carolina, Chapel Hill, NC.

Sussman, M. D. 1983. Casting as an adjunct to neurodevelopmental therapy for cerebral palsy. *Developmental Medicine and Child Neurology* 25:801-802.

Sussman, M. D., and B. D. Cusick. 1981. Early mobilization of patients with cerebral palsy following muscle release surgery. *Orthopaedic Transactions* 5:193. (Abstract)

Tardieu, C., A. Lespargot, C. Tabary, and M. D. Bret. 1988. For how long must the soleus muscle be stretched each day to prevent contracture? *Developmental Medicine and Child Neurology* 30:3-10.

Tardieu, G., and C. Tardieu. 1987. Cerebral palsy: Mechanical evaluation and conservative correction of limb joint contractures. *Clinical Orthopaedics and Related Research* 219:63-70.

Tardieu, G., C. Tardieu, P. Colbeau-Justin, and A. Lespargot. 1982. Muscle hypoextensibility in children with cerebral palsy: II. Therapeutic implications. *Archives of Physical Medicine and Rehabilitation* 63:103-107.

Truscelli, J. A., D. A. Lespargot, and G. Tardieu. 1979. Variations in the long-term results of elongation of the tendo-Achilles in children with cerebral palsy. *Journal of Bone and Joint Surgery* 51-B(4):466-469.

Valmassy, R. L. 1984. Biomechanical evaluation of the child. In *Symposium on podopediatrics—Clinics in podiatry*, edited by J. V. Ganley, 563-579. Philadelphia, PA: W. B. Saunders Co.

Watt, J., D. Sims, F. Harckham, L. Schmidt, A. McMillan, and J. Hamilton. 1986. A prospective study of inhibitive casting as an adjunct to physiotherapy for cerebral-palsied children. *Developmental Medicine and Child Neurology* 28(4):480-488.

Westin, G. W. 1980. Conservative nonoperative treatment of spastic cerebral palsy. *Orthopaedic Transactions* 4:68. (Abstract)

Westin, G. W., and S. Dye. 1983. Conservative management of cerebral palsy in the growing child. *Foot & Ankle* 4(3):160-163.

Wilson, B. D., and R. E. Allen. 1962. Splints in the treatment of cerebral palsy. *Physiotherapy* 48:41-44.

Wilson, J. M. 1984. Cerebral palsy. In *Pediatric neurologic physical therapy*, edited by S. K. Campbell. New York: Churchill Livingstone.

Yates, H. L. 1979. Personal communication. Charlottesville, Virginia. April 28.

Yates, H. L., and D. H. Mott. 1977. Inhibitive casting. In *Proceedings: First William C. Duncan Seminar on Cerebral Palsy*. Seattle, WA: University of Washington.

Zachazewski, J. E., E. D. Eberle, and M. Jefferies. 1982. Effect of tone-inhibiting casts and orthoses on gait. *Physical Therapy* 62(4):453-455.

CHAPTER 7

Splinting the Foot and Ankle—the Basics of Fabrication and Implementation

Objectives for the Reader

- To arrange the splinting area for optimum positioning, viewing of the extremity by the clinician, and diversions for the children.

- To assemble the necessary equipment and materials.

- To recall the basic considerations for fabrication of splints with elastic thermoplastics, relative to: (a) positioning the extremity; (b) holding the body segments for optimum correction of deformity; and (c) cooling the splint material before removing the mold from the child's foot.

- To prioritize the stages in molding the foot and ankle joints, beginning with the STJ/MTJ relationship and ending with ankle position.

- To explain the problems associated with molding using a copolymer or Plexiglas® "footboard" to flatten the plantar aspect of the splint.

- To define the process of posting as a method of securing proper alignment of foot structures for weight-bearing.

- To distinguish between a splint or orthosis whose features appear to meet the criteria for optimum alignment of the foot and ankle and one that does not.

- To describe the features of a desirable shoe to wear with a foot or ankle-foot splint.

- To discuss principles of progression among the varying designs of splint for the foot and ankle—for example, when to reduce support and when to increase it.

This chapter begins with a review of the process of making lower-extremity splints with low-temperature, elastic thermoplastics, such as Aquaplast-T® and Orfit® (Figure 7.1). Rather than providing step-by-step fabrication procedures for each of the existing splint designs, the principles employed in correcting soft tissue deformities during the molding process are outlined. The principles are applied to the problems of flexible pes valgus, functional equinovalgus, functional equinovarus, and crouch deformity. The fabrication techniques that implement these principles change and improve regularly and are most effectively shared in a practicum workshop setting. A discussion section follows, in which commonly asked questions are addressed.

Most of the splint fabrication techniques presented in this chapter were developed by Michael Smith, OTC, and me, as well as by participants in instructional workshops sessions who have offered their insights and experience over the past eight years. This evolutionary process will undoubtedly continue. The basic supplies and techniques of handling both the splinting material and the child are described. These methods should bring about successful fabrication of a foot- or ankle-foot splint, regardless of the specific design. Before making any splint, however, a thorough evaluation is required (see the Pediatric Biomechanical Assessment Form in Appendix 5). An alternative to goniometric evaluation of the foot and lower leg is detailed below.

Evaluating Lower Leg Structural Alignment with the Angle Finder

Until you have practiced these assessment techniques and feel confident in executing them unaided, call upon an assistant to hold the extremity for you. Undertake the open-chain assessments with the child lying prone, with the hip extended and the knee flexed. If it is necessary to raise the trunk and pelvis on pillows to alleviate lumbar lordosis and tensile strain on shortened hip flexors, then do so. The femoral condyles must remain on the frontal plane. All measures in the following assessment procedures are taken using an angle finder. (See Appendix 4 for sources.) Because of the gravity-related movement of the floating needle, the values are obtained relative to the sagittal and transverse planes. The distal leg segment must therefore be aligned precisely on the sagittal plane while you evaluate foot structures. This position is necessary to gain measures of subtalar and midtarsal joint neutrality and motion relative to the vertical bisection of the distal lower leg.

Open-Chain Assessments

To find evidence of distal varum in the lower leg:

1. Set the proximal, anterior tibial crest on the sagittal plane and hold it there (Figure 7.1).

2. Measure the angle formed by the vertical bisection of the posterior aspect of the distal lower leg. Keep the straight edge of the angle finder proximal to the Achilles tendon. Press it into the skin to blanch it, and remove it to assess skin discoloration for evidence of accurate midline placement of the bisection line (Figure 7.2).

3. Record any difference between the proximal and distal values. If the value for varum is greater than 2 degrees, it is used to position the leg and foot segments properly while molding ankle-foot splints.

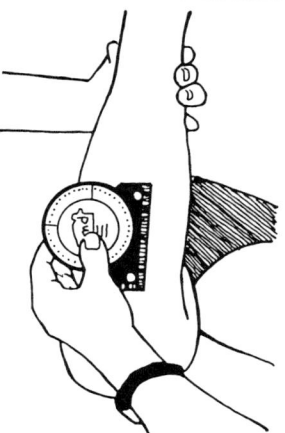

Figure 7.1 LEFT LEG. Set the proximal tibial crest on the sagittal plane and hold it there . . .

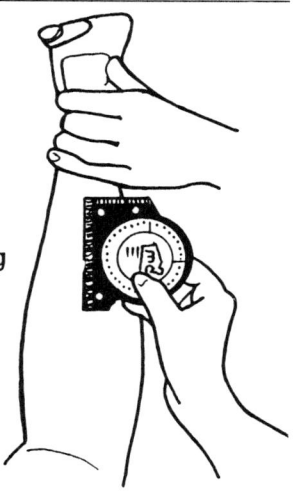

Figure 7.2 LEFT LEG. . . . while you hold the straight edge of the angle finder on the vertical bisection of the posterior distal lower leg. Record any difference in values between the distal and proximal values, indicating medial rotation or torsion.

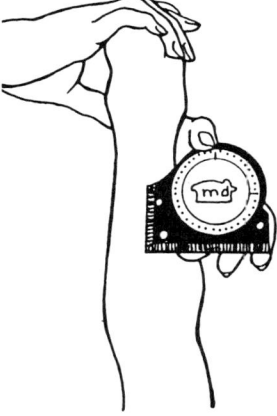

Figure 7.3
RIGHT FOOT.
STJ mobility on the frontal plane: Set the distal lower leg bisection and the calcaneal bisection on the sagittal plane and hold the leg there.

To determine frontal plane STJ mobility:

1. Set the distal lower leg on the sagittal plane and hold it there (Figure 7.3).

2. Invert the calcaneus. Note the range of excursion. Measure it if it appears abnormally limited (that is, less than 8 degrees) (Figure 7.4). Rub the posterior calcaneal ridges to blanch them. Press the straight edge of the angle finder into the skin between the ridges and remove it. Note whether the blanched line is in the center of the ridges. Repeat the process until you are satisfied that you have ascertained the midline calcaneal bisection. While the distal lower leg is held on the sagittal plane, this value equals the angle of inversion formed by the calcaneus and the lower leg.

3. Evert the calcaneus (Figure 7.5). To measure the range of excursion, longitudinally bisect the posterior calcaneus. When you are satisfied that the straight edge is placed on the calcaneal bisection, check the alignment of the distal lower leg to ascertain that it remains on the sagittal plane. Holding the leg very still, take

repeated measures of the calcaneal angle by removing and applying the angle finder until three consecutive measures are in agreement, and record (Figure 7.6).

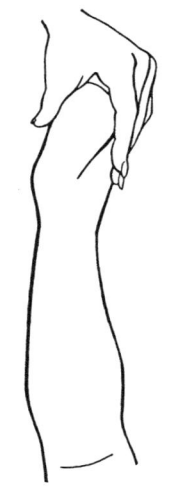

Figure 7.4
RIGHT FOOT.
Prohibit the ankle
from plantarflexing.
Invert the calcaneus
on the frontal plane.

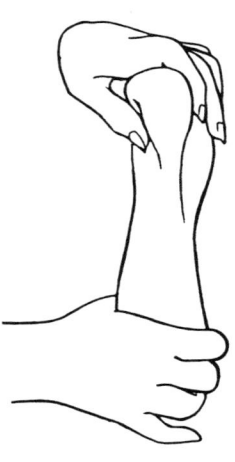

Figure 7.5
RIGHT FOOT
Evert the calcaneus
on the frontal plane.

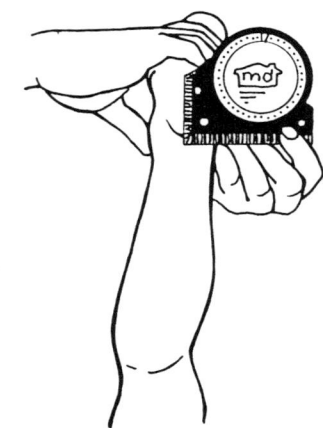

Figure 7.6   Measure the angle formed by the posterior calcaneal bisection and the lower leg bisection (which is aligned on the sagittal plane).

To determine STJ neutral position in the open chain:

1. Align the vertical bisection of the distal lower leg on the sagittal plane (Figure 7.3).

2. Palpate the talar head while supinating and pronating the lower segment of the foot. Feel also for relative dimple depth at the dorsal depressions beside the tendons of the anterior tibialis and the long toe extensor.

3. Lock the forefoot on the hindfoot when the medial talar head is congruous with the navicular tuberosity (and the dorsal depressions are equally deep) (Figure 7.7).

Figure 7.7   Neutral STJ position: Maintaining the distal lower leg precisely on the sagittal plane, palpate the talar head and the dorsal depressions until talonavicular congruity is achieved. Lock the forefoot on the hindfoot by gently loading the distal lateral pillar. Measure the calcaneal angle with the lower leg (on the sagittal plane). Proceed to forefoot assessment (Figure 7.8).

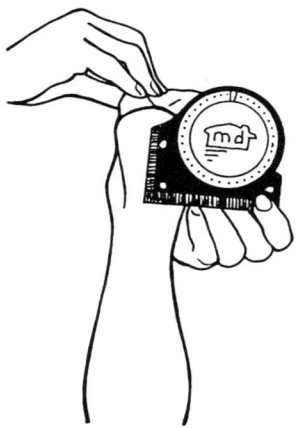

4. Check for distal lower leg alignment on the sagittal plane.

5. Use the straight edge of the angle finder to bisect the posterior calcaneus (as described above).

6. Take repeated measures of the calcaneus in STJ neutral position until three consecutive measures are in agreement.

The resulting value is the angle formed by the calcaneal bisection with the lower leg bisection. If the lower leg tilts off the sagittal plane, this reading will be altered and inaccurate.

To determine forefoot alignment with the foot in neutral position:

1. Maintain the distal lower leg on the sagittal plane with the STJ and MTJ locked in congruity.

2. Lay the horizontal straight edge of the angle finder on the plantar surfaces of all five metatarsal heads. The resulting value is the angle formed by the forefoot and the transverse plane. It represents the excursion required to bring the metatarsal heads down from congruity to full contact with the ground (Figure 7.8).

3. Calculate the forefoot varus or valgus angle relative to the hindfoot by subtracting the STJ neutral value obtained at the calcaneus from this value at the forefoot.

For example, if the value obtained at the metatarsal heads with the foot structures held in congruity is 12 degrees varus, and the calcaneal neutral value is 6 degrees varus, the forefoot/hindfoot varus relationship is 12 minus 6, or 6 degrees. When the plantar calcaneal condyles (or tubercles) lower to the ground as the calcaneus aligns in vertical position, the forefoot remains in 6 degrees of varus. If the calcaneal excursion into eversion totals 6 degrees or more, the hindfoot can evert to accomplish the lowering of the varus forefoot to the ground. This event prolongs the timing of pronation in the stance cycle. The resulting weight transfer over the flexible foot is inefficient. If the calcaneal excursion is less than 6 degrees, compensation to lower the medial metatarsal heads to the ground occurs either at the midtarsal joint, the first ray, the STJ via abduction (rather than eversion), or more proximally than the STJ. The result is active reduction of forefoot varus deviation.

Figure 7.8   RIGHT FOOT. Determining forefoot position: With the STJ aligned first in congruity and second in midposition, gently load the lateral metatarsals and lay the horizontal straight edge of the angle finder on the plantar surface of all five metatarsal heads. The resulting value equals the excursion required for the forefoot to lower to the transverse plane from a position of congruity. To calculate forefoot on hindfoot position, subtract the value for the STJ from this measure. (If forefoot value is less than calcaneal value, the forefoot position is one of valgus.)

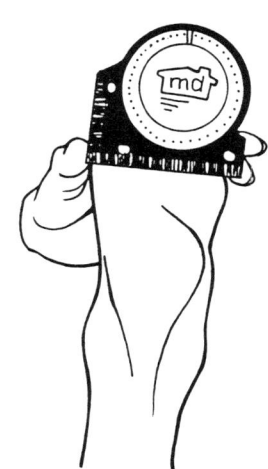

On the other hand, if the varus deviation at the forefoot is less than that at the hindfoot, then as the inverted calcaneus attempts to lower to the sagittal plane, the forefoot everts relative to the hindfoot. This forefoot valgus relationship usually occurs in the presence of abnormal limitation of calcaneal eversion mobility, and might indicate the presence of a rigid plantarflexed first ray.

Closed-Chain Assessments

To evaluate the STJ complex in the closed chain:

1. In relaxed stance, with the legs aligned in their normal base and angle of gait and the foot fully loaded, blanch the posterior ridges of the calcaneus and ascertain the location of the bisection. Take repeated measures of the angle formed by the bisection of the calcaneus until you achieve three consecutive identical readings. The resulting value represents the angle of *relaxed calcaneal stance,* which is the angle formed by the calcaneal bisection and the sagittal plane (Figure 7.9).

2. Measure the vertical bisection of the distal lower leg relative to the sagittal plane in relaxed stance. Record the resulting value (not shown). This value for apparent tibial varum represents evidence of medial rotation of the lower leg in relaxed stance.

3. Palpate the talar head while rotating the weight-bearing lower leg laterally and medially. The talar head will protrude behind the navicular in pronation, which occurs with medial leg rotation. It will protrude on the dorsum of the foot, under the tendon of the long toe extensors, in supination; this protrusion occurs with lateral leg rotation. Having gained a sense of congruity of the talar head and the navicular, particularly on the medial articulation, palpate the dimples on the dorsum of the ankle to determine relative depth. If the depth is even when you compare the two depressions, you have obtained a measure of confirmation for the position of STJ congruity. Now measure the angle of the calcaneal bisection while maintaining congruity (Figure 7.10). Compare this value with what you obtained in open-chain assessment. They should be the same. This value is the *neutral calcaneal stance position.*

4. Maintain the STJ congruity and take a measure of the distal lower leg bisection. Record the result. Varum often resolves to 0 to 2 degrees when the foot structures are aligned in congruity in the closed chain, as a result of the concurrent lateral rotation of the lower leg.

5. Reduce the STJ (calcaneal) angle to 0 degrees (the sagittal plane). Maintain the calcaneal position and take another measure of the distal lower leg. If it is greater than 2 degrees, record and use this value to tilt the lower leg medially the same amount while molding a splint with a vertical calcaneus. This value is the *functional calcaneal midstance position.*

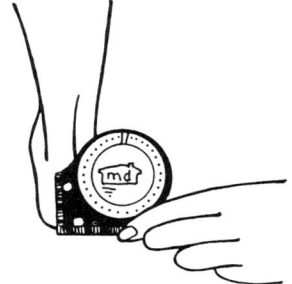

Figure 7.9 Closed-chain assessment of STJ status. Relaxed calcaneal stance: Place child in standing position at normal angle of gait. Measure the angle formed by the vertical calcaneal bisection and the sagittal plane. (Floating needle on the level finds the sagittal plane.) Check the angle at the distal lower leg bisection (not shown). Repeat the latter measurement after rotating the lower leg to align the calcaneus on the sagittal plane.

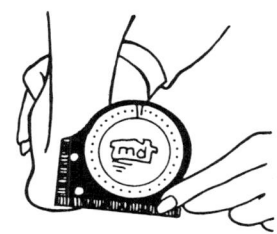

Figure 7.10 Closed-chain assessment of STJ neutrality. Shift weight onto the leg to be tested. Neutral calcaneal stance: Rotate the lower leg medially and laterally while palpating the talar head and dorsal depressions. Halt rotations and maintain the posture when talonavicular congruity is perceived. Measure the calcaneal bisection angle. (The value should concur with open-chain value.) Measure distal lower leg bisection angle in this position also (not shown).

Splint Fabrication—the Basics

Preparing the Splint Area

Have the water hot and all the splinting materials you will use—including the tools—laid out before you begin. (Each time I omit this step, I regret doing so, because the fabrication process loses its flow when I have to scramble through drawers for scissors or screw rivets.) It would also be time-efficient to precut several adhesive-backed pads in various sizes. Arrange to have mirrors in place, so you can see the foot from two or more additional perspectives and so the interested child can watch.

Entertaining the Child

Before you begin to take the mold for any device, call upon an assistant—whether a parent, caregiver, nurse, or aide—and equip that person with an assortment of developmentally appropriate toys, puzzles, picture books, paper and crayons, tortilla chips . . . whatever works to distract the child from your work. Other suggestions that have met with success include a family photo album, silly songs and well-known stories, quizzes about the morning's breakfast menu, plans for stopping at the hamburger place on the way home, and cuddling. Be prepared to entertain.

Positioning the Child

For the purpose of taking the mold, place the child in the prone position on a padded table or on a floor mat, with trunk and pelvis in midline, the knee flexed and the hips extended (Figure 7.11). This position, however disconcerting initially for the clinician who is unfamiliar with the foot from this angle, grants full visual access to

Figure 7.11
Position the child in prone
with hips extended and
knee flexed to gain visual
access to the entire foot.

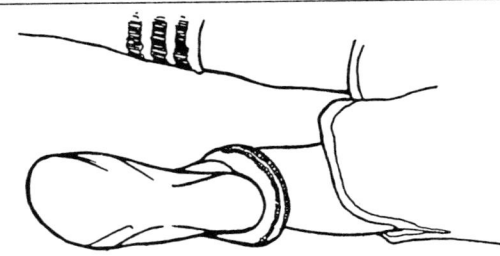

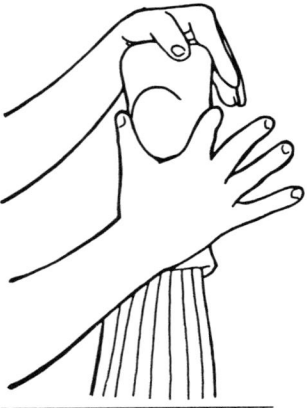

Figure 7.12
Maintain precise
sagittal and trans-
verse plane
perspectives on the
foot and leg.

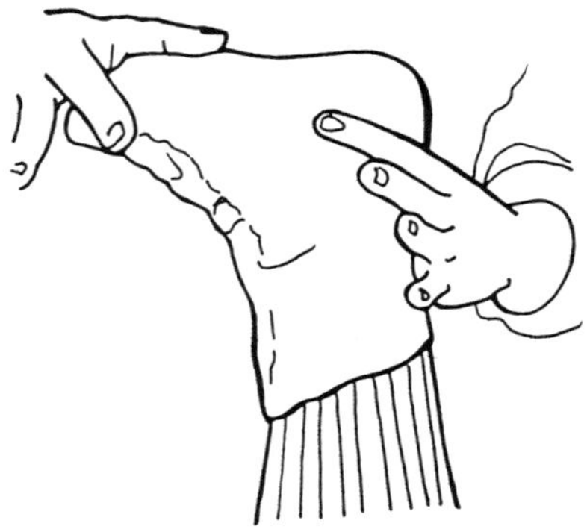

Figure 7.13 Frontal plane view reveals
talocrural joint angle.

the contour of the sole of the foot, as well as to the sagittal, transverse, and frontal plane alignment of the foot structures and the ankle (Figures 7.12 and 7.13). Well-placed mirrors aid in visualization when the assistant is not trained to recognize the significant features of alignment.

There are circumstances in which positioning in prone is difficult to manage, such as the predominance of an obligatory tonic labyrinthine reflex, severe contractures at the hips, or fear. If any of these circumstances arise, first try to gain prone position by using pillows under the trunk, head, and pelvis, to relieve tensile strain on shortened hip flexors and the lumbar spine. The important feature of lower leg alignment is the sagittal plane orientation of the lower leg, not the upper leg. The child must be comfortable, however, for the ten minutes it will take to evaluate the foot structures and to make the mold.

If adapting the prone-lying surface fails, support the child in sitting on a large chair (placed in front of a caregiver) or in the caregiver's lap. Adapt the procedure accordingly. Because visual access to the foot and ankle is significantly compromised in this arrangement, place small mirrors behind and at either side of the child's foot to improve visual access during molding.

Materials

Most splint procedures require the following supplies and equipment, or their equivalents (see Appendix 4 for sources):

- Splint material, either Orfit® or Aquaplast-T®. The thickness used most often in pediatrics is 1/8-inch (28.57 mm). However, Aquaplast-T® is also available in 3/32-inch, 1/16-inch, and 3/16-inch thicknesses, all of which have clinical application. Keep some of each thickness in stock.

- Either a temperature-regulated waterbath, a large electric skillet, a large hot-pack heating unit (with the rack in place), or a deep cookie sheet on two large stove burners. Heat the water to 160 degrees F (71 degrees C) to use Aquaplast-T®, or 135 degrees F (57 degrees C) to use Orfit®. Usually, the "W" of the "warm" setting on a thermal rheostat heats a standard electric skillet to the appropriate temperature.

- A plastic mesh guard for the bottom of any heating unit.

- Cotton stockinet. Use 100 percent cotton, not a synthetic or blended fabric, because synthetics will stick fiercely to the inner surface of the splint. For most small children, using a stockinet width of 1 to 1½ inches avoids making wrinkles in the ankle area of the splint. Keep various widths of stockinet in stock.

- Adhesive-backed Plastazote® padding, 1/8-inch and 3/16-inch thicknesses.

- Adhesive-backed moleskin (preferably made with paper backing).

- SabreGrip®—an adhesive-backed form of Velcro® hook. The mushroom loop offers three times the shear strength of a standard Velcro® hook.

- Plain-backed Velcro® loop—1½-inch or 2-inch width.

- Universal® bandage shears with protective plastic tips.

- Utility knife.

- A heat gun with a funnel-type cap for spot heating.

- A Samson® 1/4-inch hole punch, or a similar sturdy device for punching holes 1/4-inch in diameter in thick plastic material. A standard leather punch will not suffice.

- A wax marking pencil or washable crayon in a dark color.

- Edge finisher (optional).

- Vegetable shortening.

- A tape measure.

- A bucket of iced water and washcloth.

- Wax remover or splint solvent cement.

- Aluminum screw rivets (for hinged devices), 1/4-inch in length.

The clinician who has been trained in making the contoured plaster footboard may wish to use a thin, intrinsic footplate during splint fabrication. If that is the case, the following materials are needed:

- A piece of vinyl flooring with a pulp-like backing bonded firmly to the plastic and cut to a size that is 2 inches larger than the foot.

- 10 plaster splints (4 inches x 15 inches) or 1 roll of plaster bandage, cut into small stacks of squares, rectangles, and strips of varying sizes. Double the amount for two feet.
- Washable ink marker.
- Aquaplast-T® or Orfit®—1/16-inch thickness, cut to equal the size of the plantar surface of the foot plus 2 cm.

Fabrication Procedure

After gathering the materials and arranging the work space, you can expect to follow certain fabrication steps regardless of the chosen design.

Consider your assessment findings (detailed above) in determining optimal leg and foot position for molding the splint. Your goal is to align the weight-bearing calcaneus in vertical position while allowing small pronatory and supinatory excursions within the splint around that midline calcaneal orientation during the stance cycle.

If, before molding any splint that includes the entire foot, the trained clinician wishes first to make a thin, contoured, plantar interface from a plaster footboard mold, I suggest that the footboard be constructed in the following manner:

- Align the calcaneus within 2 degrees of vertical position.
- Define both medial and lateral longitudinal arches.
- Seat the calcaneus in a very shallow cup.
- Support the metatarsal arch only slightly, if at all.
- Do not build the surface of the footboard around the sides of any part of the foot (Figure 7.14). If vertical walls are evident in the footboard, even the thinnest splint material will reduce the space between sidewalls. The resulting footplate will be too narrow for the foot and will have to be heated and flared out before molding.
- For any design other than those that are used for control of crouch posture, do not post the forefoot and toes in the footboard. This postpones the decision to provide intrinsic forefoot posting and toe support of varying degrees and firmness to a later time, at fitting and checkout, or after a few days of wear (Figures 7.14 and 7.15).

The crouch-control designs are excluded from this consideration because of the need for friction-free application of the splint over the foot through the posterior opening. The footplate for these designs is molded from a plaster footboard that incorporates a hindfoot and/or forefoot varus post if one is needed. The resulting footplate is posted extrinsically before it is built into the floor of the device. The thin, contoured Aquaplast-T® or Orfit® footplate is then temporarily attached to the plantar aspect of the foot with tape or adhesive-backed Velcro®. The splint is fabricated around the footplate.

The footplate is not used for molding a stabilizing foot splint (SFS) for the following reasons: it adds bulk to the finished splint, the forefoot of the SFS is typically trimmed away, and the smallest number of variables of foot and ankle position are addressed in the SFS.

For further information regarding footboard fabrication, the reader is referred to the following clinicians:

- Susan Coram, MS, PT, Maternal and Child Therapy Center, 2332 Eastgate Blvd., Baton Rouge, LA 70816.
- Linda Yates, Director of Therapy Services, Children's Therapy Unit, Good Samaritan Hospital and Rehabilitation Center, Puyallup, WA 98371.
- Nancy Hylton, PT, Children's Therapy Center, 26461 104th Avenue, S. E., Kent, WA 98031.

Because plaster footboard fabrication falls outside the realm of this text, the following considerations for splint fabrication are presented. These techniques were developed with clinical experience gained during 10 years of fabricating splints without the contoured footboard.

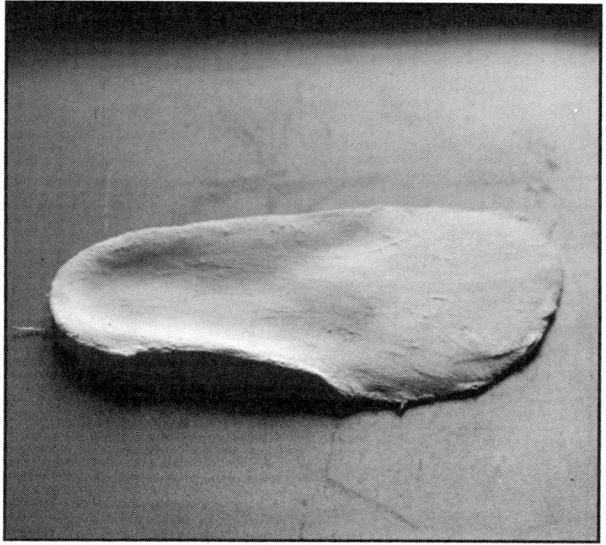

Figure 7.14   Plaster contoured footboard is useful as a positive mold for a thin, plantar footplate interface. Leave the metatarsal heads and toes unposted on the plaster mold.

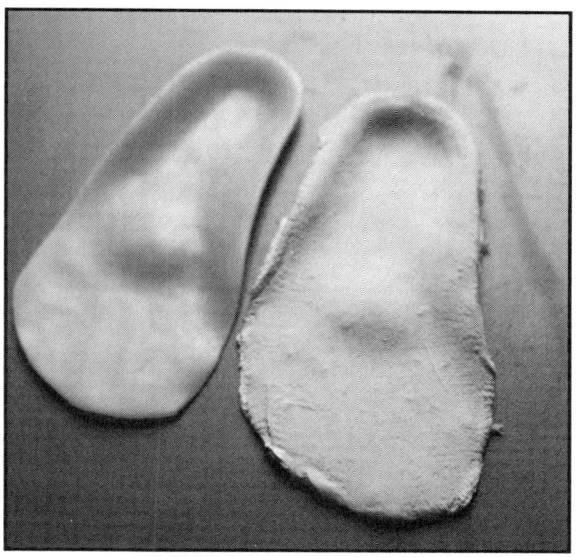

Figure 7.15   Lay heated 1/16-inch thickness Aquaplast-T® into the plaster mold. Grease your fingertips with vegetable shortening and rub the splint material into all of the contours as it sets. Remove the thin mold from the footboard and trim away any material that is broader than the weight-bearing plantar surface of the foot. Use the footplate as an interface, molding it into devices that incorporate the entire foot.

Padding for Protection and Plantar Contour

1. Apply pads to the skin to form recesses in the contour of the heated splint as it sets. The recesses in the hardened splint relieve pressure on bony prominences. For ankle-foot splints, cover the medial malleolus, the navicular, and the medial talar head with one ear-shaped pad made of 1/8-inch adhesive-backed Plastazote® (Figure 7.16). Cover the lateral malleolus and palpate for any remaining bony prominences, including the base of the fifth metatarsal, the lateral head of the talus, or the medial

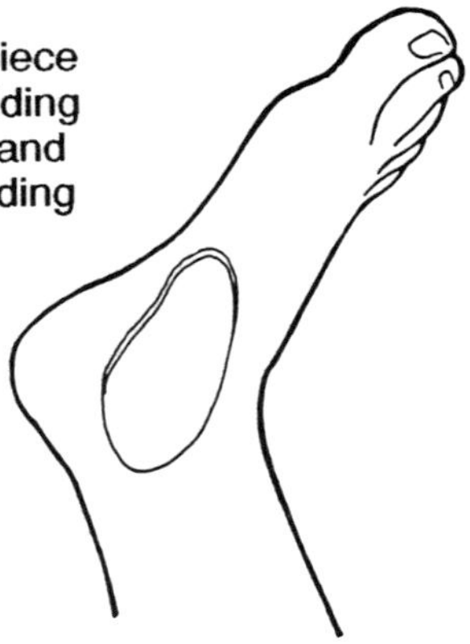

Figure 7.16
Apply one ear-shaped piece
of adhesive-backed padding
to the medial malleolus and
the navicular head. Padding
will form recesses
in the finished splint.

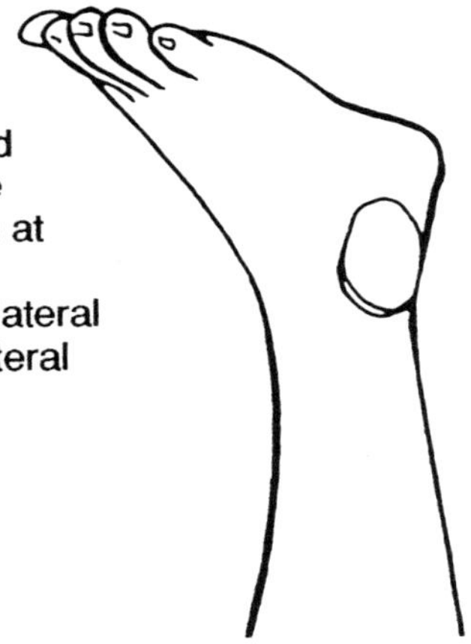

Figure 7.17
Pad the lateral
malleolus. Evaluate
the foot structures and
postures to determine
the need for recesses at
the base of the fifth
metatarsal, the dorsolateral
talar head, and the lateral
or medial
forefoot and toe.

side of the first metatarsal head (Figure 7.17). If the forefoot sweeps strongly into abduction with pronation or into adduction with supination, consider padding the distal lateral or medial forefoot accordingly. The pads are usually replaced in the finished splint and covered with moleskin.

Hinged ankle-foot devices require application of a second pad, 3/16-inch thick, to each malleolus. The extra recess afforded by the double pad allows normal rotary movement of the malleoli within the splint without abrading the skin.

Stabilizing foot splints require relief pads only for the lower segment structures, particularly the navicular tuberosity. The malleoli are not included.

If you observe more than 2 degrees of varum in the weight-bearing distal lower leg with the calcaneus aligned in midline, tilt the distal aspect of the lower leg bisection medially the same amount while molding any splint that incorporates the lower leg. Maintain the calcaneus on the sagittal plane at the same time. You can expect the resulting splint to promote a replication of the calcaneal/lower leg relationship that occurs when the calcaneus is aligned in midline.

2. If the assessment of foot structures reveals abnormal forefoot varus relative to the neutrally aligned hindfoot, reduction of varus hindfoot alignment to within 2 degrees of vertical may result in residual forefoot varus of abnormal magnitudes (that is, greater than 10 degrees after age 1 year, greater than 5 degrees between ages 2 and 6 years, or greater than 2 degrees after age 7 years). If that happens, post the plantar surface of the metatarsal heads before molding the splint (Figures 7.18 and 7.19). The result is a shell that is stable, with the plantar aspect of the forefoot and the bisection of the calcaneus aligned in an optimum perpendicular relationship. The decision to replace any or all of the forefoot posting pieces within the device is a clinical one, which is secondary to obtaining the optimally aligned shell.

This posting process, using flexible materials within a plantigrade shell, is known as *intrinsic posting* (Figure 7.20). To obtain the plantigrade shell:

- Maintain the distal lower leg in proper position and align the calcaneus on the sagittal plane or within 2 degrees of it, depending upon the correction desired (Figure 7.18).

- Use adhesive-backed Plastazote®, cut to fit the plantar metatarsal heads and stacked in beveled tiers (Figure 7.19).

- Use the angle finder to determine that the posted forefoot forms a perpendicular angle with the tibial shaft (Figure 7.19).

3. Carefully cover the lower leg and padded foot with a close-fitting sock of the thickness that the child usually wears, and add a layer of cotton stockinet in the snuggest tolerable width (Figure 7.21). Bulky socks and loose stockinet will invariably create wrinkles in the ankle joint area of the splint during molding. When molding hinged ankle-foot splints, use two thick (snug) socks under the stockinet. This creates room to allow for growth and for the calcaneus to move in small increments on the frontal plane within the device. The child wears only one pair of socks in the finished splint.

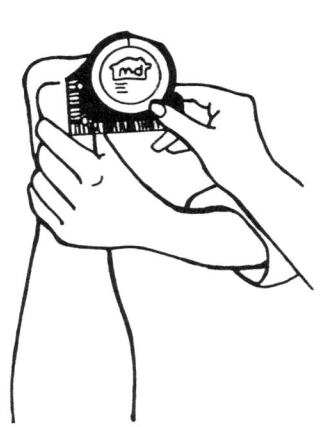

Figure 7.18
Prepost the forefoot to achieve a plantigrade metatarsal area with a vertical calcaneus. Reduce the calcaneal angle to 0 degrees, and post any remaining forefoot deviation.

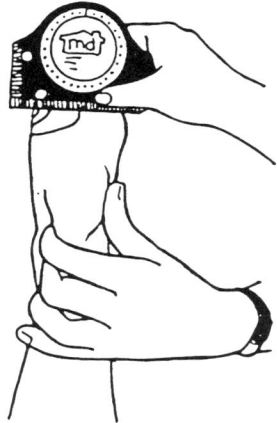

Figure 7.19
Use beveled tiers of adhesive-backed padding to post the metatarsal heads as needed to achieve a transverse-plane orientation of the metatarsal area of the shell of the splint. Use the angle finder to determine the perpendicular relationship between calcaneus and forefoot.

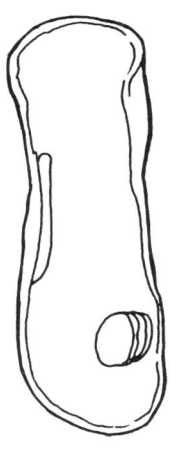

Figure 7.20
When the child's age and severity of varus deviation warrant posting in the finished splint, use beveled layers of padding materials of appropriate density and durability for intrinsic posting in the plantigrade shell. Try to avoid posting for forefoot varus, however.

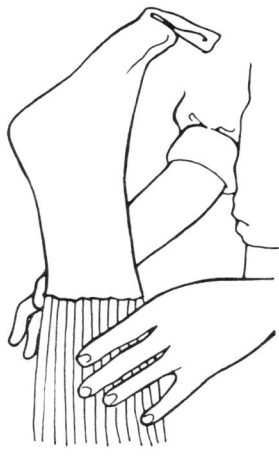

Figure 7.21
Carefully cover the padded extremity with the child's sock and cotton stockinet. Keep growth and potential shrinkage of the splint material in mind when choosing thickness of socks. Use the most snug-fitting stockinet available.

Sizing and Handling the Splint Material

1. Measure the extremity and cut the material. To size and cut an adequately sized piece of splint material, measure the length of the body segment and add 3-6 cm. Account for a small measure of longitudinal shrinkage in the 1/8-inch thickness of Aquaplast-T®. Orfit® will not shrink. By cutting the piece too short to gain ample coverage for the toes, the finishing process requires additional time and work to patch on the missing material. Take a girth measurement of the largest part of the leg and foot. This is often the greatest circumference around the plantarflexed heel and ankle. For shaft pieces, it is the calf of the leg. Do not add anything to this measurement. The 1/8-inch material stretches adequately to surround the extremity. The 3/16-inch material should be cut 1 to 2 inches narrower than this measurement. With a wax pencil, mark the resulting dimensions on a sheet of splint material. Use a utility knife to deeply score the material along the lines. Bend the material back on itself at the score line until it pops into a seam. Tear or slice it apart.

2. Place the plastic mesh pan guard in the warm water and lay the piece of splint material on top of it. Wait approximately two to four minutes for the material to turn clear. The splint material will not decompose in water that is hotter than recommended; neither will it decompose if it is left in the water for more than 20 minutes. If, when you lift the heated material from the water or the towel, it virtually falls into strings of hot plastic goo, it is defective and should be shipped back to the manufacturer for replacement. (Obtain proper vouchers for return shipments.)

3. To handle the heated material, use the plastic mesh pan guard to lift it from the water and lay it flat on a towel. Blot Aquaplast-T® dry on both sides. Use Orfit® while it is still wet. Carefully lay the soft material over your forearm or thigh so you can determine when it is cool enough to be comfortable to the child.

4. Apply the material to the child's extremity. The procedure for applying the splint material differs from devices that are molded on the posterior or anterior aspects of the extremity. For devices that encase the leg and foot segments from the posterior and/or plantar aspect, be certain that the ankle joint is totally plantarflexed at the time the material is draped over it (Figure 7.22).

- When you have draped the material over the appropriate limb segments, carefully pinch together only the edges. Do not stretch the material thin by pulling it from the center (Figure 7.22). Draw the material only enough to secure a close fit with the foot and leg, and to close down any air pockets. Avoid wrinkles by attending to the direction of pull on the material across the ankle. Look at both medial and lateral sides of the ankle and foot as you pull on the splint material.

- Flex the child's knee and move the leg and foot rapidly to dorsiflexion while the material is at its warmest. This precaution, together with use of a close-fitting sock and stockinet, will prevent the material from pleating around the ankle joint, which often happens if the ankle is dorsiflexed at the time of its application to the extremity.

5. If, on the other hand, the device encases the segments from the anterior aspect (such as crouch-control splints, both hinged and solid), the ankle should be held in dorsiflexion at the time of draping, so the material will remain smooth over the dorsum of the ankle (Figure 7.23). Failure to take this precaution will result in ridges forming across the dorsal ankle area as the material buckles into itself.

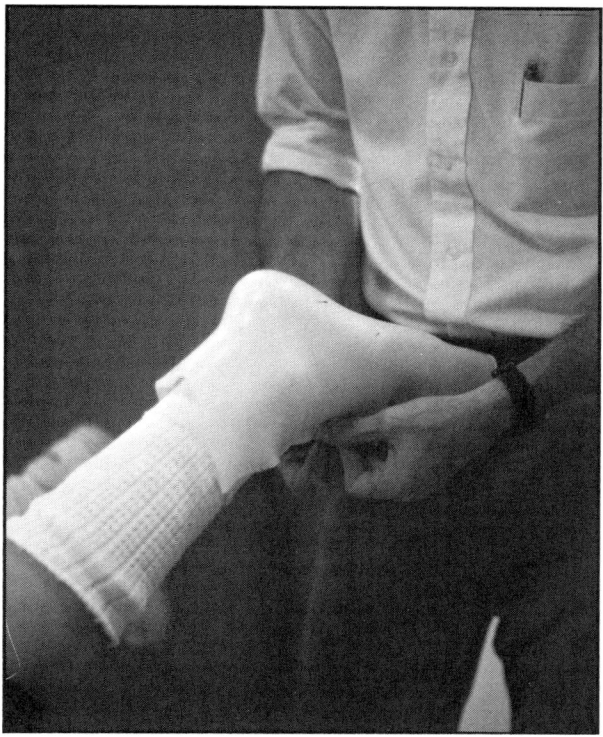

Figure 7.22 For splints that are made to contact the posterior aspect of the extremity, avoid making wrinkles in the material at the ankle area by fully plantarflexing the ankle before enclosing it with the splinting material

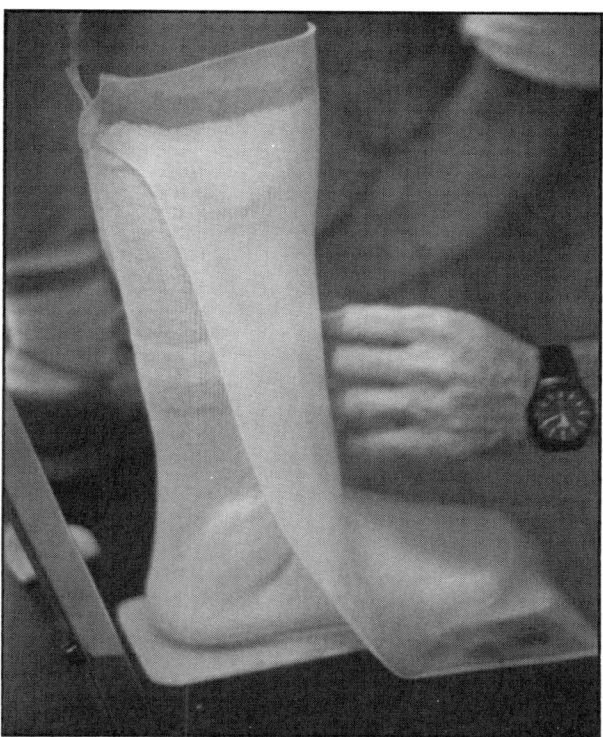

Figure 7.23 For splints that contact the anterior aspect of the foot and ankle, avoid forming wrinkles that harden into ridges by maintaining the ankle in a dorsiflexed position while enclosing it and the foot structures with the heated splinting material.

Molding and Removal

1. For precision in obtaining desired alignment of the leg and foot structures, maintain all visual perspectives precisely on the sagittal, frontal, and transverse planes (Figures 7.24 and 7.25). Do not view the foot or leg from an oblique angle.

2. Avoid pressing your fingertips into the shell of the device, because doing this will produce indentations on its inner surface. Maintain your hold on the foot by using the palmar surfaces of your hands and fingers as much as possible (Figure 7.26).

3. Maintain strict attention to the relationships between the leg and foot segments and the body planes throughout the molding procedure.

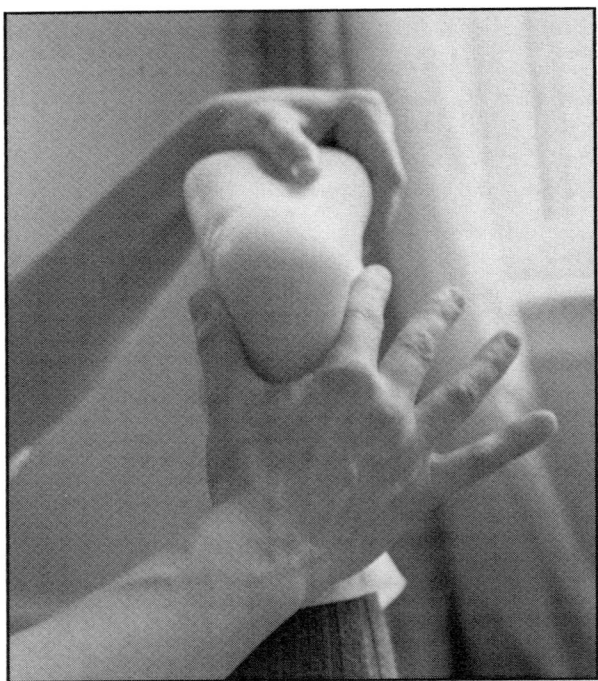

Figure 7.24 Use sagittal and transverse plane views. Mold over the contact surfaces (the "shell" of the device) by using all inner surfaces of the hand except the finger tips. Capture the posterior calcaneus. Maintain a perpendicular relationship between the forefoot and the calcaneal bisection.

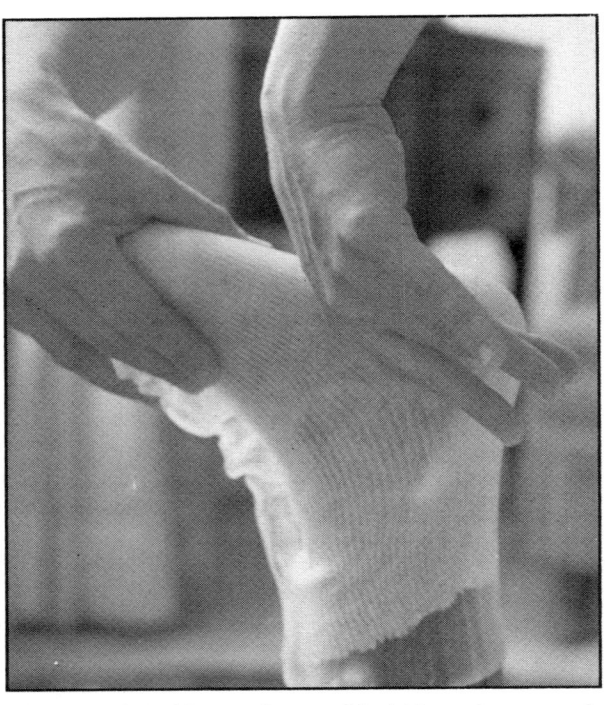

Figure 7.25 Use a diagonal hold to gain support under the sustentaculum tali on the medial side, and for the cuboid notch on the lateral plantar aspect of the foot. Mold in a shallow metatarsal bump if possible. (The bump can be done later with a heat gun.)

Figure 7.26
Define the calcaneus on the plantar aspect, molding into the medial and lateral longitudinal arches with the palms. Note the location of the metatarsal bump proximal to the metatarsal heads.

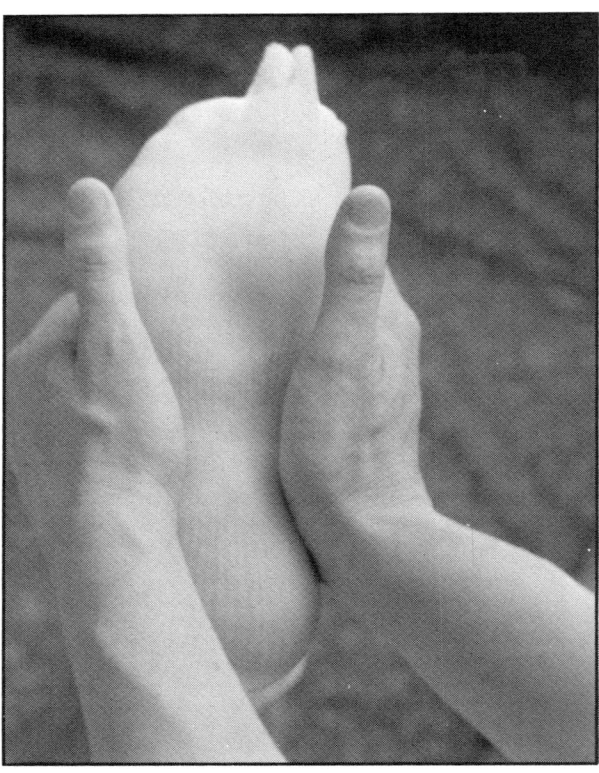

- Secure the calcaneal bisection in midposition with the lower leg aligned properly.

- If the device is for managing functional equinus deformity, carefully mold it around and above the calcaneus to define clearly all its borders within the device—including the medial, lateral, proximal, and plantar aspects (Figure 7.24).

- Mold close into the medial and lateral surfaces of the calcaneus, using a gentle, diagonal hold with the thumb and forefinger to achieve support under the sustentaculum tali on the medial side. Use this gentle hold also for the cuboid notch on the lateral plantar aspect of the foot (Figure 7.25). The calcaneal inclination is supported in some measure by these contours. Do not press in more than 6 seconds. Release the molding grip and let the material partially retract. Keep weight-bearing comfort in mind while forming plantar contours.

- Maintain the plantar surface of the metatarsal heads on the transverse plane. Be careful to avoid pulling one side of the forefoot area into more dorsiflexion than the other, or the result will be comparable to a gait extension modification, as discussed in Chapter 5 (Figure 7.24).

- Maintain the forefoot in midline relative to the longitudinal bisection of the hindfoot on the sagittal plane. Do not drag the forefoot into adduction or abduction on the hindfoot. Keep the second toe in line with the tibial crest while molding, and keep the foot at its normal thigh-foot angle (Figure 7.24).

- If desired, a shallow bump for the metatarsal arch can be molded into the plantar surface, proximal to metatarsal heads 2 and 3 (Figures 7.24, 7.25, and 7.26).

- If the ankle joint is to be included in the device, set the ankle position at the desired angle after the structures of the foot have been aligned (Figure 7.27). Avoid drawing the lateral aspect of the forefoot into more dorsiflexion than the medial aspect.

Figure 7.27
Set the desired ankle position after aligning the foot structures. Hold the ankle in 2-5 degrees of dorsiflexion to prepare for elastic retraction as the material sets.

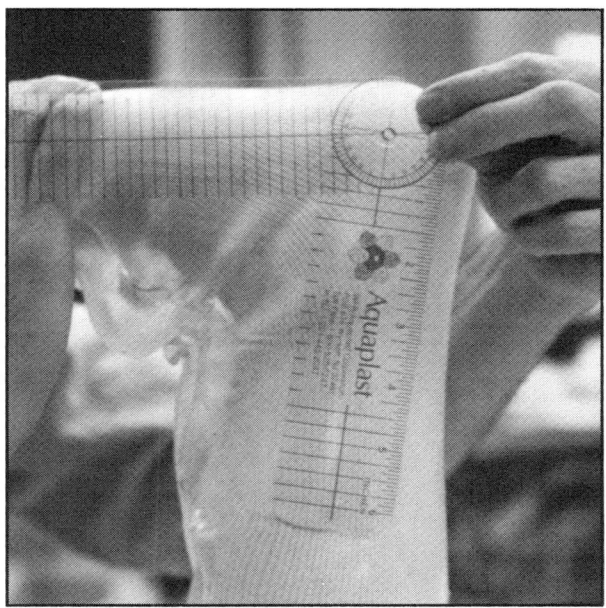

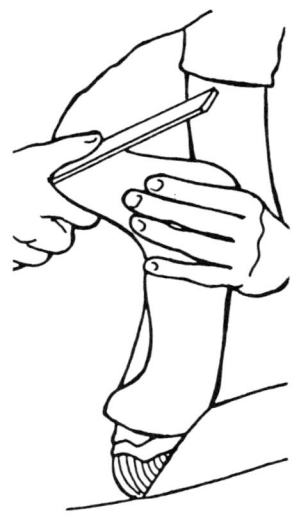

Figure 7.28
Mold a gentle toe-break into the splint while the material is clear and soft. Hold each mold for 5-6 seconds, then release. Consider the angle of progression in beveling the toe-break.

- If the splint is for ambulation and the medial or lateral walls must remain intact to prohibit abnormal transverse plane excursion of the forefoot, a small toe-break is needed for smooth forward progression (Figure 7.28). A Plexiglas® or copolymer plastic "footboard"—such as the one sold by WFR Aquaplast Corporation (see Appendix 4 for sources)—might be helpful in molding the toe-break while the splint material is very soft. Be careful, however, to consider the part of the foot that should function optimally as the final point of contact during weight transfer, and angle the toe-break (like a gait extension modification) accordingly. (See discussions of gait extension modifications in Chapters 5 and 6 and later in this chapter, in relation to altering the angle of gait.)

No limb segment should be forced into a desired alignment if the necessary joint mobility is not available. Use posting—on the interior of the device—to maintain the limited joint in its preferred position without imposing a deviating stress on the remaining joints. The therapist should subsequently attempt to restore mobility in treatment, and reduce the accommodative posting as alignment and active mobility improve.

Limitation of talocrural joint mobility into dorsiflexion, past an initial point of resistance less than 5 degrees beyond neutral, warrants consideration of a course of serial casting, or stretch splinting, or perhaps treatment for two weeks in "bioboots" or using a transcutaneous electrical nerve stimulation (TENS) unit to activate the dorsiflexors before using splints or orthoses of any design. (See Chapter 6 for discussion of conservative methods of gaining soft tissue extensibility.)

On Using the "Footboard" (A Flat Slab of Plastic) During Molding of Foot Splints

I have the following concerns regarding the use of a "footboard," which in this context is defined in the catalog and sold by WFR Aquaplast Corporation as a flat slab of plastic material (Figure 7.29).

The use of a flat footboard to gain a perpendicular relationship between the forefoot and hindfoot during the molding phase of fabrication of a splint has a certain appeal for those clinicians who believe its use simplifies the fabrication process and reduces the need to add external posting to the splint.

I do advocate placing the hindfoot and forefoot components of the shell of the foot piece in a perpendicular relationship to each other. Both the medial and lateral aspects of the forefoot section of the foot piece should contact the ground when the vertical bisection of the calcaneus is aligned in midposition. However, these relationships are better achieved by preposting the forefoot than by applying pressure into dorsiflexion on the metatarsal heads. The application of pressure with a flat "footboard" can cause the midtarsal joint (MTJ) to abduct and dorsiflex around its oblique axis rather than to evert around its longitudinal axis. The result is a flattened, pronated foot within the splint.

Figure 7.29
The copolymer or Plexiglas® "foot-board."

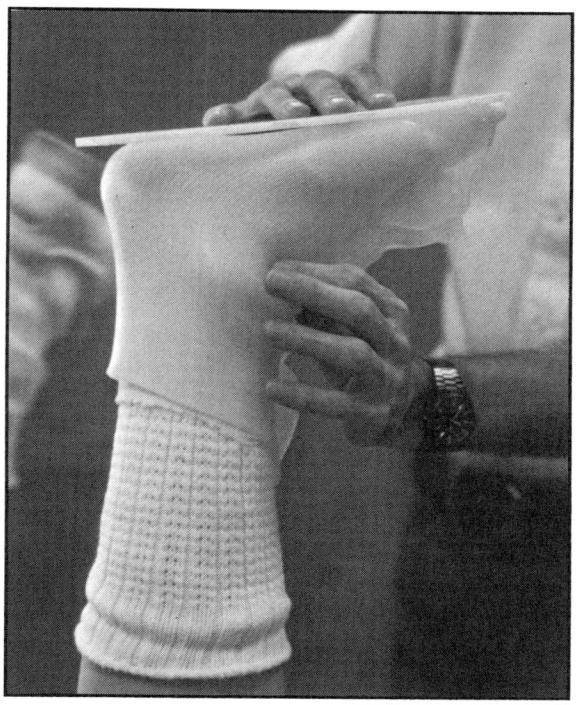

I have seen several splints made using the flat footboard molding (that is, smashing) technique, and I have been disappointed in or distressed by the design of all of them. The clue that reveals their flat board "molding" technique is a plantar surface that is pressed flat to the rounded edges, an abducted or adducted forefoot, a rounded medial wall, and an everted or inverted calcaneus. The foot structures must be pronated or supinated so abnormally to fit into the finished splints that they must be considered damaging rather than therapeutic. Luckily, the devices that were shown or given to me had been taken away from the children for whom they were made either by parents or by therapists.

By focusing primary concern on the external stability of the device and on the convenience of attempting to maneuver the forefoot onto the transverse plane using a footboard, the clinician can easily overlook the more important goals of molding. The well-made splint exhibits several contours that replicate those of the plantar surface of the foot when it is aligned in plantigrade position. The contours include the cuboid notch (lateral arch), the calcaneal inclination, support under the sustentaculum tali, the medial longitudinal arch, and the transverse arch of the metatarsal shafts. Pressing a flat board to the plantar surface of the foot while the splint material is soft prohibits the clinician from molding these plantar contours into the splint.

Pressing on the plantar surface of the forefoot with a footboard during molding can also widen the splint excessively. Because Aquaplast-T® is flexible under stress, the walls of the splint spread slightly on weight-bearing. A small degree of transverse plane expansion is desirable. But if the forefoot area is widened significantly during molding, the forefoot can shift into abnormal alignment on the transverse plane. Furthermore, the wider splint requires a larger shoe for outerwear.

The knowledgeable clinician understands the nature of the well-aligned foot and can, with practice, replicate that alignment during molding. Furthermore, the knowledgeable clinician places the intricate and dynamic structure of the foot at a higher priority than convenience of fabrication.

One way to prevent deformation of the foot structures while using a flat "footboard" is to post the metatarsal heads before applying the heated splint material, as described above (Figure 7.19). Then the need for pressure on the plantar forefoot would be minimal, because the perpendicular relationship between forefoot and hindfoot becomes established intrinsically. Nevertheless, access to the plantar contours is still prohibited by the presence of the "footboard."

Those clinicians who are trained in fabricating contoured plaster footboards might build a thin footplate as a plantar interface before molding a splint, which is discussed previously. In this case, the flat "footboard" holds less potential risk for deforming the foot structures, because the plantar contours are built into the interface and the forefoot is preposted to a plantigrade alignment. Or, as one workshop participant recently suggested, the contoured plaster footboard might be flared slightly at the heel to accommodate the thicker splint material, then chilled in the freezer and used in lieu of a flat "footboard" to obtain plantar contours in the splint, cooling the shell rapidly under the footboard at the same time.

If the clinician who is charged with making foot splints does not appreciate the nature of the foot and its structural alignment in stance and function, then I recommend that the clinician seek additional training in the areas of functional anatomy, kinesiology, and biomechanics. Until then, I recommend discarding the flat "footboard" during the molding phase of fabrication.

4. Mark trim lines. Before removing the splint, identify the trim lines you intend to use after removal and mark them with the wax pencil or washable crayon on the splint as it is setting (Figure 7.30). This will hasten and facilitate the trimming process after the mold is removed from the child. As time passes, the splint hardens, and cutting becomes increasingly arduous. Speed is essential in this process.

5. Set the mold. Once satisfactory foot and/or lower limb alignment has been achieved within the softened splint material, the limb segments should be held steady in the desired alignment. The splint material gradually loses transparency. To accelerate the setting process, apply a washcloth (dipped in ice water and wrung to eliminate any dripping) to the shell of the splint, under the

foot and on the supporting aspect of the leg (Figure 7.31). The cold cloth speeds the setting process in the supportive areas of the splint, while the portions that will be trimmed away remain comparatively soft and easy to cut with shears. The process of hardening is usually advanced enough to permit removal of the mold from the child's foot and leg within two to three minutes; less with the cold cloth.

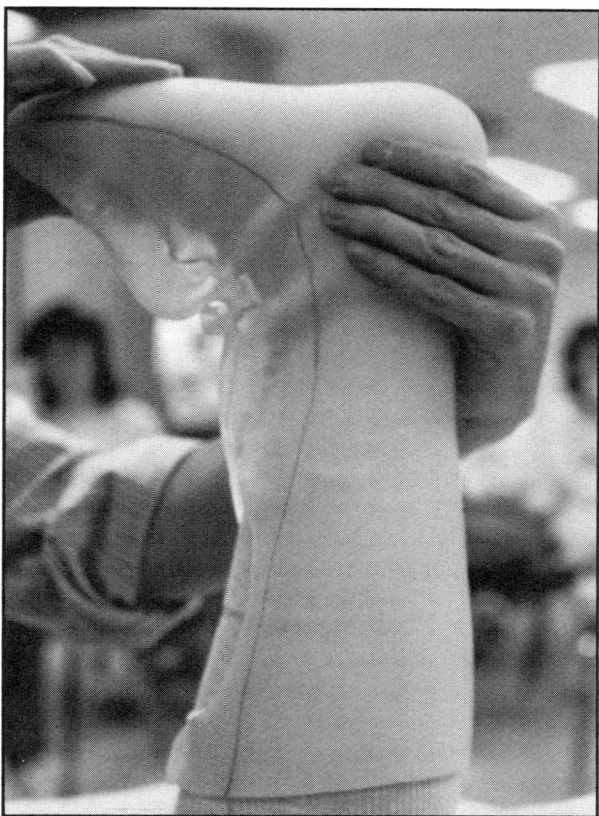

Figure 7.30   Mark trim lines as the mold sets to hasten the process of trimming out the device after removing the mold from the extremity.

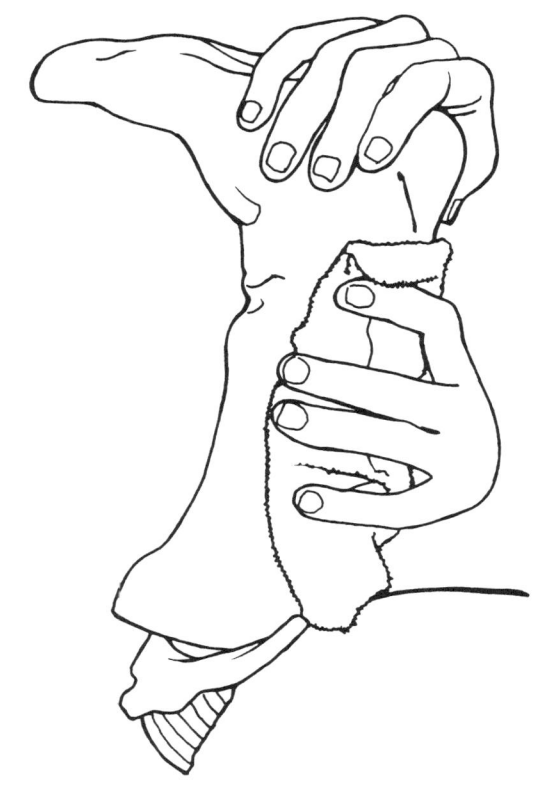

Figure 7.31   Reduce setting time by repeatedly applying a cold, dampened towel to the surface of the shell only. Do not cool the area that will require trimming. Do not drip ice-cold water on the patient's leg.

6. Remove the mold. When the pattern of the stockinet underlying the splint material is no longer visible in the area of the shell of the device, adequate hardening has occurred. You can then remove the mold without fear of deforming it, even if it remains slightly warm. Try to pull apart the flaps that form the seam, taking care not to distort the shape of the splint. Most splints require closure of the warmed splint material on the dorsal aspect of the ankle joint. For these splints, pulling apart rather than cutting the material is more comfortable for the child. While the material in that area is soft, poke a finger under the stockinet and the splint material and pull it all away forcefully from the skin before cutting it in that area (Figure 7.32). Then cut any remaining splint material, together with the adjacent stockinet, and carefully remove the splint and stockinet together.

Figure 7.32
Pull the soft splint material and the adjacent stockinet away from the dorsum of the ankle before cutting in that area, to avoid causing discomfort with the scissors.

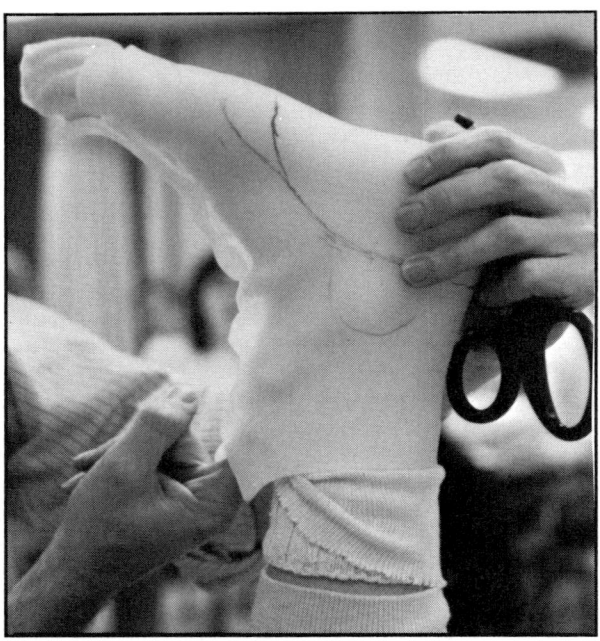

7. Trim out the device. Without delay, while the splint material is still warm near the seam, use either the Universal® bandage shears, Unlimited® scissors, Pro-Snips® or a comparable pair of sturdy shears that is capable of cutting through cold splint material to trim the splint to the desired shape. Remember, as seconds pass, the material becomes harder. In addition to reducing overall fabrication time, expedience is a labor-saving advantage in this procedure.

Finishing the Splint

1. Smooth the edges. Practice in trimming splints will probably result in minimum requirement for special procedures to trim the edges. If necessary, however, you might smooth any jagged edges by a variety of processes: whittle them carefully with a utility knife; peel them, as you would a carrot, with an edge finisher (Figure 7.33); or heat them gently with a heat gun and rub them smooth.

2. Flare the proximal border. Roll back the proximal edge of an ankle-foot splint, regardless of the style (Figure 7.34). To do this, dip the end of the splint into hot water for 30 seconds in order to soften the material, then gently work it into a flare as it hardens. If you fail to maintain pressure on the material as it sets, it will recoil into its original shape.

3. Replace the pads. To protect bony prominences from abrasion, remove the pads from the foot and replace them within the splint if the fit is adequate. If it is not, cut a new pad. Cover the pads with moleskin to keep them from peeling off.

4. Prepare the surface for the application of straps. I recommend the SabreGrip®) hook because it resists significant shear forces before separating. Brush splint solvent cement on the area of the splint where a strap will be attached. Gently heat the contact area with a heat gun only enough to soften the outer layer of the

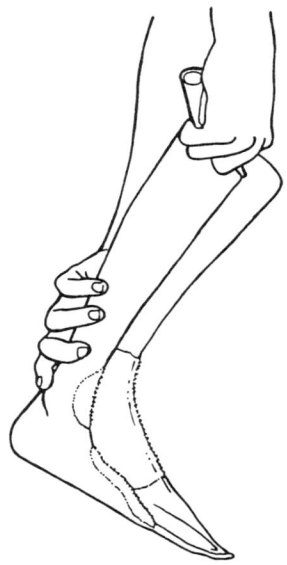

Figure 7.33
Smooth the edges.

splint material. *Do not overheat.* Then apply the hook side of the strapping fabric. Omitting this preparation step often results in the slipping of the straps away from the optimum location, after which the exposed residue of adhesive collects dirt.

5. Use extrinsic posting as needed. Sometimes added stability is needed to maintain the desired alignment of the STJ structures in a footsplint and to enhance the application of corrective floor reaction forces. When this is the case, use extrinsic posting at the hindfoot to fill any spaces between the ground and the weight-bearing sections of the shell of the device. Heel posts are used routinely to gain frontal plane stability or alignment in the stabilizing foot splint (SFS) and its modified designs.

To post the device at the heel, first use splint solvent cement on the heel area of the shell of the device, to prepare it for bonding to the posting strip (Figure 7.35). Then cut a strip of splinting material (the sticky, original type of Aquaplast® and the standard Orfit® formula work especially well for posting securely) approximately 3 cm by 18 cm. Heat the material in the water bath. When the posting piece is clear, blot it dry. Align the calcaneal bisection of the device perpendicular to the table, and maintain the alignment while filling the available space between the shell and the table top with the hot posting strip (Figure 7.36). Do not create a heel lift. Simply stabilize the calcaneus. While the post is soft and clear, trim a small bevel in the posteriolateral border for smooth contact at heel strike, and trim the sides of the post to lie flush with the side walls of the splint. The post should be no wider than the heel cup, unless the foot needs extra stability on the lateral aspect against rolling into varus.

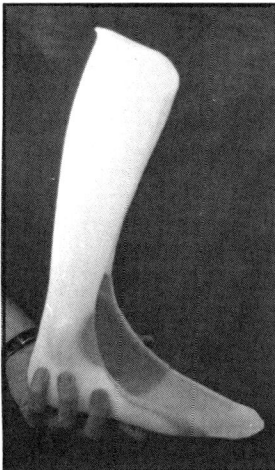

Figure 7.34
Roll back the proximal border. Replace the pads and cover them with moleskin.

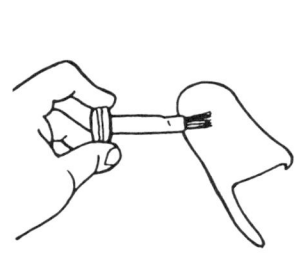

Figure 7.35
Prepare the surface of the device to bond with the post by applying solvent and heating gently until the surface is tacky but remains translucent.

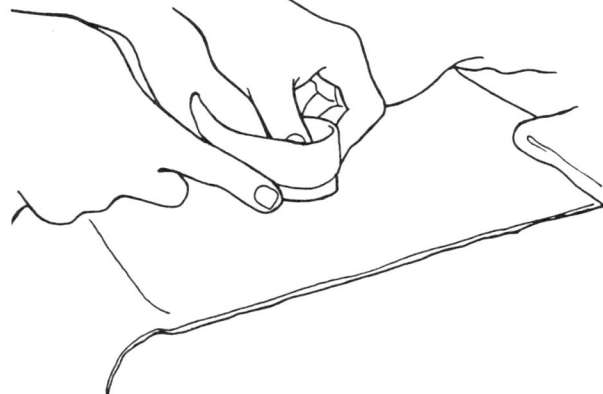

Figure 7.36 Use a hot, dried strip of splint material to fill the space between the properly aligned shell and the floor. Bring the edges of the post to a sharp angle to minimize rocking. Set calcaneal bisection on the sagittal plane.

6. Use the intrinsic forefoot post as needed. As discussed previously, I recommend using intrinsic rather than extrinsic forefoot posts in most devices for the foot or the ankle and foot (Figure 7.20). While protecting the hindfoot from the deforming influence of fixed forefoot deviation, the intrinsic post within the plantigrade shell can be altered by the compression that occurs with modeling, or by the clinician when changes are observed in the alignment of the forefoot structures.

To post at the forefoot within the plantigrade shell of a foot piece, consider the values obtained in the assessment of the foot and hindfoot and the age of the child. For example, if an angle of 6 degrees of forefoot varus remains after aligning the calcaneus in midposition, and the spastic diplegic child is 9 years of age, fill the forefoot section with PPT®, cut in a wedge or in beveled tiers, layered to form a wedge with an angle of 3 to 4 degrees with the transverse plane. This post effectively brings the floor of the device closer to the varus forefoot and removes compensatory pronatory strain on the hindfoot.

Trained therapists should use joint mobilization procedures as tolerated to remove capsular and ligamentous restrictions on correction of varus. They should reevaluate the status of the foot three or four times per year. If they note any reduction in varus deviation, they should reduce the height of the forefoot post accordingly. The primary precaution on mobilization for the pediatric foot is application of forces to epiphyseal plates in the metatarsals. Be gentle, and be precise in palpations.

As was discussed in Chapter 5, posting intrinsically for very young children requires attention to modeling possibilities. I am currently inclined to favor the idea that in a younger child, after the clinician stabilizes the hindfoot in vertical alignment, adequate forefoot mobility is usually available to allow the varus forefoot to model onto the transverse plane. In this case, the forefoot should be allowed to seek the ground without interference by a forefoot post. Close monitoring reveals the outcome of this decision within weeks of providing the splint.

If reduction potential for forefoot varus deformity is restricted by a lack of mobility into midtarsal joint eversion, plantarflexion of the first ray, and/or forefoot supination around the oblique MTJ axis, or if the initial effort to allow modeling forces to prevail causes discomfort rather than modeling, an interim, compressible forefoot post might be warranted for a young child of age 4 to 6 years. Plastazote® padding is an example of such a padding material, because it will compress with shear forces encountered in weight-bearing over a period of a few weeks. PPT® padding, on the other hand, will not bottom out for up to two years and would be contraindicated in this application. At the same time, gentle mobilization procedures to reduce capsular and ligamentous limitation on correction of forefoot varus should be instituted by trained clinicians.

To address *forefoot valgus* (eversion deformity) in a young child, I prefer to provide a plantigrade shell for the foot structures. I align the hindfoot in midline, support the lateral longitudinal arch together with the medial aspect of the forefoot, and allow the midtarsal joint

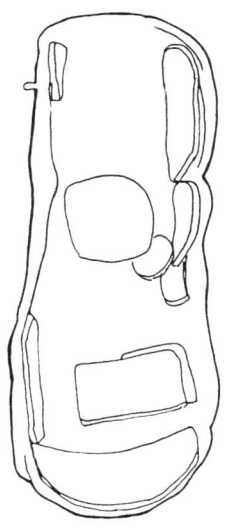

Figure 7.37
For older children and adolescents, replace padding under the lateral metatarsal heads to accommodate rigid forefoot valgus deformity within the plantigrade shell. Reduce post as mobility and control improve.

to invert around its longitudinal axis and the first ray to dorsiflex. I have no references for guidance in managing forefoot valgus in the young child, but I suspect that it would be harmful to post the forefoot into valgus to prohibit hindfoot supination. Excursion of the forefoot structures into inversion is normally significantly greater than in the opposite direction. Thus the eversion deformity at the forefoot can be expected to resolve without posting if all the following factors apply: adequate calcaneal eversion mobility; a shell that will not dorsiflex under the lateral aspect of the forefoot; and adequate stabilization of the calcaneus against inverting.

The older child and adolescent, however, might reveal a more fixed forefoot valgus deformity with perhaps a rigid plantarflexed first ray. Accommodative, rather than corrective, intervention is needed while joint mobilization procedures and therapeutic exercise are undertaken to seek improvement in forefoot alignment. The plantigrade forefoot area of the shell should be filled as needed to prevent the everted forefoot from lowering to the ground by inverting the hindfoot structures (Figure 7.37). This results in dropping the first metatarsal into a shallow recess.

Problem-Specific Fabrication Techniques

Molding to Reduce Pronation Deformity

Before making splints for the foot for any functional purpose, determine the availability of adequate extensibility of the soft tissue structures surrounding the foot and ankle. Otherwise, you must undertake alternative measures prior to splinting to gain the mobility needed for the child to achieve optimum structural alignment.

For the child whose foot shows a pronation deformity, follow the general splint fabrication procedures outlined above (Figures 7.1 through 7.37). When molding a stabilizing foot splint (SFS) for mild flexible pes planus, a supramalleolar splint (SMS) for moderate degrees of pronation, a solid ankle-foot splint (SAFS) for night splinting or for functional equinovalgus in the nonambulatory child, or the foot section of a hinged ankle-foot splint (HAFS), remember Valmassy's (1984) rule for allowing for calcaneal valgus deviation in relaxed stance (the child's age subtracted from the number 7), and consider these factors:

- The splint is flexible under body weight; thus it will allow a small degree of excursion of the calcaneus and forefoot structures.
- For reasons of rapid growth and possible shrinkage of the splint material as it sets, the splint is made over one or two socks of typical thickness. (The HAFS is made over two layers of thick socks. The SFS, which is more easily replaced with growth, is made over one sock.) The child wears one sock under the splint. The calcaneus can move within the remaining space at the heel cup area of the shell as the thick sock compresses.

The goals of molding for pronation include the following:

- Reduction of excessive calcaneal eversion in weight-bearing positions. Secure the medial and lateral aspects of the calcaneus, molding under the sustentaculum tali and into the medial and lateral longitudinal arches.

- Reduction of calcaneal plantarflexion, MTJ dorsiflexion around the oblique axis, and first ray dorsiflexion. Gently support the calcaneal inclination via the posterior aspect of both the medial and lateral longitudinal arches. Do not force correction beyond age-appropriate expectations. If a fat pad is still present, accommodate it.

- Reduction of excessive forefoot abduction. Adduct the forefoot into parallel alignment with the hindfoot. Keep the second toe in line with the tibial crest.

- Modeling down from forefoot varus to within 2-3 degrees relative to the vertically aligned hindfoot. For the very young child without adequate mobility within the foot structures, align the calcaneus in vertical position and prepost the medial forefoot to plantigrade at molding. Then refrain from replacing the forefoot post when finishing the splint.

- Protect the soft tissues supporting the transverse arch. Mold gently into the metatarsal notch, which lies proximal to the second and third metatarsal heads. The resulting shallow bump defines the midline orientation of the forefoot and prevents the central metatarsal heads from dropping excessively with pronation. This bump is not intended to maintain a transverse arch across the metatarsal heads. In stance in the normal foot, all five metatarsal heads lower to the ground and take weight.

Molding to Reduce Equinovalgus Deformity

All measures described for reduction of pronation deformity (see above) apply to this problem and are addressed in molding any ankle-foot splint prior to adjusting the ankle position. If there is full passive extensibility in the muscles and connective tissue of the posterior compartment and the talocrural joint, consider using the following approach to reduce the added component of functional equinus and its associated difficulties:

- Aquaplast-T® and Orfit® materials possess the characteristic of elasticity, or "memory." They recoil slightly as they cool, evidently returning to their original state before stretch was imposed. Therefore, it often happens that the angle at which the ankle joint was held during molding is greater than what is evident in the finished splint. A few degrees of dorsiflexion are lost. The material is soft and clear, but to be certain of maintaining an angle of between 90-95 degrees of dorsiflexion in the finished ankle-foot splint, set the angle of ankle dorsiflexion at 2 to 3 degrees more than desired while molding. Night splints should set at an angle that maintains a gentle stretch on the plantarflexors (Figure 7.27).

- While the material is warm, press in along the grooves on both sides of the Achilles tendon, in the depressions posterior to the malleoli and in the area of the tendo-Achilles insertion on the calcaneus. These contours will catch the calcaneus and prevent it from slipping proximally with activity in the plantarflexors, as long as the foot does not shear forward in the device.

- If proximal torsional forces are strong, add an anterior shell to strengthen the structure of the device (Figure 7.38).

Molding to Reduce Equinovarus Deformity

Functional equinovarus deformity is usually a powerful deformity and demands the application of corrective forces to the foot in the direction opposite from those applied to reduce pronation. The following corrective measures are suggested on the presumption that full passive mobility of the involved structures is available. The following components of correction should be implemented as the splint mold sets:

- Reduce calcaneal inversion. Align the calcaneus in vertical, or slightly everted, position (within 5 degrees). Then, if necessary, reinforce the lateral forefoot of the splint with a low vertical wall to prevent it from dorsiflexing, and buttress the lateral heel box of the splint with extra layers of splinting material. If more stabilization is needed, ask an orthotist or cobbler to reinforce the lateral heel box and midfoot area of the shoe to prohibit the foot and leg from deviating laterally in stance.

- Reduce the height of the medial longitudinal arch. Gently dorsiflex and abduct the forefoot around the oblique axis of the MTJ, and dorsiflex the first ray.

- Prevent shortening in the medial plantar fascia. Prepad the medial surface of the first metatarsal head and great toe. Apply a gentle force into abduction with dorsiflexion at the forefoot. Be careful not to stairstep the metatarsals, bunching one on the other.

- Prohibit stress-induced forefoot eversion around the longitudinal axis. Prepost the rigidly everted (valgus) forefoot to achieve a plantigrade shell while molding. Maintain a low lateral vertical wall in the forefoot of the splint, to prevent it from dorsiflexing under stress. Depending upon the age of the child, while you are finishing the splint, do either of the following: 1) refrain from replacing the post in the shell and allow the forefoot to attempt to model into correction, or 2) accommodate forefoot valgus deviation by replacing the post intrinsically to recess the first metatarsal head (for the older, more fixed deformity).

Functional Considerations

- Prohibit abnormal knee hyperextension. Evaluate the status of equinus deformity before attempting to manage this problem with splints of any type. There will be no favorable result if knee hyperextension occurs secondary to fixed or strong rather than to mild functional equinus deformity (Molnar 1986; Rang et al. 1986). Serial casting might be needed to reduce the influence of the equinus pattern on knee hyperextension.

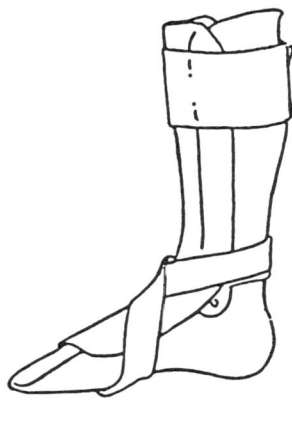

Figure 7.38
To gain strength against torque within the shaft and foot sections, use an anterior shell.

If there is a manageable degree of functional equinus deformity or a simple problem of ligamentous laxity at the knee joint, try using a knee hyperextension splint (described in Chapter 5) with a splint for the foot or for the ankle and foot that meets the specific requirements for alignment of those structures. The combined splinting systems allow a more normal ankle motion to occur in gait than does a single system that prohibits normal ankle plantarflexion as a means of getting floor reaction forces into flexion at the knee joint.

At times, the knee hyperextension splint is either not used appropriately or not tolerated, or the forces of knee hyperextension are too great for the knee splint to be an effective control system. In either of those cases, if supination of the foot is associated with knee hyperextension, facilitate pronation in early stance in the foot splint. Then, if necessary, build a hinged ankle-foot splint and set the posterior stop to prohibit plantarflexion past a point of 5 degrees of ankle dorsiflexion. The dorsiflexed ankle causes floor reaction forces to reduce knee hyperextension during stance.

The knee hyperextension splint and the dorsiflexed ankle-foot system of controlling knee hyperextension are training mechanisms. The child must wear them consistently for several weeks or months, and the clinician should monitor closely to determine their effectiveness in promoting the achievement of better knee control in stance with the system removed. Rarely is knee instability great enough to warrant prolonged orthotic intervention, unless the instability was induced surgically via posterior capsulotomy.

• Reduce pelvic lateral rotation and elevation. Prohibiting knee hyperextension and equinovarus can also reduce pelvic retraction (lateral rotation) on the ipsilateral side in gait. The mechanism is as follows: Equinovarus typically creates a rigid, supinated, plantarflexed foot and ankle. The distal deformity rotates the lower leg posterolaterally, induces knee hyperextension, and effectively lengthens the weight-bearing leg. The rigid, longer leg pushes the pelvis proximally and posteriorly.

When the clinician intervenes to reduce knee hyperextension and the equinovarus components distally, the foot pronates, the knee flexes, the dorsiflexed ankle reduces the length of the leg, and the flexing knee draws down and forward on the same side of the pelvis over the loaded, plantigrade foot. (Downhill skiers demonstrate this mechanism as they walk in tall, rigid ski boots.)

This chapter has thus far reviewed the general techniques used in the fabrication of foot and ankle-foot splints for children. In the next section, we will use the criteria and principles discussed in this and previous chapters to determine the features of an acceptable pediatric lower-extremity splint. The implementation of the device is considered, along with correct splint application procedures and some commonly asked questions.

Checkout Procedures and Discussion

We have observed the course of development of the structural features of the lower extremities in relation to forces imposed by normal and abnormal biomechanics, muscle action, and motor skills. We have seen how problems of alignment within the foot structures can contribute to proximal structural deviations and increased functional limitation in children with abnormal muscle tone. We have discussed some of the conservative intervention measures that are available to the management team for reducing certain components of the more common foot and ankle deformities. And we have addressed some of the underlying principles of alignment and deformity correction that are implemented in molding casts and the more commonly used splints.

Now, let us apply these perspectives to the analysis of a splint or orthosis for the pediatric foot and ankle; we can then determine whether it meets the criteria for optimum biomechanical alignment and functional advantage. The principles of assessment are illustrated in the context of examining a solid ankle-foot splint or orthosis, although they apply (with modification) to splints and casts of varying design. We will conclude with a discussion of some of the questions that are asked frequently by seminar participants.

The checkout process involves several facets of intervention: the structure of the device, its proper application, and its functional impact in standing and, if appropriate, in gait. We will consider each factor separately.

Evaluating Structural Components

We begin to assess the features of a device by considering the familiar solid ankle-foot splint or orthosis. Presume the child for whom it was made is 5 years of age, reveals functional equinovalgus deformity, and stands only with assistance. She has received the device illustrated in Figures 7.39 and 7.40. Several questions need to be addressed:

*   Is the device in Figure 7.39, which might be either a splint or an orthosis, molded to hold the calcaneus securely in age-appropriate alignment? [Note: For a child 5 years of age, Valmassy (1984) allows up to 2 degrees of calcaneal valgus, disregarding evidence of distal varum in the lower leg, which is usually resolved to within 2 degrees by age 5 years.]
    *   — No. In fact, the calcaneal angle is 13 degrees. Furthermore, the plastic overlying the medial malleolus protrudes abnormally, and the plastic overlying the lateral malleolus is flattened. These problems indicate that significant medial rotation of the lower leg, which accompanies excessive calcaneal eversion in pronation, was molded into the device. Refer to Figure 7.41 for a desirable alternative.

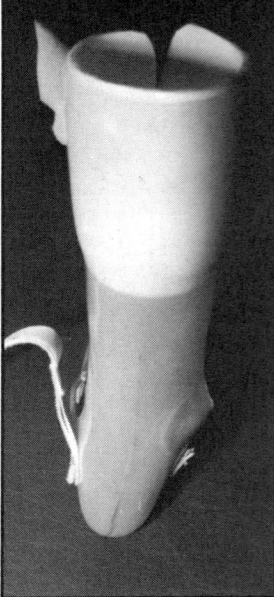 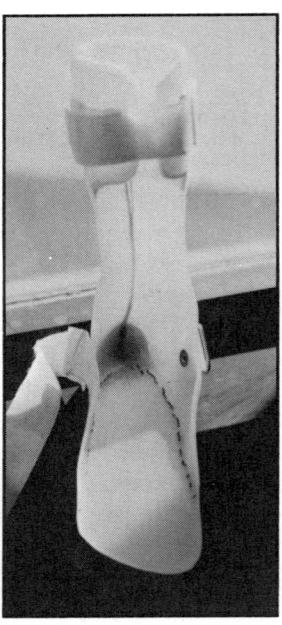 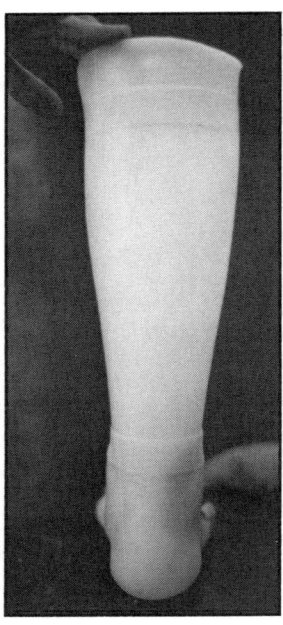

Figure 7.39
Solid AFO or SAFS—
posterior view.

Figure 7.40
Solid AFO or SAFS—
anterior view.

Figure 7.41
Solid AFO or SAFS—
posterior view.

• Is the device featured in Figure 7.40 trimmed to be deep enough along the medial and lateral walls of the ankle and foot sections to cover the malleoli and to stabilize the tarsus and metatarsals on the frontal plane?

— No. The walls are trimmed low, half-covering the malleoli and undercutting the navicular. The walls are trimmed to the floor on both sides of the metatarsal heads, leaving the job of prohibiting abnormal forefoot abduction and adduction to the soft upper of a shoe. Children with abnormal tone regulation and neuromotor control often require ample stabilization to gain adequate structural alignment for optimum muscle function. Refer to Figures 7.42 and 7.43 for comparison.

• Is the floor of the foot support section in Figure 7.40 appropriately contoured to conform to and support the calcaneus and the medial and lateral longitudinal arches in functional alignment?

— No. There is no contour that conforms to the plantar aspect of the foot. The floor of the device is flat. The medial edge of the floor of the orthosis resembles the lateral edge, because there is no incurvation where the arch would rise off the base. Refer to Figures 7.42 and 7.43 for a more appropriate plantar configuration.

• Is age 5 years old enough to reveal evidence of the arches?

— Yes. This child began to lose the fat pad that covered the longitudinal arch at the age of 3 years. However, at 5 years, the height of the arch is lower than an adult's, so the device should reveal a low arch.

Figure 7.42
SAFS—anterior view.

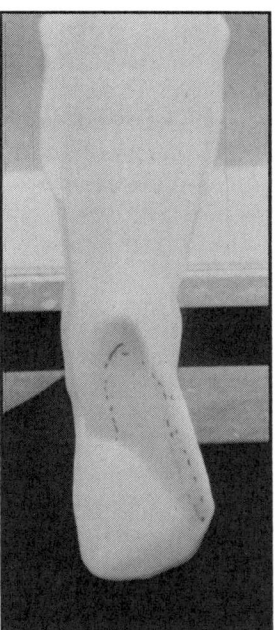

Figure 7.43
SAFS.

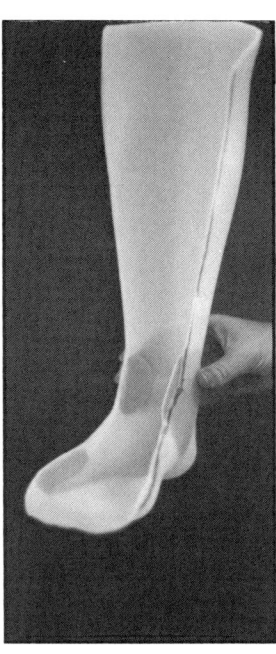

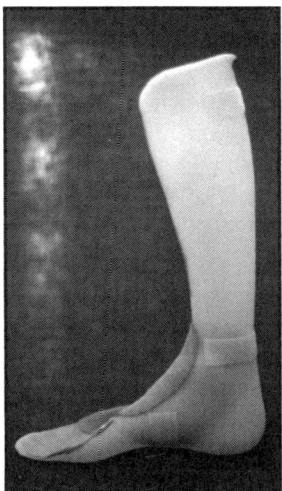

Figure 7.44
SAFS—medial view.

- Is the device contoured in the area of the heel cord to capture the calcaneus from above, so it will not slide up the shaft? (The same concern applies to the hinged AFS and to the cast boot.)
  - No. Inspection of the device in Figure 7.39 reveals no evidence of measures having been taken to capture the calcaneus and define the Achilles tendon. Refer to Figure 7.44 for comparison.

Other questions about structural assessment include the following (which are not illustrated):

- When the vertical bisection of the calcaneus is aligned with the sagittal plane within the 2 degrees of valgus allowed for this child, and the existing distal lower leg varum is accommodated, does the floor of the entire metatarsal section lie on the ground?
  - If it does not, and the only component of the splint that is malaligned is the metatarsal floor, then consider altering the alignment of the metatarsal area by heating it and molding it on a greased table top to lower the elevated side to the floor. At that point, consider the child's age, the available mobility in the forefoot structures, and the modeling potential before deciding to provide a forefoot post intrinsically with layers of padding of varying density and durability.

Orthoses that are made without regard for achieving a plantigrade forefoot on a vertical hindfoot cannot be adjusted. They should be refabricated. While awaiting the corrected orthosis, provided that the hindfoot and shaft pieces do not deviate when the forefoot position is corrected, add an extrinsic post to the metatarsal area of an orthosis with PPT® padding and moleskin.

- In order to promote a functional, slightly flexed knee position and forward progression in ankle-foot devices made to manage functional equinus, the shaft piece should form an angle of 2-5 degrees of dorsiflexion with the floor of the device.

On the other hand, in managing calcaneus deformity and related crouch posture, the hinged crouch-control ankle-foot splint (HCAFS) requires that the ankle joint of the device be set at 5 to 7 degrees of dorsiflexion. This angle allows forward progression over the splinted foot in gait, and the gradual introduction of the correction for crouch deformity. Then this angle can be reduced in increments of 1 or 2 degrees by filling the space between the proximal dorsal extension on the foot piece and the distal shaft piece.

Proper Application and Assessment of Fit

Apply the devices to the child and look for the following features of fit both without socks and with socks and shoes on.

Instruct the child's caregivers to apply the splint or orthosis correctly, to ensure its optimum effectiveness. Improper donning techniques, rather than inadequacy of the device, often causes poor tolerance. For example, many adults seem to think that if the straps are loose, the splint is more comfortable. They do not seem to understand that a foot that slides up in the splint is in positional argument with the contours of the device, which results in far more discomfort than snug strapping. The clinician can, however, easily meet these caregivers halfway by lining the straps with thin foam padding.

Equinus-related splints are most easily applied while the child sits comfortably, supported from behind. (If the children are small enough, I prefer to teach caregivers to apply splints while the children sit on their laps, allowing the affected legs and feet to be seen and handled from above.) Before trying to slip the foot into the device, whether it is solid or hinged at the ankle, attend to the following two considerations (Figure 7.45):

1. Fully flex the child's hip and knee so ankle dorsiflexion is easier to achieve.
2. Simultaneously, fully dorsiflex the ankle and supinate the foot so the great toe is higher off the floor of the device than the little toe.

With these steps accomplished, proceed as follows:

3. Slide the heel into the heel pocket of the device (Figure 7.45).
4. Lay the forefoot down onto the floor of the device, tucking the lateral aspect into the lateral wall.
5. Secure the proximal foot with a wide strap, padded if needed and feathered (snipped at short intervals along the proximal edge) to relieve binding. This strap holds the heel down in the heel pocket of the device (Figure 7.46).
6. Secure the distal tibia with a wide strap to hold the heel back in the device (Figure 7.46).
7. Secure the proximal tibia with a wide strap (Figure 7.46).

To apply a crouch-control device (CAFS/HCAFS), pull the walls apart behind the malleoli, tip the shaft medially while sliding the foot piece over the foot, and align the shaft section with the tibia (Figures 7.47 and 7.48). Failure to use the tipping maneuver results in an unnecessary struggle to don and doff the splint.

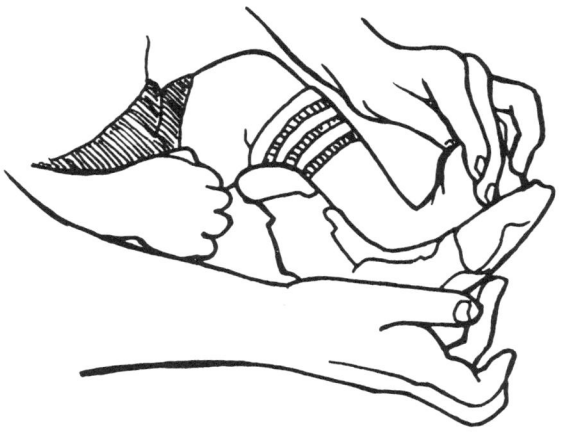

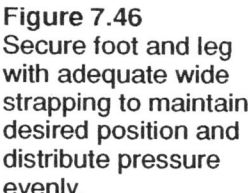

Figure 7.46
Secure foot and leg with adequate wide strapping to maintain desired position and distribute pressure evenly.

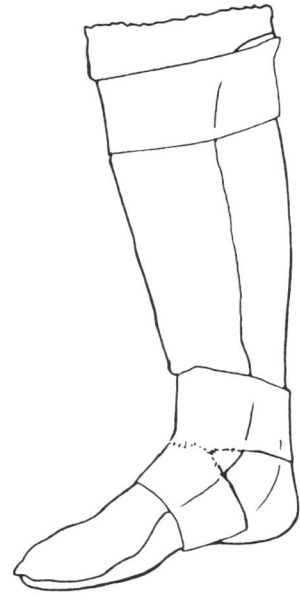

Figure 7.45 Application procedure—posterior contact AFS/AFO: Flex the knee and ankle, maintain neutral STJ, slide heel in first, medial forefoot last.

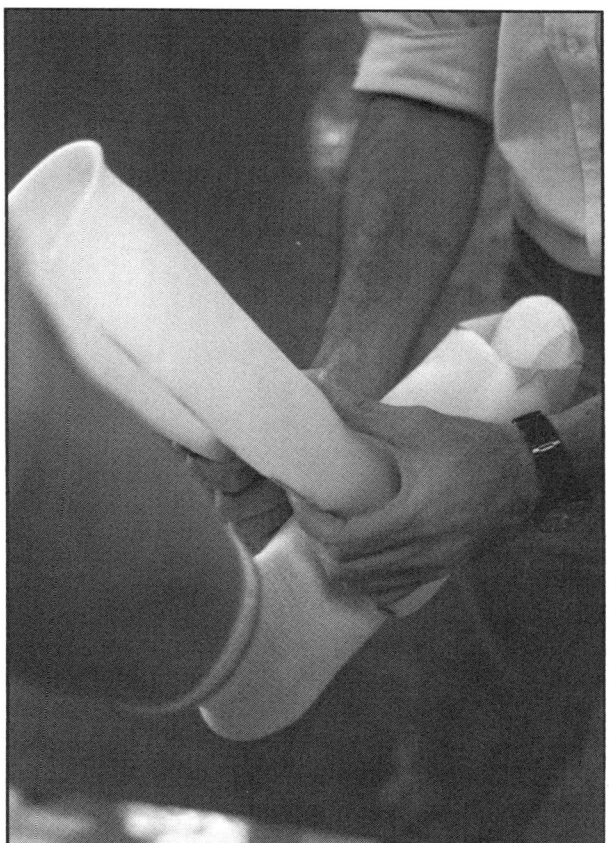

Figure 7.47 Application procedure—crouch-control AFS: Tip the shaft medially before slipping foot into foot section . . .

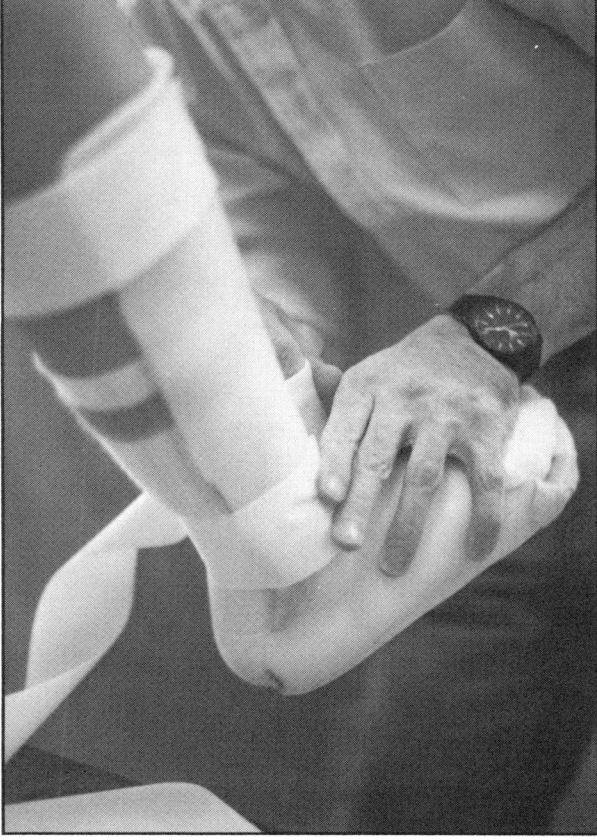

Figure 7.48 . . . then realign shaft portion after foot is inserted.

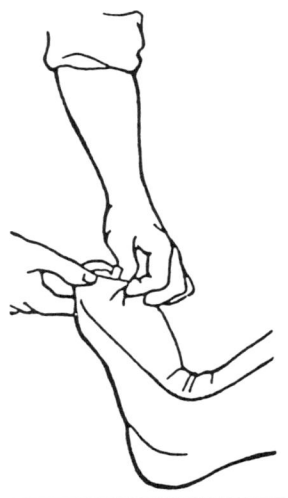

Figure 7.49
Toes are all supported
with .5 cm to spare.

After applying the device appropriately, continue with the check-out procedure.

- Does the distal anterior portion of the floor of the device support the full length of all toes, extending beyond them by .5 cm? (Figure 7.49)
  — Growth, forward shear, and spreading of the foot in standing will occur, so a little extra length is desirable (Figure 7.49).

This feature of support for the toes is important for children with developmental disabilities, particularly those who rely on primitive toe-grasping mechanisms to stabilize. If this section of the floor of the splint is available, the therapist can work with the device to try to reduce toe-grasp. (See suggestions below.) If the distal floor has been cut off, either proximal to the toes across the metatarsal heads, or proximal to the metatarsal heads, the respective outcomes include the following: The toes tend to claw over the distal edge and become tight in flexion; painful callouses form on the metatarsal heads, usually resulting in complaints and refusal to wear the device; or the lever arm for support for the foot and ankle is reduced, resulting in minimal influence on equinus posturing. Consequently, I refuse approval of any ankle-foot orthosis made for a child with neuromotor disorder if the anterior edge of the foot section stops short of the full length of the toes, or if it cuts across the metatarsal heads. If the device will not be replaced, I modify it to reestablish the minimum adequate toe support by posting with an extension made of splint material or PPT® padding covered with moleskin.

- Is there evidence that any of the trimmed edges bind on the surface of the foot, ankle, or leg?
  — If so, mark them and relieve the constriction by heating to flare, or by trimming. The foot and leg should slide easily into and out of the splint.

Assessment of Function—Standing

Place the child in standing, with support as needed, and continue check-out procedures.

- Does the foot pronate abnormally within the device? Is it likely that the shoe will contribute the needed support to achieve proper alignment?
  — If the foot pronates abnormally, and the structural assessment indicates that it was built with adequate alignment features, then consider two courses of modification:

1. Reduce available room for pronatory excursion by inserting Plastazote® padding within the splint, beginning at the lateral calcaneus, medial tarsus, and lateral forefoot.

2. If pronation persists after reducing the space, consider posting under the plantar surface of the medial calcaneus and/or medial metatarsal heads, if the child's age and modeling potential warrant this decision. Refrain from posting for two or three weeks in very young children to see if some modeling begins to occur within the splint after gaining adequate hindfoot stabilization.

Toe Grasp—Approaches to Management

Check for evidence of persistent toe grasping. If it is present, the following methods of minimizing the problem are suggested.

- Evaluate for shortening of the long and intrinsic toe flexors. Use serial casting to regain true muscle length and extensibility in the toe flexors before attempting to reduce toe grasp as a functional compensation. If functional toe grasp persists after full extensibility has been achieved, and this extensibility allows 90 degrees of great toe hyperextension and 65 degrees of hyperextension at the other metatarsophalangeal (MTP) joints, do the following: Keep 50-60 percent of body weight aligned over the hindfoot because when the center of gravity is displaced forward, toe grasp is a normal equilibrium response. If toe grasp persists, look again at the available support for midline hindfoot and midtarsal joint alignment, and adjust them accordingly. Toe grasping often accompanies abnormal pronation because the long toe flexors gain a mechanical advantage for contracting at the toes. This advantage occurs because of the altered orientation of the axes of the foot joints. If the splint design appears adequate, and toe grasping persists, take any of the following actions:

  — Post under the medial calcaneus with 1/8-inch Plastazote®, to increase STJ congruity.

  — Elevate the lateral four toes slightly: Add an elevation for the full length of all the toes, raising the lateral four toes onto a slightly higher surface than the great toe. Build the toe pad on the floor of the device from the crease that separates the ball of the foot from the proximal phalanges, but to the distal edge of the device. Use one or two layers of 1/8-inch Plastazote® or PPT® padding to lift the toes. Cover the padding with moleskin. A thin, wide metatarsal strap can help secure the toes in extension by prohibiting elevation of the metatarsal heads. (The 2-inch-width SabreStrip® loop is a good choice because it is thin and soft.)

  — Separate the proximal toes by using a silicone elastomer such as Otoform-K®, which molds like putty into a firm but slightly compressible substance (see Appendix 4 for sources); or use a light foam toe spreader. The elastomer must be cleaned with its specific solvent and bonding agent before it will attach to the splint.

- If functional toe grasping persists, consider the possible influence of an abnormal toe grasp reflex in response to application of pressure to the plantar surface of the metatarsal heads. If evidence exists for toe grasp reflex activity, try to relieve pressure under the metatarsal heads. This action will diminish sensory input to the reflexogenous area for toe grasp, which would presumably thus be diminished. There are two ways to relieve pressure under the metatarsal heads when making splints:

1. At the time of splint fabrication, build a recess into the splint in the designated area by applying a Plastazote® pad, 1/8- or 1/4-inch thick, cut to fit the plantar surface of the metatarsal heads.

Bevel all edges for smooth contour. Then apply the socks, the stockinet, and the splint material. Mold the splint material carefully under the distal, central metatarsal shafts while the splint material is setting. This prevents the central metatarsal heads from lowering into the recess formed in the sole of the device. Replace the pad in the finished splint to protect the structures of the longitudinal arch from abnormal weight-bearing forces. The soft pad under the metatarsal heads can be expected to lessen the proprioceptive and tactile input into the receptors in that area of the foot.

2. If you have already made the device or want to increase the depth of the metatarsal depression, do the following: Apply a Plastazote® pad to the plantar aspect of the metatarsal heads, cover the padded foot with a sock and stockinet, heat the area of the metatarsal heads with a heat gun until it is clear, and apply the splint to the foot. The padding will create a recess in the area of the metatarsal heads as the splint material sets.

These and the following approaches to management of the tonic toe grasp reflex are derived from the rationale used in the inhibitory casts developed by Yates, Mott, and Duncan at Good Samaritan Hospital in Puyallup, Washington.

• Draw the great toe medially, abducting it away from the second toe. Apply a thin, soft strap through a slot in the floor of the device, between the great toe and the second toe. Connect it with Sabre Grip® hook and Velcro® loop to the outer surface of the distal medial wall or floor of the device. When the strap is fastened, it draws the great toe medially, away from the other toes. By separating the great toe, the lateral deviation of the remaining toes and forefoot can be discouraged (presumably through the ligamentous connections), and the global pattern of toe grasp can be broken. Yates (1979) and Hylton (1988) have advocated this technique as a feature of their casts and orthoses. I have tried using the toe strap, but I met with resistance due to discomfort every time, despite selecting soft strap material. Keep this idea available as an option and implement it as needed. Maintain maximum concern for the child's comfort and explore the effectiveness of any and all more comfortable alternatives, such as elastomer.

Both of these systems for relief of toe grasp (metatarsal pressure relief and the hallux-adductor strap) may be combined as well as used separately. There would be a better understanding about their immediate and long-term biomechanical consequences if research were undertaken to explore their effects on alignment and function.

Features of Appropriate Outerwear for the Splinted Foot

Most of the splints for the foot and ankle demand shoes sometimes two or more sizes larger than the child normally wears. Because the splint provides the main support for the foot structures, it is not necessary to purchase expensive "orthopedic" shoes to wear over them. However, the outer and inner dimensions of any shoe or sneaker can influence the functional effectiveness of the splint. For this reason, I shop for appropriate models of outer athletic shoes and try to keep several sizes in stock. I can save the caregivers the trouble of shopping for them after the therapy session, and I can see for myself that the functional requirements of the outer shoe, as an adjunct to the splint, have been met.

The optimum support for most splint designs is provided by a sneaker or shoe with the following characteristics (Figure 7.50):

- Flat and stable sole: no heel wedge, no bumps on the surface. The thickness of the sole is the same at the heel and toe. The edges of the sole contact the floor on all sides of the shoe, prohibiting rocking.
- The toe box is flexible and wide.
- The heel box is reinforced and, in tennis shoes, edged in rubber or plastic.
- The tennis shoe insole is removable.
- The lacing panels are not stitched together across the forefoot; instead they can be opened to expose the entire tongue. Basketball-style sneakers, both low-cut and high-cut, open closer to the toe than other styles. They are particularly useful as outerwear for wider feet and bulkier splint designs.

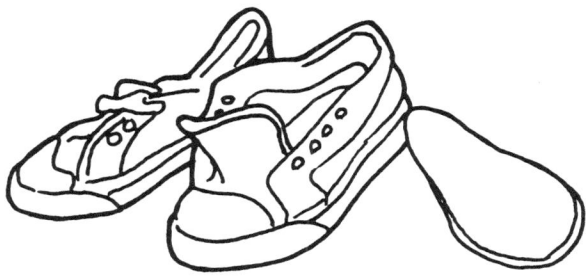

Figure 7.50   Shoes are a significant feature of the support system. They must be stable, flexible, deep, and wide at the toe box. Remove the insole.

Some therapists suggest that a high-cut heel box (such as a high-top basketball style sneaker) offers greater support for holding the splinted foot in the shoe. I question the decision to use any splint that will not stay down in the shoe. Alternative interventions may be needed, such as a series of casts to increase mobility at the ankle and possibly the knee joints, or the application of a more dynamic device such as a hinged ankle-foot splint. A thorough assessment of contributing factors is needed.

I do find use for the high-cut style sneaker if, in a hinged device, the hinge happens to fall close enough to the upper edge of the heel box in a standard sneaker that its operation is hindered, or if the hinge does not seat properly in the shoe. The flexible cloth upper of the high-top sneaker does not impede the motion needed at the ankle.

These features appear in tennis shoes sold by many discount department stores. However, some children have such wide feet that special shoes are required after the application of splints.

For some children, a sneaker causes problems related to tripping on carpeting or rough surfaces. For them, a leather sole may be more feasible. I advocate initially complementing the splinting system with a well-designed inexpensive tennis shoe. If tripping is a problem, then the caregiver will need to shop for a suitable leather shoe.

When the shoe fits well over the splint, the functional influences of the complete system can be evaluated. Continue functional checkout procedures by applying the splints with socks and shoes.

- Is the device too tight with socks on?
  - If so, try heating and flaring open the anterior edges. It is not necessary to clamp the foot into a circumferential grip in most devices. The edges should be trimmed back enough to allow easy access without a struggle. By using wide Velcro® straps, you can achieve a circumferential fit, if desired, after applying the splint.

Place the child in standing position with the splint(s) and appropriate shoe(s) on. Play together for several minutes to allow areas of pressure to become apparent.

- Note whether the complete system realigns the foot, ankle, and lower leg for optimum weight-bearing efficiency and stability.
- Evaluate the control that the sneaker or shoe offers relative to medial or lateral deviations of the splinted leg. If the child needs a closer fit or greater stability, either line the inner walls of the heel box with adhesive-backed padding, or add a post to the splint to stabilize the heel against rolling.

Allow the child to wear the splint around the department for 10 to 15 minutes. Watch for evidence of discomfort while you review splint care and management instructions with attending caregivers. (See Appendix 1: Splint Care Instructions and Precautions.)

Functional Assessment—Ambulation

Observe changes in gait pattern or alignment in standing, and note undesirable manifestations. These might include one or more of the following signs:

- Knee hyperextension or "back-knee."
- An apparent compulsion to walk backwards rather than to stand still.
- Toe-stepping.
- Limping or refusal to take weight on the splinted foot.
- In-toeing (beyond your expectations).
- Out-toeing beyond 10 degrees.
- Spin (or whip) upon heel-strike or at toe-off.

If any of these problems are evident, try the following measures:

Knee hyperextension—As discussed previously in the context of management of equinovarus deformity and in Chapter 5, try first to influence the foot to pronate slightly at the STJ. If knee hyperextension does not diminish, add a knee hyperextension splint to the management system. Interfere with normal ankle motion only as much as is necessary to assure safe toe clearance in swing. Use night splinting to maintain extensibility into dorsiflexion.

These measures may fail for reasons related to effectiveness, tolerance, or compliance. If that is the case, reduce the available plantarflexion provided in the hinged AFS to stop at 5 degrees of dorsiflexion. Prepare the surface with splint solvent cement and add a small patch of heated splint material to the proximal posterior outer edge of the foot section to increase its height (Figures 7.51 and 7.52). The resulting range of plantarflexion should end in a position of 5 degrees of dorsiflexion (Figure 7.53).

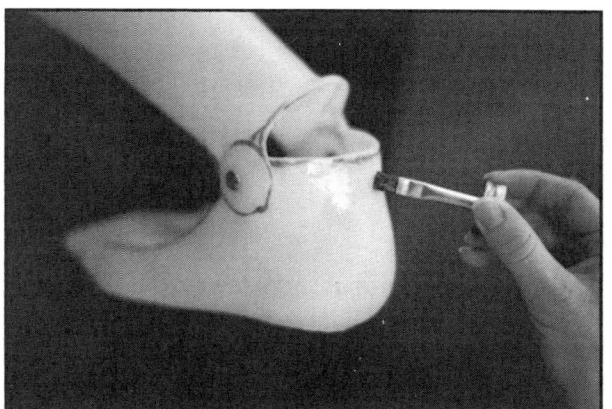

Figure 7.51   Revise HAFS to alter (or strengthen) the angle of the plantarflexion stop: Apply solvent to proximal posterior heel section . . .

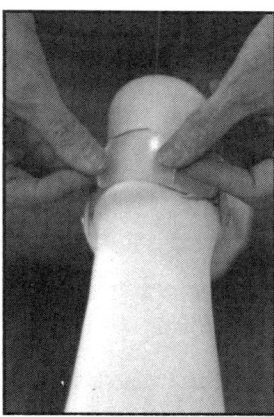

Figure 7.52
. . . then apply a small patch of heated splint material. To increase angle of dorsiflexion, extend the patch above the rim of the heel piece.

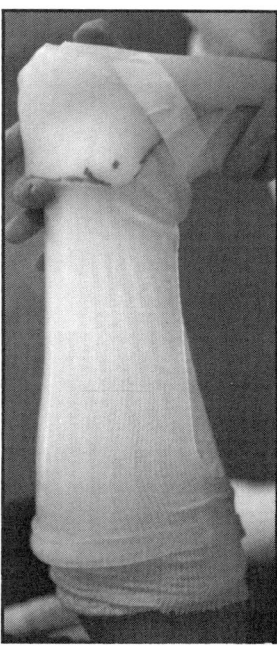

Figure 7.53
HAFS, modified for knee hyperextension: Set the ankle stop at 5 degrees of dorsiflexion.

Backward stepping—The angle of dorsiflexion between the shaft of the device and the floor is set at 90 degrees or less, which is inadequate to facilitate forward progression. This problem occurs only in solid-ankle devices, such as the SAFS, a solid AFO, or a cast boot. The addition of a heel lift usually corrects this problem.

Persistent toe-stepping—Some children continue to walk on their toes, even while wearing a solid AFS, an AFO, or a cast boot. The cause might be inadequate ankle dorsiflexion structured into the device, which induces a mandatory knee hyperextension that the child avoids by remaining on toes.

Persistent toe-stepping often indicates a lack of knee extension range of motion and/or control of the timing needed to establish full knee extension just prior to heel strike. Persistence of knee flexion through both swing and stance phases results in an obligation to step on the toe, regardless of the position of dorsiflexion maintained at the ankle (Rang et al. 1986). In treatment sessions and home programs, work on the following objectives: to mobilize any tight hip joint capsules and ligament structures, particularly the anterior ligaments on the opposite side; to strengthen knee extensors in combination with hip flexion, in both the closed and open chain; and to supplement therapeutic exercise with night splinting and positioning systems, with an emphasis on maintaining hamstrings mobility.

If these measures do not result in a significant gain in knee extension mobility and function within four months, I advocate conservative intervention with long-leg serial casts, combined with weight-bearing and therapeutic exercise. (See Chapter 6 for discussion of progressive long-leg casts.) Surgical lengthening remains a viable (though last) alternative for regaining adequate knee extension mobility, but only if surgery follows dynamic EMG analysis to determine the need for concurrent distal rectus femoris transfer (Perry 1987; Gage et al. 1987).

Increased in-toeing—Abnormal femoral antetorsion is common among children with a history of movement and tonus abnormality since birth. As the structure of the femur aligns the femoral condyles in medial rotation, the uncompensated lower leg and foot are similarly aligned. As discussed previously, however, many children gain positional stability in stance via forefoot abduction, as a component of pronation. In the latter case, the rearfoot structures are rotated medially on the fixed, abducted forefoot. Uncorrected pronation of the foot dampens the kinetic chain that normally features lateral rotation in stance. The angle of gait appears more normal when this compensation is operating. However, as the pronated foot absorbs and promotes proximal medial torque forces, the switch from shock-absorber to rigid lever, and from pronation to supination, fails to occur (Figure 7.54).

When compensatory pronation at the subtalar and midtarsal joints is prohibited, or corrected, the proximal torsional components become evident. The result, then, of restoring the joints of the foot to their proper alignment, either in splints or casts, is often a sudden manifestation of in-toeing, or an increase in its severity, particularly if the child is ambulatory (Figure 7.55).

As was discussed in Chapter 4, a second factor that often produces in-toeing is medial genicular position, which entails excessive medial rotation of the tibia and fibula on the femur and a lack of soft tissue capacity to allow excursion of the lower leg into lateral rotation. Treatment must be aimed at restoring a balance of ligament extensibility and muscle power—between the medial and lateral knee flexors—to allow the tibia to rotate laterally with extension.

I advise the child's caregivers to accept a nondebilitating increase in in-toeing while the ambulatory child wears the splints. I have clinically observed a reduction in in-toeing after as little as three months of splint wear in some children, and over a period of several years in others. (Compare the same child in Figures 7.54 and 7.56.) Reducing pronation in the foot structures seems to restore the operation of the closed kinetic chain in favor of the normal moment of lateral rotation in stance. Rapid resolution of in-toeing in this case is most likely the result of repeated application of lateral torque forces to the shortened soft tissues at the knee joint. Therapeutic exercise focuses on supporting this same adjustment by facilitating strengthening and mobility into lateral rotation with hip and knee extension, combined with weight-bearing.

For children who use foot splints and orthoses and do not require control at the ankle joint, another approach to the problem of in-toeing is to adjust the trim lines on the sole of the device in the order of the gait extension modification. (See Chapter 5 for a thorough discussion of gait extension modifications of the SFS.) The rationale for the gait extension modification is the facilitation of forward progression by imposing a path of least resistance at the forefoot that favors lateral rotation of the foot. This modification is useful for children up to 12 years of age (Spencer et al. 1984).

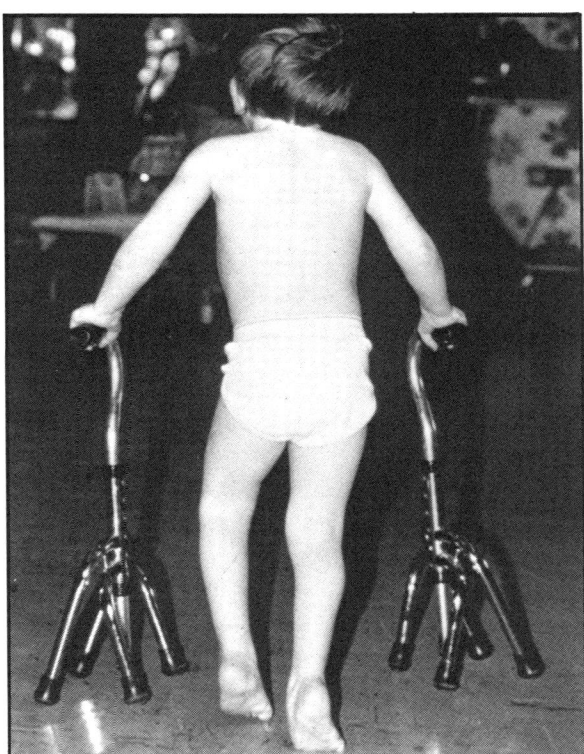

Figure 7.54 Evidence of medial torsional and rotary deformity prior to prolonged application of foot and ankle support devices, unilateral proximal hamstrings release and bilateral TALs at age 4 years, and many years of therapeutic exercise and ambulation.

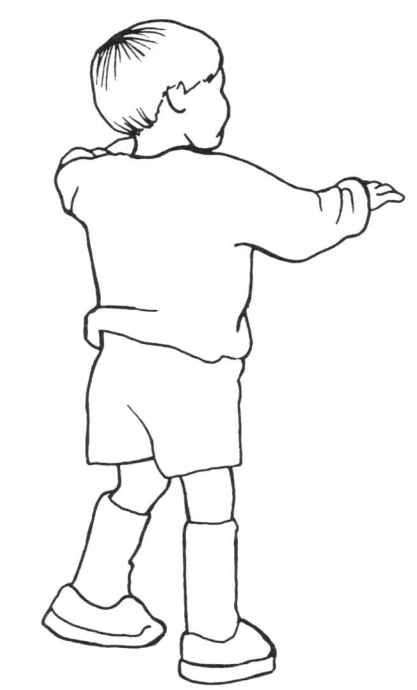

Figure 7.55 Application of control system for the foot pronation often results in increased in-toeing. Reducing compensatory foot pronation reveals proximal torsional and rotary deformities.

Figure 7.56
Note eventual reduction of medial torsional and rotary deformity and evidence of in-toeing in gait six years later. (Compare with Figure 7.54.) (This child moved away during the year this picture was taken. At age 14 years, gait analysis revealed that he had developed severe calcaneal—crouch—deformity with marked lateral torsion of the lower legs and knee flexion contractures. His posture at hips and pelvis was within normal limits.)

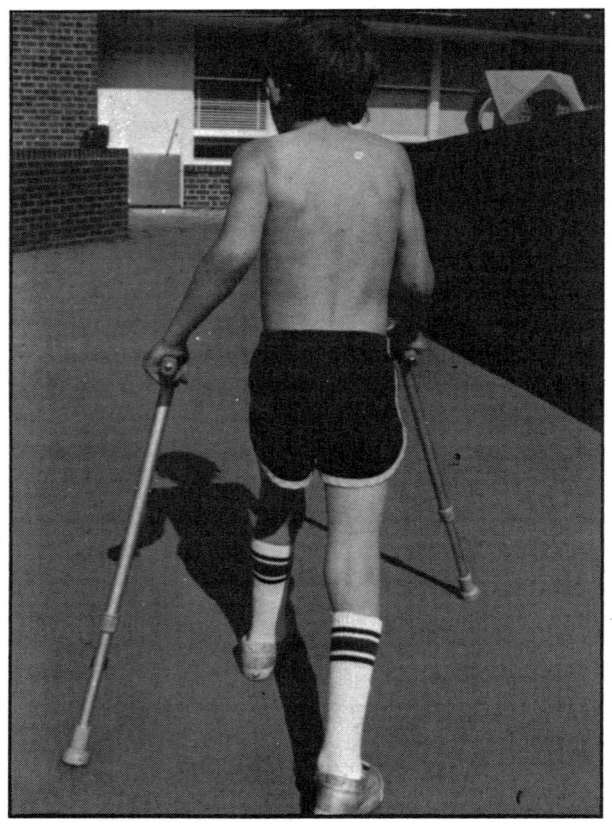

Out-toeing beyond 15 degrees—In the same context as the gait extension modification discussed above and in Chapter 5, a rigid medial extension of the floor of the foot support device presents the child who walks with toes turned out with a hindrance to forward progression over the medial aspect of the forefoot. This modification is contraindicated in children older than 8 years (Spencer et al. 1984).

Limping or a refusal to take weight on the splinted foot—If you observe evidence of discomfort, remove the splint immediately and check the skin for any dark red, well-defined spots. If you observe these spots, check the edges and the interior aspect of the splint for corresponding sharp ridges or lumps or for a poverty of relief or of padding over a bony prominence. Then carve, heat, and flare, or recess and pad accordingly. If binding is evident near the toes and the sneaker appears to be too tight, create more room for the splint by snipping the stitching in the sneaker at the areas where the lacing meets the tongue, until a larger shoe can be obtained.

If there is no evidence of localized pressure as a cause for refusal to take weight, consider using desensitizing and joint mobilization techniques. Prepare the plantar surface for weight-bearing by applying deep pressure to the heel and lateral borders and firmly stroke the plantar surface of the foot. Use simple tone-reduction handling techniques for generalized relaxation, if needed. Then, reapply the splints and reassess.

Heel spin in the stance phase—Some children with hypotonia and/or developmental delay demonstrate ligamentous laxity resulting in genu recurvatum exceeding 15-20 degrees. These children may contact the floor only with the corner of the heel of the shoe, in which case a spin of the foot and leg occurs. If a child with this type of problem uses an AFS, either hinged or solid, even when it is set in 5 degrees of dorsiflexion, the problem of heel-standing usually persists.

The first line of intervention for these children should be a knee hyperextension splint (a simplified Swedish knee cage). (See Chapter 5 for a thorough discussion of knee hyperextension splints.) If the knee splint is tolerated, evaluate the remaining foot and ankle structures for significant deviation or functional problems.

Another simple approach to this problem is to build up the posterior outer wall of the shoe, extending its lever arm in order to block the heel from rocking back. This buttress cannot be flexible and is best applied by an orthotist or cobbler.

If the knee hyperextension splint and/or the buttress fails, I recommend using a knee-ankle-foot orthosis, hinged at both the knee and the ankle, with two artificial hamstring straps connecting the posterior thigh cuff to the shaft of the leg section. The straps, which are made of nonstretch Dacron® or nylon webbing with a tooth type of buckle, are infinitely adjustable and are generally set to limit knee extension to a maximum of five degrees of flexion. Extension beyond that setting is prohibited by the tension on the strap, which functions as an artificial hamstring muscle. This device can be effective for training and for quadriceps strengthening if used consistently and monitored closely. I have yet to succeed in building one with splinting material. When made of copolymer, it may be used for a three- to six-month training period. Consistency seems a key feature in the success of this temporary intervention.

The expense of high-temperature orthoses of this type may be prohibitive, warranting further exploration of alternative designs with splinting materials. Years of sessions of therapeutic exercise devoted to reducing the problem of knee hyperextension, however, are also expensive.

Forefoot spin or heel whip—If the foot spins on the metatarsal heads after midstance, the floor of the device may be too flat at the toes and rigid enough to prohibit toe hyperextension with forward progression. Alternately, children might be flexing their toes, effectively fusing their forefeet. In either case, the toe-support area of the splint, orthosis, or cast should be beveled upward slightly at the medial corner, which facilitates smooth forward progression over the foot at the end of the stance phase. Such a beveled floor also facilitates hip extension on the stance leg after midstance.

Whips in midstance to terminal stance also suggest the presence of a forefoot varus deformity or an abnormally short first metatarsal, necessitating a foot spin to accomplish push-off over the medial aspect of the forefoot. Evaluate the child and the splint closely for either of these problems, and intervene accordingly with age-appropriate posting of optimal density and durability.

Note: Whether or not you have seen evidence of functional problems, remove the splint and examine the leg and foot for pressure areas.

The "Break-In" Period

Evidence of pressure is not necessarily a problem sign. A large pink area over the medial tarsus and lateral forefoot, for example, reveals that a new distribution of support forces has been applied. In this instance, apply alcohol to the pink areas to help to accelerate the formation of a callous on the skin, and wait for the pink area to fade to normal color before reapplying the splint. Instruct caregivers to continue to use this procedure as a means of gradually building tolerance for the support system without raising a blister or causing the child unnecessary discomfort. The time that elapses between skin checks is gradually increased from one to two hours to four or more, over a period of one to two weeks. (See Appendix 1: Splint Care Instructions and Precautions.)

Discussion: Questions and Considerations

Participants in splint and cast workshops often ask the following questions during the discussion session.

On Aligning the Foot Structures in Children Under 5 Years of Age

Should the clinician try to build 4 degrees of calcaneal valgus position into a splint designed to support the foot and ankle of a child age 3 years?

I appreciate the clinician's concern for the normal developmental features of the foot and lower leg, because I share the same concern. However, the clinician must remember that we are working with splinting material of low durability and significant flexibility. The splints are simply not so well constructed or rigid that they prohibit small calcaneal excursion on weight-bearing. I therefore typically set the calcaneus on the sagittal plane, incorporating varum in the distal lower leg if greater than 3 degrees. I assume that the cartilaginous calcaneus, any fatty tissue, the thick sock, and the flexibility of the material will allow the child of 3 years to gain 4 degrees of calcaneal eversion in weight-bearing within the splint. Because the ankle-foot devices are less apt to allow frontal plane excursions of the calcaneus than the foot splints, I sometimes mold them over a double layer of thick socks. The finished splint is worn with one sock.

Some clinicians suggest using semisoft intrinsic varus posting under the foot to allow for pronation within the HAFS. They propose that this posting will help to minimize adverse reaction to wearing the device. The intrinsic post is made of Plastazote® and Aliplast® materials, heated in a convection oven, molded to the plantar surface of the child's foot, and ground on a grinding wheel to post into varus or valgus as needed at the forefoot and hindfoot (Jenkins and Turner 1988).

In the event that a child fails to tolerate a HAFS molded over a thick sock, or in the presence of a strong tonic grasp reflex or severe tactile hypersensitivity in the foot, the intrinsic post offers a feasible management alternative. Furthermore, to a limited extent, the intrinsic post can be replaced or revised and the HAFS shell retained when growth occurs. However, I have not yet experienced a failure to tolerate a HAFS in my clinical experience whenever I have implemented the appropriate selection criteria. Any failures to tolerate the HAFS have occurred because of limitation of mobility in the talocrural joint; they have resolved after a course of serial casting to regain mobility. I also have concerns about varus posting the foot of a young child in any device, because of the modeling possibilities that such posting might prohibit at the forefoot and first ray.

On Constructing the Hinged Devices

How can the hinged ankle-foot splint be built to minimize the forces that cause the shaft piece to crack next to the hinge joint?

The hinged AFS cannot express the rotary motions that normally occur between the leg and foot in the stance phase of gait. The hinges are simple axes, allowing one direction of motion around them. Rotary motions must occur in subtle excursions within the device while the device guides the leg forward over the plantigrade foot. When the hinge joints are placed directly over the malleoli in the splint, the shaft piece rotates medially over the weight-bearing foot piece after heel strike and laterally over the same fixed foot piece after weight assumption until toe-off. These rotary excursions of the shaft piece over the fixed foot piece cause the splint material in the area of the hinge to fatigue and eventually break. Torque forces are the cause of the fatigue.

In fact, we walk over an axis at the talocrural joint that differs markedly from the anatomical axis of motion. The ankle joint axis normally lies at 20 to 30 degrees lateral to the frontal plane. In order to walk on a sagittal plane line of progression around that axis, it would be necessary to adduct the foot (in-toe) 20-30 degrees to dorsiflex the leg over the foot.

In fact, we typically use an angle of gait that lies on or within 10 degrees lateral to the sagittal plane, suggesting that the functional talocrural joint axis lies within 10 degrees *medial,* rather than lateral, to the frontal plane.

Therefore, to gain durability in the HAFS (both standard and crouch-control types) and to facilitate forward progression over the plantigrade foot in stance, I advocate setting the medial hinge on the peak of the medial malleolus and the lateral hinge proximal and anterior to the lateral malleolus, so that a line connecting the two hinges lies on the frontal plane or rotated slightly medial to it (Figure 7.57). The result is a relatively torque-free progression of the shaft over the plantigrade foot in a normal line of progression (Figure 7.58).

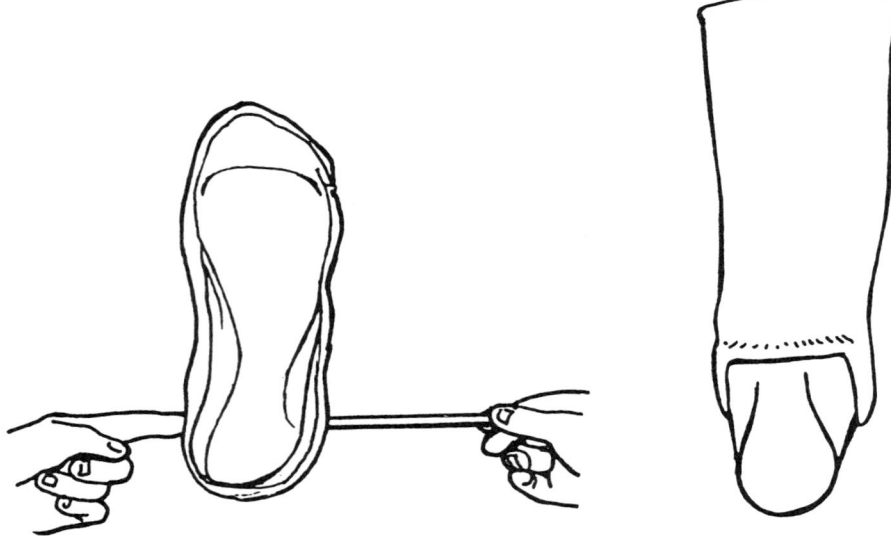

Figure 7.57 Locate hinges on an axis that lies on, or medially rotated relative to, the frontal plane. Medial hinge is centered on the peak of the medial malleolus. Lateral hinge is aligned anterior and proximal to the lateral malleolus. The hinges are parallel relative to the transverse plane.

Figure 7.58 Dorsiflexion occurs within the splint on a smooth sagittal-plane line of progression over the plantigrade foot.

On Treatment in Splints and Orthoses

Do you think it is appropriate to use splints during treatment sessions, or should the child remain barefoot and rely on the devices for carry-over?

I always remove all foot devices and socks during a portion of the treatment session, at which time I attend to such concerns as tactile hypersensitivity, joint mobility limitations, and floor mobility skills that do not require full loading on the foot. I definitely advocate using splints as needed during treatment, however, such as when the therapist cannot successfully maintain optimal alignment in the joints of the foot and ankle while facilitating more proximal weight shifts and responses. Ligamentous laxity in the foot structures can defeat even the cleverest therapist.

When already stressed and lengthened ligaments are forced to bear continued abnormal stresses, the therapist who fails to protect them during weight-bearing activities undermines the goal of achieving a relative shortening of those ligaments as the child grows. The supporting tissues must be consistently protected from inordinate stresses while the child grows in height if the chain of deforming events is to be broken. In addition, the therapist who hopes to facilitate normal closed-chain biomechanical events is likely to experience increased success by providing adequate support for the distal joints involved in that chain. If the soft tissue support structures gain strength and their slack is absorbed by bone growth, the foot support devices can, of course, be removed.

The key to using splints in treatment is to minimize any unnecessary constriction on desirable motion. For this purpose, the therapist may construct a foot support system for use in therapy sessions, although the same child uses ankle-foot devices at school and at home. When it is time to introduce the child to a less restrictive support system under supervised conditions, the therapist can come to an informed judgment regarding the child's readiness to progress to such a system.

Although night splints are useful in maintaining extensibility of muscle and connective tissue, they do not eliminate the need for daytime splints or orthoses. Well-made splints and orthoses can arrange the architecture of the foot and ankle to effect optimum loading through the extremity, efficient weight transfer, and forward progression. They can also prohibit compensations related to inadequate dorsiflexion in swing. The result is a proprioceptive experience of a more normal lower extremity function than the child can gain independently. The therapist is always prepared to move to less controlling systems when the child shows readiness to discard a component of the splinting system and assume a more active control.

On Progression

How do you decide what to use next as a splint design? Is there a group of devices that are used in sequence in management?

I follow the principles and indications stated in Chapter 5 in determining the appropriate splint design. I suggest reevaluating the design in use at whichever of the following points comes first: the foot changes; three months; when the splint cracks; or when the child outgrows it. I regard the limited durability of the device as an advantage in this context, because I must reassess the child's status relative to the chosen intervention when the device breaks.

I do not map a course of progression according to splint designs, although there are increments of support and control available within the varying models. I prefer to try to offer the child the most dynamic, least restrictive device possible without compromising the alignment of the foot structures. I also feel that less support for the foot and ankle is better than more only when the quality of antigravity function is retained in the less restrictive devices. I supplement dynamic splint use during the day with night splinting to maintain joint and muscle mobility whenever possible. When a dynamic system fails to offer functional improvement because stability is a more pressing requirement, I limit available motion to provide greater positional stability, and I work with the child to gain the proximal control needed to function effectively with less support.

I accept that growth spurts and illness and family stresses of all sorts can bring on joint contractures, despite the efforts of all the child's caregivers to prevent them. I do not consider a return from foot support splints to serial casting followed by ankle-foot splints to be a failure. The problem at hand should be managed appropriately, and growth-induced recurrence of contracture is a fact of management in children with hypertonus. The thoughtful clinician should be prepared to move in either direction of control as needed, and to offer caregivers a logical rationale for doing so.

The relative cost-effectiveness of splints also offers clinicians and families the opportunity to provide different support systems for different circumstances. It is not necessary to select a single device for all purposes when different activities present different functional requirements. It is possible to provide the child with foot splints for formal occasions, special celebrations, and therapy sessions; ankle-foot splints for school; and stretch splints at night. In this way, the child has the opportunity to apply some foot and ankle-control skills in short-term, less-supported circumstances, and to demonstrate readiness for progression.

On Using Casts and Splints for Children with Hemiplegia

I've been told that a child with hemiplegia should be managed with bilateral, identical interventions, particularly casts, so the sensory-motor experience will be symmetrical. Is this always necessary?

I don't agree with that idea. I do not concur with the notion that the two abnormal experiences of walking with both feet and ankles immobilized are better than one. I would rather facilitate the most natural and efficient weight-bearing progression possible. Because of this, I begin casting only the more affected side.

I do agree with the concern that children with hemiplegia demonstrate compensatory deformities in the less affected foot and leg; sometimes they reveal hamstrings contracture or pronation deformity on that side. The possibility for bilateral involvement is worth investigating in all children with hemiplegia, in my opinion, and adequate and specific support and intervention for both sides should be offered.

If valgus deformity is evident in the less affected foot, I usually apply a stabilizing foot splint (SFS) to correct the alignment and, if needed, glue a lift to the sneaker to level the pelvis while the cast is worn on the more affected leg. There are exceptions to this approach, however, including the two following:

1. **Inadequate weight transfer onto the casted foot.** If the hemiplegic child maintains the more involved hip in an abducted position, the clinician must examine to rule out pressure sore and leg length discrepancy as precipitating problems. If they are not present, the team may attempt to intervene with a second cast for the less involved extremity. The second cast may be made with a wedged sole designed specifically to facilitate the desired weight transfer. The wedge should be built with the thickest edge at the posteriolateral aspect of the sole of the cast. The thinnest edge is anteriomedial. This posting angle throws the child's weight forward and laterally during the stance phase, toward the more affected side.

2. **Hamstrings contracture on the less affected side.** I advise long-leg casting to regain mobility, combined with weight-bearing activities and therapeutic exercise (Westin et al. 1983).

I do not use identical splinting devices for any child with hemiplegia, because the problems at the feet are not identical. I usually attempt to stabilize the less involved STJ complex in neutral alignment with a foot splint (SFS) if I note any deviation. On the more affected side, I prefer the dynamic ankle-foot devices—the hinged AFS or AFO—for the child who lacks toe clearance in swing or spontaneous and timely ankle dorsiflexion in gait. The amount of toe-drop in the swing phase is a significant factor in selecting these interventions. I gradually revise the plantarflexion stop to allow increasing degrees of plantarflexion to occur. Sometimes toe-drop resolves in swing and heel contact occurs with greater than 70 percent consistency in early stance with the foot unsupported in any device. If that happens, a supramalleolar splint (SMS) or SMO or modified SFS is considered next on the line of progression to minimal support systems.

I recommend consistent night splinting with the foot structures aligned and the ankle in at least 5 degrees of dorsiflexion throughout skeletal growth in an attempt to maintain extensibility in the triceps surae group of muscles. I often return to solid casting, however, if the child reveals after a growth spurt that previously gained ankle joint mobility and control have been lost to soft tissue shortening. I do not regard these episodes of cast use as failures, but rather as appropriate management.

On Treating Leg-Length Discrepancy in Hemiplegia

What about maintaining a shorter leg on the affected side as an aid to achieving clearance of the toe in swing?

As was discussed in chapter 5, I disagree with that idea, too. The child who wears an AFS or an AFO is in no need of assistance in clearing the toe; rather, this child needs a level pelvis for the transfer of weight from one leg to the other. The child with leg-length discrepancy and functional equinus deformity who walks without an ankle-foot support device will attempt to preserve the level alignment of the pelvis by toe-stepping, which minimizes vertical displacement during gait. This compensatory maneuver can accelerate the recurrence of fixed equinus deformity on the shortened side. I feel that the stance phase is far more important than swing when considering the issue of leg length. My first concern is maintaining a level pelvis.

When only one splint is used because the foot on the opposite side aligns normally, assess for leg-length discrepancy as a result of the thickness of the splint. If a discrepancy is present, attach a lift to the sneaker on the shorter side to restore a level pelvis. As a trial, tape a lift cut from 1/4-inch crepe sole material to the entire sole of the appropriate shoe. Evaluate the effect on pelvic alignment and function. If satisfactory, glue the lift on with contact cement or call upon a cobbler for professionally made lifts to be applied to all the shoes that the child normally wears.

Because a structural deficit in leg length of 1 cm or more can be expected with congenital hemiplegia, the application of a splint to the more affected side often levels the pelvis adequately.

Check leg lengths regularly. Deficits might not persist.

On Managing the Older Child

What about children with foot deformity who are older than 8 or 9 years of age? Are they too old for these interventions?

I have a couple of suggestions for this age group, and limited expectations for their success. Many factors contribute to the status of the foot and its correctability at this age. If the foot has been allowed to fall into deformity since infancy, the bones have formed and ossified in deformity as well. The deformed structures are not limited to soft tissue as the child ages. If the deformity is pliable and can be corrected with handling, however, a measure of benefit may be derived from intervening conservatively. The problem with tolerance in older children relates to the conflict between the need for rigid support for a pliable deformity and the status of bony development. Ultimately, the aim of intervention for the foot that exhibits rigid, unyielding deformity shifts to accommodation, maintenance, and prevention of further progression of deformity.

With these conditions in mind, here are some suggestions to consider:

- Trained therapists should implement joint mobilization techniques within the limits of contraindication, in an attempt to regain a normal mobility within the joints of the foot.

- The child of 8 to 15 years is not too old to undergo a serial casting course to try to regain lost mobility in soft tissue structures. Extend the time limit on the course before choosing to resort to surgery. Each cast may be worn for up to two weeks and/or the course of casting may span up to eight weeks. Allow for some complaints of aching discomfort that suggest that bone realignment (and possible reformation) is occurring. In my experience, these complaints do not occur consistently, and if they do, they pass within two or three weeks. If not, or if the child is debilitated by discomfort, remove the cast and recast with less correction. If complaints persist, discontinue the course.

- The heavier child with hypotonia and neuromuscular disorder will show a diminished response to the floor reaction forces applied by a foot splint. The pressure applied to key areas of the foot can become a problem rather than a facilitator of improved alignment, because the child's motor skills and consequent responses to the corrective forces are depressed.

Forefoot varus or valgus posting should be provided, using PPT® or other durable foam materials, in any device that is meant to restore a more normal STJ alignment and function.

- If a suitably posted foot splint fails to provide adequate or comfortable support for pronation, try gaining stability on the frontal plane while distributing the pressure over a larger skin surface by applying a hinged ankle-foot device. Adjust the plantarflexion stop to allow use of needed and available sagittal plane ankle motion. Use a splint first (posted as needed at the forefoot) to determine its effectiveness and the child's tolerance. Then, if satisfied, provide a comparable and more durable orthosis. Use this device consistently as the child grows taller, with the hope that laxity in the supportive ligaments will diminish. An ankle-foot support system may be needed for 6 to 12 months, or for the duration of its appropriate fit, or even for several years. The child's functional status will determine the need for this type of continued support.

- Biomedical engineering groups, podiatrists, and many therapists who specialize in sports-related problems are developing a rapidly expanding assortment of orthoses for adults of all ages. These orthoses are modified to meet the needs for age and activity-related support and comfort, though they do not claim to address the needs of the developmentally disabled population. Most of these devices are fabricated from a positive plaster mold and are poured from a negative impression cast of the patient's foot (Figure 7.59). Qualified clinicians can order these devices by sending to orthotic laboratories the negative cast mold taken in supine or prone positions with the foot structures aligned in either calcaneal midposition or STJ neutral position with the fourth and fifth metatarsal heads gently loaded. A completed prescription form and a detailed description of the functional ability, activity level, alignment features in and above the foot must accompany the negative cast mold(s). Most of these devices are designed to stabilize the flexible foot structures and to prevent pain, injury, or further deformity. They are not generally expected to correct existing deformity. I often use these devices for older children who require maintenance and comfort but for whom the SFS has proven unsuitable.

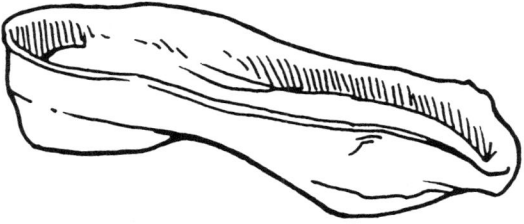

Figure 7.59 "Neutral position" cast molds are used to fabricate a variety of shoe inserts and "sporthotics" for older children and adults, and for children with mild hypotonia. Set this mold within 2 degrees of calcaneal midposition if STJ neutrality exceeds 3 degrees varus.

Summary

Among the most exciting features in this area of pediatric management are its vitality and fluidity. New considerations will come with new materials, new designs, and new information. We can expect that continued use of critical assessment skills will encourage us to consider how these interventions can be improved and refined or restructured. The main skills needed are detailed observation and problem solving, supported by objective data.

The final chapter is devoted to raising questions about these methods, their various rationales, and their effectiveness that require answers that can be derived only from further clinical research.

References

Agnew, P., DPM. Personal communication. 1988. Richmond, VA. December 8.

Coram, S. 1989. Personal communication and course handouts, Springfield, OH, January 16.

Gage, J. R., J. Perry, R. Hicks, S. Koop, and J. R. Werntz. 1987. Rectus femoris transfer to improve knee function in children with cerebral palsy. *Developmental Medicine and Child Neurology* 29:134-159.

Hylton, N. 1988. Personal communication and course handouts. First Annual Conference—Neurodevelopmental Treatment Association, Kansas City, MO. May 23.

Jenkins, W., and D. Turner. 1988. *AFO enhancement with the pediatric patient: Articulating AFOs with intrinsic posting.* Seminar, June 24-25. Cited in in-service training by J. LaVonne Jaeger, November 29, Lexington, KY.

Jordan, R. P. 1984. Therapeutic considerations of the feet and lower extremities in the cerebral palsied child. In *Symposium on podopediatrics—Clinics in podiatry*, edited by J. V. Ganley, 547-561. Philadelphia, PA: W. B. Saunders.

Jordan, R. P., J. Cusack, and B. Resseque. 1983. *Foot function and its relationship to posture in the pediatric patient with cerebral palsy and other neuromuscular disorders.* Symposium, sponsored by the Neurodevelopmental Treatment Association, NY: May 20-22.

McCrea, J. D. 1985. *Pediatric orthopedics of the lower extremity—An instructional handbook.* Mount Kisco, NY: Futura.

Molnar, G. E. 1986. Orthotic management of children. In *Orthotics, etcetera, 3d ed.*, edited by J. B. Redford, 352-387. Baltimore, MD: Williams and Wilkins.

Perry, J. 1987. Distal rectus femoris transfer. *Developmental Medicine and Child Neurology* 29:153-158.

Rang, M., R. Silver, and J. de la Garza. 1986. Cerebral palsy. In *Pediatric orthopaedics, 2d ed.*, edited by W. W. Lovell and R. B. Winter, 345-396. Philadelphia, PA: J. B. Lippincott.

Spencer, A. M., and V. A. Person. 1984. Casting and orthotics for children. In *Symposium on podopediatrics—Clinics in podiatry*, edited by J. V. Ganley, 621-629. Philadelphia, PA: W. B. Saunders.

Tax, H. R. 1985. *Podopaediatrics, 2d ed.* Baltimore, MD: Williams and Wilkins.

Valmassy, R. L. 1984. Biomechanical evaluation of the child. *Symposium on podopediatrics—Clinics in podiatry*, edited by J. V. Ganley, 563-579. Philadelphia, PA: W. B. Saunders.

Westin, G., and W. S. Dye. 1983. Conservative management of cerebral palsy in the growing child. *Foot & Ankle* 4(3):160-163.

Yates, L. R. 1979. Personal communication. Charlottesville, VA. April 28.

CHAPTER 8

Research Considerations

Objectives for the Reader

- To discuss the potential usefulness of clinical research into splinting and serial casting as a means by which current methods and materials might be improved, validated, or discarded.

- To generate research questions whose answers lie in radiologic assessment procedures.

- To identify features of posture, gait determinants, and sagittal-plane joint motions of the lower extremities in gait that might be modified by the use of splints or casts of varying designs.

- To promote and participate in the continued search for objective measures to support or refute the efficacy of these and similar intervention methods.

In this chapter, I look to the reader and to the future for ways to obtain objective data that will contribute to a greater understanding of the mechanisms at work in modifying and controlling joint alignment in the distal lower extremities. Clinicians should always be alert to ways to improve the methods and materials described in this and related publications. Presumptions emerge from new concepts regarding modeling of bone and fibrous tissues, from studies of the biomechanics at work in the closed chain, and from the differences in structure and alignment between children and adults collectively. These new concepts raise enough questions to keep the most facile of grant applicants at their keyboards for a long time.

It is an exciting time to begin to ask these questions. Technology is rising to the challenges by providing radiologic methods such as single-exposure weight-bearing roentgenograms using lead acrylic wedges, high resolution magnetic resonance imaging (MRI), and improved interpretation of structural findings on computerized tomography (CT scan). These techniques offer alternative means of ascertaining the torsional declination angles in the femur and tibia (Petersen et al. 1987; Murphy et al. 1987). This country is experiencing a steady rise in the number of facilities sponsoring sophisticated gait analysis laboratories with dynamic electromyography (EMG) and computerized video data collection capability. These evaluation procedures are expensive, and their use requires substantial financial support by interested funding sources. But when these procedures are used, the risks to the child are negligible and the potential for learning is monumental.

Rose (1962), Bleck et al. (1977), and others present quantitative roentgenographic evidence that shoe inserts of various sorts are effective in reducing pes valgus (flexible pes planus) deformity. Their studies, however, do not address the circumstances of the child with developmental delay.

Rosenthal (1984) used roentgenographic studies and measurements to address the question of whether well-designed AFOs and shoe inserts are quantitatively effective in managing structural foot deformity in cerebral palsy. His findings were positive.

Harris et al. (1986) used a single-subject research design to determine the efficacy of "inhibitive orthoses." They quantified the time that a quadriparetic child was able to maintain standing balance and compared his performance with and without the supportive devices. (The devices in this article feature Hylton's supramalleolar and ankle-foot orthoses.) They noted significant improvement in standing balance duration when the subject used the devices.

Watt et al. (1986) evaluated the effects of a three-week period of solid-cast wear on several features of physical and functional status of 28 children with spastic cerebral palsy who were between 18 months and 5 years of age. Prior to cast application, two weeks after cast removal, and five months later, they gathered data. Evidence of static-muscle tonus was gathered using standard neurological techniques for determining deep tendon reflexes at the knee and ankle, the Babinski response, and clonus. The researchers assessed performance of 12 developmental skills, including equilibrium responses and independence in gait. They took measures of passive range of motion at the ankle. They used clinical observation and films or videotapes to evaluate gait pattern, accounting specifically for early stance posture of the ankle and foot and midstance knee alignment.

Bertoti (1986) investigated intervention with bivalved cast boots for 16 children with spastic cerebral palsy. She compared features of gait—such as stride length, width, and angle—with and without cast boots and found a significant improvement in stride length when the children wore the casts.

Hinderer et al. (1988) explored comparative effects of bivalved casts with and without a contoured plaster footboard on features of gait in a single-subject research study. These researchers used footprint data to measure stride length, step length, foot progression angles, and base of support. They took videotapes at regular intervals to compare other functional skills.

The process of collecting and analyzing quantifiable data has not yet been implemented to study the effectiveness of the splints described in Chapter 5 for children with neuromotor disorders. The nature of management of developmental disabilities is such that dividing a population into control and study groups would disregard the multiple variables of daily routine, components of the management program, weight-bearing demands, and compensatory skills inherent in such a population. The single-subject research design proposed by Harris and Riffle (1986), however, offers the clinician an alternative approach to this research effort.

Answers to the following questions lie in precise video gait analysis, dynamic EMG, and radiologic assessment. The data should be collected to compare at least four circumstances:

- Status prior to applying splints.
- Status immediately upon providing splints.
- Status within three to six months of providing splints.
- Status two, five, and ten years later.

Questions About Skeletal Alignment

The first group of questions relates to the impact of splints on structural alignment. As discussed in Chapter 3, Bleck et al. (1977) determined that the average normal angle of talar plantarflexion relative to the transverse plane is 26.5 degrees (S.D. 5.3 degrees) in children ages 18 months to 16 years. A more recent study reveals that the same angle shows a slow, linear decline from a mean of approximately 34 degrees at birth (nonweight-bearing) to approximately 25 degrees at age 9 years (presumably in weight-bearing) (Vanderwilde et al. 1988).

The normal mean calcaneal inclination increases from approximately 12 degrees at birth to approximately 23 degrees by age 5 years (Vanderwilde et al. 1988). McCrea (1985) states that the calcaneal inclination angle normally lies between 15 and 30 degrees.

As also discussed in Chapter 3, on dorsoplantar view of the foot, Bleck et al. (1977) intersected a line drawn adjacent to the lateral border of the calcaneus with another line drawn adjacent to the medial border of the neck of the talus. They refer to the resulting angle as the dorsal talocalcaneal angle and have determined that it lies at 18 degrees (S.D. 5.6 degrees) in the average child (age range 18 months to 16 years).

Vanderwilde et al. (1988) use longitudinal bisections of the talus and calcaneus to obtain measurements of the dorsal talocalcaneal angle. Their study of normal children graphically shows a linear decline from an approximate mean of 42 degrees at birth to 22 degrees at 9 years of age.

Drawing again from Chapter 3, clinical—as opposed to radiological— assessment reveals the calcaneal stance angle when comparing the vertical bisection of the calcaneus with the sagittal plane (Valmassy 1984; McCrea 1985). This angle should decline from 6 degrees of valgus at age 1 year to 2 degrees by age 5 years and thereafter (Valmassy 1984). Root et al. (1971) suggest that after age 6 years, any calcaneal stance deviation greater than 2 degrees into varus or valgus exceeds the limit for optimum biomechanical balance of the foot structures.

The normal angle for the transmalleolar axis (at the ankle joint) gradually increases from 6 degrees at age 1 year to 20-30 degrees at age 7 years (Root et al. 1971; McCrea 1985).

Researching the Stabilizing Foot Splint

With the values discussed above, and related values, it is possible to generate a research effort by investigating the influence on skeletal alignment of the various designs of the stabilizing foot splint (SFS). If the study population consists of children with hypotonia, developmental delay, adequate mobility into fully corrected alignment, and a calcaneal stance deviation exceeding the age-appropriate maximum normal angle (I suggest using Valmassy's values), it is possible to ask many of the same questions posed by Bleck and Berzins in 1977.

- Do children who stand while wearing an SFS show immediate improvement in talocalcaneal and talar-transverse plane alignment when radiologic evaluation compares the foot structures before and after its application?

- If change occurs in the weight-bearing angles of the talus and calcaneus by applying the SFS, do the values reduce to within the reported norms?

- Does the degree of change, if any, in talar and calcaneal angles increase or decrease when modifications for enhancing support such as forefoot post or malleolar extension are added to the devices?

- If correction of the talar and calcaneal angles is evident on application of a new splint, is it retained throughout the duration of use?

- When assessing the hindfoot alignment from a posterior view, does the radiographic angle of relaxed calcaneal stance change both before and after application of the posted SFS?

As an alternative to roentgenographic procedures, Rose (1962) used a pronanometer to study the effect of shoe inserts on the rearfoot complex. This single-subject study measured the subsequent rotary adjustment in the tibia and fibula. The pronanometer consists of a standing frame (with recesses for aligning the feet) and a stick mounted on a flat wooden base to project perpendicular to the surface. This stick is then strapped securely onto the proximal lower leg. A large protractor is located on the transverse plane at the level of the stick when the subject stands in the frame. The stick rests on the protractor (Figure 8.1). As the foot pronates and supinates, closed-chain kinetics dictate that the lower leg must rotate. This action causes the stick to move on the protractor.

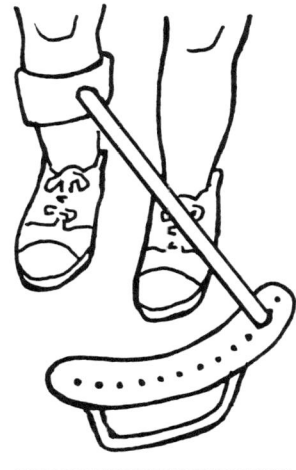

Figure 8.1
Pronanometer.
The point of the stick
moves toward the cen-
ter of the protractor as
the foot supinates.
(Rose 1962).

If the extensibility and integrity of the ligaments supporting the rearfoot complex are adequate to elicit these closed-chain responses, this device can be used to retrieve quantifiable evidence of change in the foot structures as the change is communicated proximally. The data collected will reveal alteration in talar position by deduction rather than by direct measurement, so corrective talar displacement will also be presumed but not quantified. This type of research would fit the single-subject format, provided it is fully replicable by other researchers.

The use of the pronanometer to establish age-related norms for the tibial rotation angle would help in comparing any changes observed in children with flexible pes planus to the expected or normal value for children of the same age. Such normative information would be useful in assessing the significance of the data. The nature of the pronanometer as an evaluative instrument might interfere with adequate replicability in gathering normative data, however. This is because specific points of reference, such as the tibial tuberosity, must be determined to locate the stick and the strap in precisely the same place for each child, anatomical differences notwithstanding.

Nevertheless, a single-subject analysis comparing the data collected in a single session would illuminate many quantifiable differences. The researcher should compare the values obtained when the child is in bare feet, in tennis or athletic shoes, in leather shoes, and in the same shoes with inserts. Any shoes used in the study would have to be a standardized design.

Valmassy (1984) suggests that intervention with an orthosis is appropriate after the age of 3 years, when the normal foot is no longer pronated and apropulsive. Bleck et al. (1977) report that intervention with the UCBL shoe insert and the Helfet heel seat for the younger age groups in their study resulted in a greater degree of improvement in talocalcaneal alignment than was observed in older children. Their study group included children as young as 18 months. This diversity of professional opinion leads me to ask the following questions:

- Is early intervention with the SFS—at or before the age of 18 months—quantifiably advantageous in protecting the foot structures in the children who exhibit excessive STJ pronation?
- If improvement is noted, how much time is needed to bring about lasting adjustment in structures of the foot in the presence of mild, moderate, or severe degrees of hypotonia or of laxity?
- What is the optimum daily wearing schedule for the SFS in children with hypotonic neuromotor impairment?
- Is it possible to wean away from and ultimately remove the SFS and still retain any notable correction after a predictable number of years of intervention in children with neuromotor impairment?

As was discussed in Chapter 5, Valmassy (1984) claims that the varus forefoot in children is not correctable and should be accommodated. Spencer et al. (1984) and D'Amico (1984) disagree and warn that early posting (before school age) to maintain the forefoot in varus interferes with the modeling process that normally reduces talar torsion and varus deviation. Agnew (1988) and I agree with the latter authors on the basis of acquired knowledge of developmental biomechanics. This difference of clinical opinion, however, raises some important questions for researchers who use splints and orthoses for children with neuromotor dysfunction:

- When there are problems of sensorimotor control and weight transfer over the foot, can the normal modeling process at the forefoot be expected to proceed in order to reduce varus deviation after providing functional support for the subtalar joint?
- If so, at what ages?

- When is it clinically appropriate to provide a permanent forefoot post for a child with hypotonia?
- Do associated interventions, such as joint mobilization to improve the range of plantarflexion of the first ray and of the talonavicular joint, affect the process of correcting forefoot varus deformity with stabilizing foot splints?

Researching the Ankle-Foot Splints

The group of questions listed above may also be applied to investigation of ankle-foot splints. In addition, the following questions might be asked:

- How do splints compare to "well-built" high-temperature orthoses of similar design, in the restoration of the talus and calcaneus to their normal measures of alignment?
- How do the different ankle-foot splint styles compare to each other in restoring alignment?
- How do the different splint styles affect the predominating angles at the knee and hip in stance, such as the angles of knee flexion, knee hyperextension, rotary deviation of the condyles from the frontal plane, hip flexion, hip adduction, hip rotations, pelvic tilt angle, and sacrofemoral angle?
- What is the influence on proximal joint alignment of posting at the forefoot?

Questions About Functional Influence of Splints

The writings of Ogg (1963), Bauman et al. (1963), Boenig (1977), Sutherland et al. (1980), Rose-Jacobs (1983), Hoffer et al. (1983), Holden et al. (1986), Norlin et al. (1986), Bertoti (1986), Watt et al. (1986), and others offer many methods of measuring—and thus quantifying—components of gait that span several levels of sophistication.

The studies by Holden et al. (1986) and Norlin et al. (1986), the latter of which was described in Chapter 4, drew the following conclusions, which will help the researcher identify results of biomechanical interventions:

- The variable in the data derived from spastic gait patterns in cerebral palsy that most deviates from the control data is stride frequency (cadence), which typically reveals a decline with increasing age (Norlin et al. 1986).

- As a single measurement, velocity is a good indication of gait ability (Norlin et al. 1986; Holden et al. 1986).
- Repeated measurements of gait velocity, stride length, and stride frequency should help describe changes in the gait ability of a patient.

Gait studies can be implemented to address such concerns as the functional differences that can be identified in children who first walk without, then with, splints of varying design. These differences might include measures such as any of the following.

Gait Determinants

- Walking velocity.
- Duration of single-limb stance.
- Cadence.

Distribution of Loading Forces across the Foot

- Using a force plate in a gait lab to derive quantitative data.
- Documenting such postural features as the positions of the ankle and foot at foot contact, and the angle of the knee and ankle in midstance, from a videotaped evaluation.
- Using footprint studies.

Functional Features of Efficiency and Balance

- Frequency of stumbling or falling.
- Dependency on external support, such as a walking aid or an adult's hand, to take six to ten (or any number of) independent steps.
- Energy consumption (that is, heart rate and oxygen uptake).

Features of Gait Pattern

- The timing and ranges of sagittal plane motions of the pelvis, hip, knee, and ankle at specific points in the gait cycle.
- The timing and ranges of rotary excursions of the femur and lower leg at various points in the gait cycle.
- The ranges of frontal plane excursions of the femur, tibia, and calcaneus during the stance phase.
- Step length.
- Stride length.
- A ratio of length of stride to leg length.
- The width of the supporting base.
- Angle of foot progression.

Features of Muscle Activity in Gait

Electromyographic (EMG) analysis reveals such information as the following:

- The timing and relative activation of the gluteus maximus and medius, the adductors, the hamstrings, the rectus femoris and various quadriceps muscles, the triceps surae, the anterior tibialis, the peroneals and the posterior tibialis singly or in combination throughout the gait cycle. Data might be collected before and after donning splints, then during a period without splints, followed by the reapplication of splints. The researcher should maintain long-term follow-up.

The data collected (while maintaining all the other aspects of daily management unchanged) would generate evidence of the influence of various splints on magnitude and phasic activation of specific muscle groups. Such studies might compare the following:

- The solid to the hinged ankle-foot splints for bilateral and unilateral problems of functional equinus deformity.

- The solid crouch-control splint to the anterior floor reaction orthosis for managing crouch posture. (Here, too, is an opportunity to compare radiologically the alignment of the foot structures in each device. Does either device affect the magnitude or timing of EMG activity in the triceps muscle group? If so, how?)

- The solid crouch-control splint to the hinged and supramalleolar crouch-control splints as they affect the activity of the triceps surae muscle group and of the quadriceps in children who demonstrate calcaneal deformity crouch gait.

The clinician might also measure the effect on circumferential measurements of the calf musculature before, and at two to six months after, using hinged crouch-control, hinged ankle-foot (with various settings of the posterior stop), and solid ankle-foot splints.

Other dimensions of functional impact may be explored by posing questions such as these:

- How soon after introducing an ankle-foot device for children of comparable age and ambulatory capability can one expect to see quantifiable improvement in gait with the device removed?

- If the child's knee extension mobility is full, what is the relationship between strengthening activities for the triceps surae group in stance position—as on a BAPS® (Biomechanical Ankle-Platform System) board or a replica—and persistence of, or reduction in, crouch deformity?

- Do strengthening activities produce a lasting influence on postural alignment, gait determinants, or gait pattern?

- If so, is there an average or minimum duration of training, or a threshold number of repetitions of specific activities required for significant, spontaneous adjustment posture or adjustment of the gait pattern?

- Is age a feature of these expectations?

- What are the minimal requirements for a maintenance program of exercise after a child with either hypotonic or hypertonic neuromotor disorder has achieved postural improvement?
- Is there a relationship between degrees of severity of involvement—measured in terms of standardized motor quotient, radiologic assessment of foot deformity, and/or cognitive level—and functional outcomes using splints?

Questions About Managing Deformity with Casts and Alternative Conservative Measures

Chapter 6 devoted considerable discussion to the evidence of the effectiveness of night splinting to maintain or gain muscle tissue extensibility, either following or in lieu of serial casts. The writings of Westin et al. (1983), Tardieu et al. (1987), Tardieu et al. (1988), Tardieu et al. (1982), Hayes et al. (1970), and Baumann et al. (1985) were cited among the pertinent literature regarding this issue. In considering these findings regarding night splinting, questions arise:

- During serial casting, what is the effect of setting the subtalar and midtarsal joints of the pronated foot in neutral (that is, fully congruent) position on the rate of lengthening of the soleus muscle belly? (Resting muscle belly and tendon length is determined at the initial point of resistance to passive stretch. The muscle's passive excursion is determined as the difference between initial and final points of resistance.) (Tardieu et al. 1987)

- What is the effect on muscle extensibility of using a stretch-style, hinged ankle-foot splint, in which the foot is aligned in congruity and the foot and shaft pieces are connected with TheraBand® or surgical tubing? (Carpenter 1989)

  — How does this splinting method, in which a gentle, persistent, tolerable stretch is applied for six hours daily or at night, compare with serial casting to gain mobility?

  — How many hours of wear would be required to maintain adequate muscle extensibility in children with hypertonus using a stretch splint? How does this time compare with the six hours recommended by Tardieu et al. (1988)?

- What is the effect on soleus muscle hypoextensibility of using treatment boots during therapeutic exercise, such as the "bioboots" designed by Coram (1989) to maintain the weight-bearing foot structures in full congruity (neutral position)?

  — If proven effective, is daily treatment necessary to regain extensibility?

— What is the optimum content of therapeutic exercise activities in the boots?

— What effect do they have on maintaining extensibility after it is regained? How often must they be used in maintenance? For how long?

— Is night splinting required if neutral boots are part of a maintenance program?

— Does contracture recur within five months of discontinuing the use of the neutrally aligned treatment boots? Does night splinting affect this outcome? Is age a factor?

• How does daytime wear of a foot support system that permits ankle plantarflexion affect the rate of recurrence of contracture following serial casting?

— In this case, does night splinting provide maintenance of extensibility longer than five months?

Bertoti (1986) and Hinderer et al. (1988) recorded footprint ambulation patterns in ink or chalk, as a pretest and post-test for children with hypertonus wearing bivalved plaster casts. They then evaluated the patterns to determine stride length, width of base, and angle of gait with and without the cast boots.

Using this method of assessing footprint patterns:

• How do bivalved below-knee casts compare quantifiably with splints and orthoses as they influence these footprint characteristics? If a significant difference is detected, could the clinician deduce that the weight of the cast is a significant factor?

• What is the effect of using fiber glass casting material rather than plaster and fiber glass?

• How are footprint characteristics affected after removing the casts?

Using the single-subject design proposed by Harris et al. (1986):

• How do bivalved casts compare quantifiably with ankle-foot splints and orthoses of varying designs, with regard to the achievement of independent standing balance?

• Are any of these differences retained after cast removal? Immediately? If so, how long do they persist?

Questions About the Influence of Therapeutic Exercise on Bone Structure

Research Related to Femoral Antetorsion

Bleck (1987) suggests that the earlier the hip flexion contracture is reduced, the greater the reduction in femoral antetorsion. Bleck also suggests a relationship exists between the application of lateral hip rotation in extension and the reduction of neonatal femoral antetorsion. Considering the high incidence of both abnormally increased femoral antetorsion and pronation deformities in children with neuromotor disorders, I propose a program of therapeutic exercise that is designed to elongate the anterior soft tissue structures of the hip joint, which prohibit extension and abduction. This program should also activate the oblique abdominal muscles for pelvic stabilization and activate the gluteus maximus. It should be judiciously instituted as early as the first four to 12 months of life. The aim of such intervention is the effective application of lateral torque forces to the proximal femoral shaft to reduce the normal angle of neonatal antetorsion.

Research efforts to obtain quantifiable evidence of femoral antetorsion—including both hip rotation tests for antetorsion and CT scans, or other sophisticated radiologic assessments—should provide data to support clinical impressions of the effectiveness of early therapeutic intervention. For example, if computerized tomographic measures are taken prior to and at six-month intervals following the initiation of a prescribed therapeutic exercise program (using the techniques suggested by Murphy et al. 1987), does the data collected show a significant reduction in the torsional declination angle of the femur?

- Do variations in the program alter the findings?
- Do variations in the child's age alter the findings?

I would like to encourage rehabilitation engineers to design and produce a climbing machine for young children of age 2 years and more, built on the same principles as those often seen in commercial fitness centers. A computerized video game could be operated by the pedals, perhaps. Such a machine might offer an effective mechanism for strengthening the hip extensors, lateral rotators, and quadriceps, and for reducing femoral torsion.

Associated functional and postural considerations might affect the data. These include such questions as the following:

- What is the incidence of W-sitting among these children?
- What are the torsional and rotary features of the lower leg and knee joint?
- What is the incidence and degree of pronation deformity?

Until researchers obtain and present objective data, clinical evidence cannot be overlooked. If a child who has been given a supportive device for the feet appears to function with greater balance and efficiency in the upright position than was possible prior to its application, the clinician can presume to have proceeded correctly. As research efforts generate more information about these and related interventions and methods, and technologies evolve to meet new challenges, clinicians will redefine expectations and designs accordingly.

Summary

Most children with developmental disability have orthopedic problems. Preventing or minimizing deformity requires a long-range effort spanning the child's entire growth period. The structures of the foot and leg, in the context of tonus abnormality and compensatory balancing mechanisms, require mandatory protection from excessive stresses until the child achieves bone maturity after adolescence (Regnauld 1986; Salek 1977; Salek 1981; Westin et al. 1983; McCrea 1985; Jordan et al. 1983; Baumann et al. 1985). Although clinicians may have provided therapeutic and orthotic intervention in the child's early life, the alignment and function of the foot and ankle should remain a management issue either until the child completes bone growth or the clinician can observe and sustain alleviation of the deforming forces when the child is barefoot. Many patients need shoe inserts throughout adulthood (Jordan et al. 1983).

The decision to postpone splinting, casting, or orthotic intervention until research either supports or denies clinical evidence—or to wait until the neurologically involved child "outgrows" alignment deviations—overlooks the role that muscle action and loading forces (both normal and abnormal) play in sculpting the body structure (Frost 1986). A "wait and see" position denies the dysfunctional influence of prevailing problems of postural adjustment and motor control on foot deformity. I regard the decision to offer adequate, protective support for the structures of the foot as a first choice among intervention alternatives.

This area of pediatric management has taken to its feet and begun to toddle. When we undertake to substantiate or refute our observations with data, the resulting information will advance our current concepts and methods by long and graceful strides, bringing us all closer to the highest order of effective intervention for children with neuromotor disorders.

References

Agnew, P., DPM. Personal communication. 1988. Richmond, VA. December 8.

Bauman, J. H., and P. W. Brand. 1963. Measurement of pressure between the foot and shoe. *The Lancet* (March 23):629-632.

Baumann, J. U., and M. Zumstein. 1985. Experience with a plastic ankle-foot orthosis for prevention of muscle contracture. *Developmental Medicine and Child Neurology* 27:83. (Abstract)

Bertoti, D. B. 1986. Effect of short leg casting on ambulation in children with cerebral palsy. *Physical Therapy* 66:1522-1529.

Bleck, E. E. 1987. *Orthopedic management of cerebral palsy—Clinics in developmental medicine nos. 99/100.* Philadelphia, PA: J. B. Lippincott.

Bleck, E. E., and U. J. Berzins. 1977. Conservative management of pes valgus with plantarflexed talus, flexible. *Clinical Orthopaedics and Related Research* 122:85-92.

Boenig, D. D. 1977. Evaluation of a clinical method of gait analysis. *Physical Therapy* 57:795-798.

Carpenter, D. 1989. Personal communication. Scranton, PA. February 4.

Coram, S. 1989. Personal communication. Springfield, OH. January 15.

D'Amico, J. C. 1984. Developmental flatfoot. In *Symposium on podopediatrics—Clinics in podiatry,* edited by J. V. Ganley. Philadelphia, PA: W. B. Saunders Co.

Frost, H. M. 1986. *Intermediary organization of the skeleton, vol. 2.* Boca Raton, FL: CRC Press.

Harris, S. R., and K. Riffle. 1986. Effects of inhibitive ankle-foot orthoses on standing balance in a child with cerebral palsy: A single-subject design. *Physical Therapy* 66:663-667.

Hayes, N. K., and Y. R. Burns. 1970. Discussion on the use of weight-bearing plasters in the reduction of hypertonicity. *Australian Journal of Physiotherapy* 16:108-117.

Hinderer, K. A., S. R. Harris, A. H. Purdy, D. E. Chew, L. T. Staheli, J. F. McLaughlin, and K. M. Jaffe. 1988. Effects of "tone-reducing" vs. standard plaster casts on gait improvement of children with cerebral palsy. *Developmental Medicine and Child Neurology* 30(3):370-377.

Hoffer, M., and J. Perry. 1983. Pathodynamics of gait alterations in cerebral palsy and the significance of kinetic electromyography in evaluating foot and ankle problems. *Foot & Ankle* 4:128.

Holden, M. K., K. M. Gill, and M. R. Magliozzi. 1986. Gait assessment for neurologically impaired patients: Standards for outcome assessment. *Physical Therapy* 66:1530-1539.

Jordan, R. P. 1984. Therapeutic considerations of the feet and lower extremities in the cerebral palsied child. *Symposium on podopediatrics—Clinics in podiatry,* edited by J. V. Ganley, 547-561. Philadelphia, PA: W. B. Saunders.

Jordan, R. P., J. Cusack, and B. Resseque. 1983. *Foot function and its relationship to posture in the pediatric patient with cerebral palsy and other neuromuscular disorders.* Symposium, sponsored by the Neurodevelopmental Treatment Association, New York: May 20-22. Unpublished lecture notes and instructional materials.

McCrea, J. D. 1985. *Pediatric orthopedics of the lower extremity—An instructional handbook.* Mount Kisco, NY: Futura.

Murphy, S. B., S. R. Simon, P. K. Kijewski, R. H. Wilkinson, and N. T. Griscom. 1987. Femoral anteversion. *Journal of Bone and Joint Surgery* 69-A(8):1169-1176.

Norlin, R., and P. Odenrick. 1986. Development of gait in spastic children with cerebral palsy. *Journal of Pediatric Orthopaedics* 6:674-680.

Ogg, H. L. 1963. Measuring and evaluating the gait patterns of children. *Journal of the American Physical Therapy Association* 43:717-720.

Petersen, T. D., and W. Rohr. 1987. Improved assessment of lower extremity alignment using new roentgenographic techniques. *Clinical Orthopaedics and Related Research* 219:112-116.

Regnauld, B. 1986. *The foot: Pathology, aetiology, semiology, clinical investigation and therapy.* New York, NY: Springer-Verlag.

Root, M. L., W. P. Orien, and J. H. Weed. 1971. *Biomechanical examination of the foot, vol. 1.* Los Angeles, CA: Clinical Biomechanical Corporation.

Rose, G. K. 1962. Correction of the pronated foot. *Journal of Bone and Joint Surgery* 44-B:642-647.

Rose-Jacobs, R. 1983. Development of gait at slow, free and fast speeds in 3- and 5-year-old children. *Physical Therapy* 63:1251-1259.

Rosenthal, R. K. 1984. The use of orthotics in foot and ankle problems in cerebral palsy. *Foot & Ankle* 4(4):195-200.

Salek, B. 1977. *The significance of the structural and functional development in the normal foot and therapeutic implications thereof in the child with neuromotor disorder.* Unpublished monograph. Suffolk Rehabilitation Center, Commack, NY.

Salek, B. 1981. *Corrective footwear in young children with neuromuscular disorders.* Presentation—Neurodevelopmental Treatment Association Eastern Regional Conference, Philadelphia, PA, November 8. Unpublished lecture notes and instructional materials.

Spencer, A. M., and V. A. Person. 1984. Casting and orthotics for children. In *Symposium on podopediatrics—Clinics in podiatry,* edited by J. V. Ganley, 621-629. Philadelphia, PA: W. B. Saunders Co.

Sutherland, D. H., R. Olshen, L. Cooper, and S. L-Y. Woo. 1980. The development of mature gait. *Journal of Bone and Joint Surgery* 62-A:336-353.

Tardieu, C., A. Lespargot, C. Tabarz, and M. D. Bret. 1988. For how long must the soleus muscle be stretched each day to prevent contracture? *Developmental Medicine and Child Neurology* 30:3-10.

Tardieu, G., and C. Tardieu. 1987. Cerebral palsy: Mechanical evaluation and conservative correction of limb joint contractures. *Clinical Orthopaedics and Related Research* 219:63-69.

Tardieu, G., C. Tardieu, P. Colbeau-Austin, and A. Lespargot. 1982. Muscle hypoextensibility in children with cerebral palsy: II. Therapeutic implications. *Archives of Physical Medicine and Rehabilitation* 63:103-107.

Valmassy, R. L. 1984. Biomechanical evaluation of the child. *Symposium on podopediatrics—Clinics in podiatry,* edited by J. V. Ganley, 563-579. Philadelphia, PA: W. B. Saunders.

Vanderwilde, R., L. T. Staheli, D. E. Chew, and V. Malagon. 1988. Measurements on radiographs of the foot in normal infants and children. *Journal of Bone and Joint Surgery* 70-(a):407-415.

Watt, J., D. Sims, F. Harckham, L. Schmidt, A. McMillan, and J. Hamilton. 1986. A prospective study of inhibitive casting as an adjunct to physiotherapy for cerebral palsied children. *Developmental Medicine and Child Neurology* 28:480-488.

Westin, G. W., and S. Dye. 1983. Conservative management of cerebral palsy in the growing child. *Foot & Ankle* 4(3):160-163.

Splint Care Instructions and Precautions

Caregivers receive copies of this instruction sheet, which the clinician should review with them. The reader is invited to revise or adapt this form as needed or to run copies for use in a clinic.

The splint provider has the responsibility to explain fully splint care considerations to the child's caregivers. A thorough explanation beforehand may prevent damage such as that caused by exposure to strong heat sources.

Splint Care Instructions and Precautions

Child's Name _____ Date _____

Type of Splint _____ Number of Splints ____

This splint was custom-made for your child. Please read the following instructions to prevent problems related both to your child's comfort and to the properties of the splint.

When Your Child Should Wear the Splint

Build up wear time gradually. If your child spends most of the time in standing and walking activities, start by applying it for 30 minutes at a time. Then remove it, check the skin, and use alcohol on pink areas. Replace the splint when normal skin color is restored. Children who stand and walk only intermittently or occasionally may wear the splint(s) for one to two hours between skin checks.

Double the wear time if evidence of pressure is minimal.

When tolerance for the splint has been established and it can be worn comfortably for four hours, use the splint according to the schedule that your clinician recommends:

- ☐ During sleep.
- ☐ Daytime, all of the time.
- ☐ Daytime, as needed to manage the deformity for which it was designed. (Alternate with a less supportive device if available if there is an apparent need for control of the foot and leg.)
- ☐ Night and day, all the time, except for therapeutic exercise and hygiene.

Change the child's socks often enough to keep the skin dry. Use cotton socks only, to reduce skin irritation due to perspiration. (During the summer, talcum powder or foot antiperspirant might be helpful.)

Precautions for Splints Made of Aquaplast® or Orfit® Materials

- • Keep the splint away from open flames because it will burn.
- • Be careful not to allow the splint to lose its shape by placing it in places where the temperature goes above 100 degrees F. For example, don't lay it on a radiator, don't let the child take a hot bath or shower while wearing it, and don't lay it on a sunny windowsill or on the front or rear dashboard of a car. Don't leave a splint in a tennis shoe when laundering the shoe.

Splint Care Instructions and Precautions

Cleaning

- Your child's splint can be cleaned by using soap and water.
- Towel dry it. Don't immerse it in water over 135 degrees F.

Use a cleaner with a chlorine base or another commercial spray cleaner for spots that won't dislodge with soap and water. Be careful to rinse the splint thoroughly. (Disregard this suggestion if your child has an allergic sensitivity to cleaning products such as these.)

Adjustments

Please discontinue use of the splint and contact us immediately if you notice any of the following:

- Swelling
- Pain
- Broken or missing parts
- Pressure areas (red spots that don't go away in 20-30 minutes)
- Rash

Phone Number   Therapist(s)

_____   _____

_____   _____

_____   _____

_____   _____

Consent to Undertake Serial Casting Procedures

If your facility requires preauthorization from legal guardians for such procedures as a course of serial cast applications, the following form (or an adapted version) might be useful. Make copies of the signed form for your facility's files and for the child's legal guardian.

Consent to Undertake a Series of Solid Cast Applications

I, _____(parent or legal guardian),

hereby authorize or direct _____(clinician)

or associates of his/her choosing, to undertake to apply a series of plaster casts to

_____(patient).

I understand that this process may involve repeated cast removal and reapplication whereby the affected body segments are gradually and repeatedly set in more normal alignment. I also approve any accompanying services deemed reasonably necessary to the anticipated success of this procedure, such as an increased schedule of standing episodes and therapeutic exercise sessions, both at home and at the clinic.

I understand that the purposes of attempting this procedure include the following:

1. Conservative (nonsurgical) reduction of soft tissue contracture by physiologic addition of muscle cells and lengthening of tendon ligament and fascia.
2. Restoration of optimum biomechanical alignment of affected segments as a preparation for management of deformity with splints or orthoses and for continued strengthening and functional training.
3. Facilitation of optimum function of the involved segments by reducing undesirable restriction of movement in the casted joints.
4. Provision of more appropriate sensory experiences related to postural alignment, relative to weight distribution through the foot and lower leg structures.

I understand that every precaution has been taken against the following events, but that the risks involved with this procedure include the following:

1. Muscle spasm, which may require cast removal or muscle relaxant medication for relief.
2. Pressure sore(s).
3. Allergic reaction to the materials used.
4. Swelling or other signs of circulatory constriction (for example, numbness or tingling sensations, or discoloration of nail beds).

Consent to Undertake a Series of Solid Cast Applications

I have been instructed to remove the cast(s) or to have them removed promptly when there is any evidence of spasm, allergy, circulatory restriction, or pressure sores.

This process will be terminated within six weeks, or after two cast changes, if evidence of significant improvement in joint mobility is not observed, or if an open pressure sore develops.

I hereby acknowledge that _____
(Attending Clinician(s))
has (have) provided adequate information concerning this procedure and its benefits and risks, as well as alternative measures.

I have read and fully comprehend this consent form. I sign it freely and voluntarily and expect to receive a copy of this form.

_____ Date _____
(SIGNATURE—PARENT/LEGAL GUARDIAN)

Time _____

I hereby certify that I have personally reviewed the contents of this consent

form with _____.

_____ Date _____
(SIGNATURE—ATTENDING CLINICIAN)

Time _____

Care and Management Following Cast Application

This form is intended for distribution to caregivers at the time of application of a cast. There should be several copies on hand in the casting area. Each point should be reviewed orally with the child's caregivers prior to termination of the session.

Care and Management
Following Plaster or Plaster and Fiber Glass
Cast Application

During the first 24 hours, **prohibit weight-bearing** and alert the nursing staff (including the night shift, if in the hospital) and/or other caregivers and the child's family to **check the following signs every one to two hours:**

1. Pulse at toes.
2. Circulatory status, via capillary refill.
3. Color of nail beds.
4. Veins, for duskiness.
5. Swelling.

For relief of symptoms 1 through 5, try flaring the edge of the cast at the top and bottom to relieve constriction. If the sign(s) (#1-5) fail to subside after flaring the ends, contact the attending clinician and/or remove the cast.

6. Evidence of pain.
7. Evidence of muscle spasm.

These signs (#6-7) indicate that stretch has been applied to the muscle fibers, or there is a ridge on the interior of the cast. The most cautious course is cast removal to inspect the skin or to reduce the degree of tension on the muscle fibers.

After the initial drying period, continue to check for:

1. **Refusal to bear weight on (either) casted foot.**
2. Unusual odors coming from the cast.
3. Cracks or dents in the plaster.
4. Changes for the worse in sleeping patterns or general affect (particularly if the patient is nonverbal or comatose).
5. Wetness that could cause softening of the cast.
6. Knowledge of objects, such as coins, dropped into the cast.

All of these signs warrant prompt cast removal.

Bathing

Plaster casts are not waterproof even when fiber glass cast tape covers them. The cast must not get wet. Use sponge bathing techniques or apply a rubber cast cover (commercially available) or thick plastic bags over the cast(s), taped securely to the leg, for bathing. If possible, keep the casted leg out of the water altogether; for example, place the leg on the kitchen counter while bathing the child in the sink. Use a tub-seat in the sink for support.

Care and Management
Following Plaster or Plaster and Fiber Glass Cast Application

In case circumstances develop that suggest the occurrence of skin breakdown, muscle spasm, or circulatory constriction, contact the attending clinician to **arrange for prompt removal of the cast(s).** If the cast is made of Gypsona® plaster, try to soak it off at home. Otherwise, go to your local emergency room to facilitate intervention.

Call me immediately if you see any of the trouble signs.

Attending Clinician: _____

Phone number: Work _____

Phone number: Home_____

Resources for Materials and Assistance

Resources for Materials and Assistance

Sources of Materials for Splinting

The source for Orfit®, which is discussed below, is
SePro Health Care, Inc.
140 Domorah Drive
Montgomery, PA 19836
800-523-3660
(In Pennsylvania: 215-646-6606)

Orfit® is a low-temperature splinting material, neutral or flesh-colored. It comes in five types, two degrees of stiffness, and two thicknesses (1/16-inch and 1/8-inch), with a three-year shelf life. It possesses properties of uniform elasticity and transparency when heated; it heats at 130 degrees F. It loses transparency as it cools and hardens. It is self-adhesive—no need for solvents—and does not shrink.

The stiff formula of Orfit® is in strength comparable to Aquaplast-T® in 1/8-inch thickness. The cost of Orfit® and Aquaplast-T® is also comparable.

The source for the materials listed next is
WFR Aquaplast Corporation
P.O. Box 635
Wyckoff, NJ 07481
800-526-5247
(In New Jersey: 201-891-1042)

- Aquaplast-T® (nonsticky) and Aquaplast® (sticky) are low-temperature splinting materials. They are available in various colors and in three types, three degrees of stiffness, and four thicknesses (1/16-inch, 3/32-inch, 1/8-inch, and 3/16-inch). Each product possesses properties of elasticity and transparency when heated at 140 degrees F. The distributor does not mention shelf life. Aquaplast-T® requires the use of solvents to assure bonding with posts and other materials. It demonstrates shrinkage, which increases in severity with increases in the thickness of the material.
- Temperature-regulated water bath (and timer)
- Cotton stockinet—in a variety of widths
- Aluminum screw rivets (1/4-inch)
- Samson® hole punch (1/4-inch)
- Plastic-tipped Universal Shears®
- Left- and right-handed Unlimited Scissors®
- Pro-Snips®
- Adhesive-backed moleskin with paper rather than plastic backing
- Adhesive-backed Plastazote® padding (1/8-inch and 3/16-inch thickness)
- Molestick® padding (foam-lined moleskin)

- Utility knife
- Deburring tool (edge finisher)
- Splint solvent cement
- Crepe sole (1/4-inch thickness)
- Heat gun
- Standard Velcro® (plain- and adhesive-backed, various widths)
- Plain-backed SabreStrip® in various widths (Velcro® loop)
- Adhesive-backed SabreGrip® in 1-inch width only (a mushroom-shaped form of Velcro® hook)
- Tooth-buckles (1-inch width)
- Nylon webbing for straps (nonstretch)
- Otoform-K Silicone Elastomer®
- Theraband®

The source for the next six items is
Fred Sammons Orthopedic Catalog
Box 32
Brookfield, IL 60513-0032
800-323-7305

- PPT® padding 12 inches by 42 inches (1/8-inch and 1/16-inch thicknesses)
- Softskin® padding (foam-lined moleskin)
- Otoform-K Silicone Elastomer®
- Cast protectors (for bathing)
- Posting pads for forefoot deviations
- Large splinting water bath

The following splinting supplies are available through
Alimed, Inc.
297 High Street
Dedham, MA 02026
800-225-2610

- AliCover®
- Aliplast®
- Molestick®
- Nickelplast®
- Self-Stick Plastazote® in various thicknesses (1/16-inch to 1/4-inch)
- T-Stick®
- AliBrite® padding
- TheraCork® sheeting
- PPT® in various thicknesses
- PQ Viscoelastic Polymer
- Aquaplast®
- Polyflex®
- Stockinet
- Tubigrip®

- Velcro®
- Velfoam®II
- Webby

Sources of Materials for Casting

Any local supplier of orthopedic supplies should be able to provide the following items. The attending orthopedists will have the names of reputable dealers.

- Cotton stockinet of various widths
- Cotton Webril®, or similar flat cotton roll padding
- Cast saw (the average cost is $500—less for the noisier, less durable models, more for those with a vacuum attachment)
- Replacement blades for the cast saw
- Orthopedic felt—1/4-inch thick
- Extra fast plaster splints (5 inches x 30 inches)
- Extra fast plaster bandages (3-inch and 4-inch widths)

The following items are available through
Smith & Nephew/Rolyan
N93 W14475 Whittaker Way
Menomonee Falls, WI 53051
800-558-8633
(In Wisconsin: 800-722-0442)

- Polyflex II® (for forming low-cut shoe inserts from plaster footboard molds)
- Various splinting materials
- Various types of stockinet and Tubigrip®
- Gypsona® specialty plaster casting bandages and splints. Among the advantages of this cast material are rapid setting time (two minutes) and easy removal of the cast by soaking it for 20-30 minutes in warm water. This eliminates the need for a cast saw for those casts that are made entirely of this plaster material. (Protective measures for plumbing are necessary, however, wherever the cast is removed.)

This company also sells a large splinting water bath and various types of Tubigrip® and casting materials.

A source for the following items is
WFR Aquaplast Corporation (address above)

- T-Stick® padding—adhesive-backed
- Cotton padding (similar to, but not exactly the same as, Webril®)
- Adhesive-backed felt padding (1/4-inch width)
- Extra fast setting plaster splints (4-inch width)
- Extra fast setting plaster bandages (various widths)
- Latex gloves (for use with fiber glass cast tape)
- Caraglas® fiber glass cast tape (clear, blue, red, and green)
- Nylon webbing strap, nonstretch (1-inch width)

The source for Pudgee®, which is listed next, is
Dynamic Systems, Inc.
Development Facility
Route 2, Box 182-B
Leicester, NC 28748
704-683-3523

Pudgee® orthopedic foam pads are made of 100 percent open-cell gel-foam with soft, doughlike consistency. These pads protect against heel sores in solid serial casts. They are not recommended for protection of a thinly covered bony prominence or calcaneus, however, unless supplemented with 1/8-inch felt or another, firmer cushioning material. They can be used as a thin underlayer for the firmer paddings and are excellent for pressure relief in splints. The material comes in 1/2-inch to 3-inch thicknesses, with or without a coated surface.

Additional Suppliers of Products for Managing Foot Deformity

Level and angle finder: 3-inch and 4⅛-inch diameter

Mackanburg-Duncan, Inc.
Oklahoma City, OK 73118
800-654-8484

Contact the company for the name of a local hardware dealer. The company requires a minimum order of $50.00 from distributing hardware stores. The 3-inch angle finder costs less than $10.00.

Apex Foot Products
170 Wesley
S. Hackensack, NJ 07606
800-526-APEX
(In New Jersey: 800-237-APEX)

Velcro® in bright colors

Aplix, Inc.
12300 Steele Creek Rd.
Charlotte, NC 28217
800-438-0424
(In North Carolina: 704-588-1920)

Surgical Supply Service (podiatric supplies)
1235 Vine Street
Philadelphia, PA 19107
800-523-0706
(In Pennsylvania: 800-462-1598)

Johnson & Johnson Products, Inc.
Hospital Services
P.O. Box 4000
New Brunswick, NJ 08903
800-255-2500

Foot & Ankle Orthopedics
4 Columbus Avenue
Mt. Kisco, NY 10549
800-431-7801

Feiner Brothers—Elkay Supply
Orthotic & Prosthetic Supplies
20 East Second Street
Mineola, NY 11501
800-645-3256

Custom Orthoses

G. R. Laboratories
130 West High Street
Topton, PA 19562
215-682-6334

Bergmann Orthotic Laboratory
1730 Holder Lane
Northfield, IL 60093
800-323-8267

Extra-Depth Shoes and Adapted Shoes

Alden Shoe Co.
Taunton St.
Middleborough, MA 02346

Miller Shoe Co.
4015 Cherry St.
Cincinnati, OH 45223

Musebeck Shoe Co.
Forest and Westover
Oconomowoc, WI 53066

P. W. Minor & Sons
3 Treadeasy Ave.
Industrial Park
Batavia, NY 14020

Odd Shoe Exchange
Attention: Geane Sallman
2242 West Kelm Drive
Phoenix, AZ 85015

Biomechanical Ankle Platform System (BAPS)

Camp International, Inc.
P.O. Box 89
Jackson, MI 49204
800-492-1088
In Michigan, call collect: 517-787-2720.

Tri-Wall®

Tri-Wall Containers Co.
Butler, IN 46721
219-868-2151

APPENDIX **5**

Pediatric Biomechanical Assessment Form

Pediatric Biomechanical Assessment Form

PELVIS	Left	Right
Sagittal plane alignment (tilt)—standing		
Sagittal plane alignment (tilt)—sitting		
Sacrofemoral angle (X-Ray)—standing		
Sagittal plane motion—total range in standing		
Frontal plane alignment		
Frontal plane motion—total range in standing		
Transverse plane alignment		
Transverse plane motion		

HIP JOINT	Left	Right
Staheli's prone hip extension test		
Knee tuck for hip flexion mobility (supine)		
Hip (femoral) rotation:		
1. Prone with hips extended and knees flexed		
Medial rotation		
Lateral rotation		
2. Supine with hips and knees extended		
Medial rotation		
Lateral rotation		
3. Sitting with hips and knees flexed		
Medial rotation		
Lateral rotation		
4. Sitting with knees extended		
Medial rotation		
Lateral rotation		

FEMUR	Left	Right
Hip rotation test for femoral torsion:		
Medial rotation		
Lateral rotation		
Ryder's test for femoral torsion:		
Medial position		
Lateral position		

KNEE JOINT	Left	Right
Flexion:		
Supine with hip flexed		
Prone with hip extended		
Flexion contracture (popliteal angle):		
Initial end range		
Final end range		
Varum:		
Space between the femoral condyles		
Tibiofemoral angle		
Valgum:		
Space between the medial malleoli		
Tibiofemoral angle		
Iliotibial band		
Rotary status (in knee flexion):		
Medial tibiofibular rotation (in hip flexion)—sitting		
Lateral tibiofibular rotation (in hip flexion)—sitting		
Medial tibiofibular rotation (in hip extension)—supine		
Lateral tibiofibular rotation (in hip extension)—supine		

KNEE JOINT (continued)	Left	Right
Thigh/foot angle:		
Medial foot position		
Lateral foot position		
Transmalleolar axis/foot alignment		
Talar torsion:		
Foot abduction		

TIBIA AND FIBULA	Left	Right
Tibiofibular torsion (in knee extension)		
Distal varum (open chain):		
Relaxed calcaneal stance		
Neutral calcaneal stance		
Calcaneal midposition		

ANKLE (TALOCRURAL JOINT)	Left	Right
Dorsiflexion in knee flexion:		
STJ neutral:		
Initial end range		
Final end range		
Calcaneal midposition:		
Initial end range		
Final end range		
Dorsiflexion in knee extension:		
STJ neutral:		
Initial end range		
Final end range		
Calcaneal midposition:		
Initial end range		
Final end range		
Plantarflexion		

SUBTALAR JOINT	Left	Right
Radiologic assessment:		
Calcaneal inclination		
Lateral talocalcaneal angle		
Talar declination		
First ray inclination		
Dorsoplantar talocalcaneal angle		
STJ clinical assessment: *The examiner must maintain true sagittal-plane perspective and must align the posterior border of the calcaneus on the frontal plane.*		
Frontal-plane STJ mobility:		
Inversion		
Eversion		
Relaxed calcaneal stance		
Neutral (congruent) STJ position		
Method I—Palpating the head of the talus:		
Open-chain		
Closed-chain		
Method II—Palpating the dorsal depressions:		
Open-chain		
Closed-chain		

MIDTARSAL JOINT (TRANSVERSE TARSAL)	Left	Right
Oblique axis—dorsiflexion mobility:		
STJ neutral		
Calcaneal midposition		
STJ maximally pronated		
Oblique axis—plantarflexion mobility:		
STJ neutral		
Calcaneal midposition		
STJ maximally pronated		

MIDTARSAL JOINT (TRANSVERSE TARSAL) (continued)	Left	Right
Longitudinal axis—frontal plane (rotary) mobility:		
STJ neutral:		
Inversion		
Eversion		
Calcaneal midposition:		
Inversion		
Eversion		
STJ maximally pronated:		
Inversion		
Eversion		
Longitudinal arch—footprint configuration:		
Broad		
Normal		
High-arched		
Lateral border:		
Straight		
Concave		
Convex		
Heel oval:		
Medial		
Midline		
Lateral		
Feiss line:		
Open-chain		
Closed-chain		
Great toe hyperextension (windlass effect):		
Open-chain		
Closed-chain		
Forefoot alignment on the hindfoot:		

MIDTARSAL JOINT (TRANSVERSE TARSAL) (continued)	Left	Right
Forefoot varus:		
STJ neutral		
Calcaneal midposition		
Forefoot valgus:		
STJ neutral		
Calcaneal midposition		
Forefoot alignment to the transverse plane:		
STJ neutral		
Calcaneal midposition		
STJ maximally pronated		

METATARSAL SYSTEM	Left	Right
Tarsometatarsal alignment on the transverse plane (using relaxed weight-bearing footprint):		
Metatarsus adductus		
Forefoot adductus		
Forefoot abductus		
Relative metatarsal length (describe abnormality)		
First ray:		
Dorsiflexion		
Hypermobile		
Plantarflexion		
Rigid		
Semi-rigid		
Flexible		
Metatarsophalangeal (MTP) joints:		
Flexion mobility		
Hammertoe		
Extension mobility with metatarsals free		
With metatarsals stabilized in dorsiflexion		

METATARSAL SYSTEM (continued)	Left	Right
Hallux valgus		
Hallux adductus		
Proximal interphalangeal joints (PIPJ):		
Flexion mobility		
Extension mobility		
Hammertoe		
Claw toe		
Distal interphalangeal joints (DIPJ):		
Flexion mobility		
Extension mobility		

LEG LENGTH *Keep the pelvis level in all open-chain tests of leg length.*	Left	Right
Supine position:		
With hips and knees flexed (knees at 90 degrees):		
Knee height (lower leg)		
Femur length		
With hips and knees extended:		
Anatomic length		
Clinical length		
Prone with knees flexed 90 degrees:		
Plantar calcaneal plane		
Malleoli		
Standing position		
Shoulder line		
Pelvic obliquity		
Hip flexion contracture		
Genu valgum		
Genu varum		
Knee flexion (abnormal)		

LEG LENGTH (continued)	Left	Right
Knee extension (abnormal)		
Talocrural dorsiflexion (abnormal)		
Talocrural plantarflexion (abnormal)		
STJ pronation		
STJ supination		
MTJ pronation		
MTJ supination		
First ray plantarflexion		
First ray dorsiflexion		

Glossary
of Acronyms

Glossary of Acronyms

AFO	Ankle-foot orthosis
AFRO	Anterior floor reaction orthosis
AFS	Ankle-foot splint
CAFS	Crouch-control ankle-foot splint
CGFR	Chondral growth/force response
CT	Computerized tomography
EMG	Electromyography
FNI	Femoral neck isthmus
HAFO	Hinged ankle-foot orthosis
HAFS	Hinged ankle-foot splint
HCAFS	Hinged crouch-control ankle-foot splint
KAFO	Knee-ankle-foot orthosis
LGP	Longitudinal growth plate
MES	Minimum effective strain or signal
MRI	Magnetic resonance imagery
MTJ	Midtarsal joint
MTP	Metatarsophalangeal
SAFS	Solid ankle-foot splint
SCAFS	Solid crouch-control ankle-foot splint
SFS	Stabilizing foot splint
SMO	Supramalleolar orthosis
SMS	Supramalleolar splint
STJ	Subtalar joint
TCA	Transcondylar axis
TGP	Trochanteric growth plate
TMA	Transmalleolar axis, or axis of mortice
TMTJ	Tarsometatarsal joint